THE EMPOWERED WOMAN'S
GUIDE TO BETTER HEALTH

TAKING CARE OF YOU

MARY I. O'CONNOR, M.D.
KANWAL L. HAQ, M.S.

MAYO CLINIC PRESS

MAYO CLINIC PRESS

200 First St. SW
Rochester, MN 55905
mcpress.mayoclinic.org

To stay informed about Mayo Clinic Press, please subscribe to our free e-newsletter at MCPress.MayoClinic.org or follow us on social media.

For bulk sales to employers, member groups and health-related companies, contact Mayo Clinic at SpecialSalesMayoBooks@mayo.edu.

Proceeds from the sale of Mayo Clinic Press books benefit medical education and research at Mayo Clinic.

Art Direction and Design: Mayo Clinic Press
Cover and Production: Creative Management Partners, LLC
Illustrations: Margot Sarkozy except for *Vaccines* on page 430, created by Alyssa Clapp, and the *Vicious Cycle Pandemic Circle* on page 452, courtesy of Movement is Life.

ISBN: 978-1-945564-14-7

Library of Congress Control Number: 2022934406

Printed in Canada

To my husband Thomas and our children Moira Kathleen, Roarke Patrick and Riona Carlin. Divine Mother has blessed me beyond measure with you.

Mary I. O'Connor

To my whole heart, my husband Shiraz and our pillars: Mama, Papa, Mom, Dad, Iqbal, Namara, Isra, Emad, Zuhair, and our entire family (past, present, and future). Blessed to have your love.

Kanwal L. Haq

Contents

PART 1 Women and the current health landscape

PART 2 Common conditions impacting women

Why we wrote this book

Our mission in writing this book is to support women in becoming better advocates for their own health. We want this book to be a "what-you-need-to-know" resource on women's health and a tool that can assist you in asking questions and communicating your health concerns. We know that women do not always receive the same health care as men. Women of lower socioeconomic status and women of color, in particular, experience health care disparities. This is unacceptable, and we want to help change that by empowering all women to be actively engaged with their health care team.

Women's health is vast in scope. It includes but is not limited to topics such as reproductive, sexual and maternal health. These topics, while important and widely covered, are only a fraction of women's health. In this book, we did not include subjects such as pregnancy that have many available resources; rather, we focused on conditions that impact women more than men or differently from men, as well as other areas important to women across their lifespans.

At different stages in life, we have distinct health needs and face different health challenges. However, many of us are not prepared for (or even informed about) our health journey ahead. For many of us, middle school health class was the last time we learned about our changing bodies. But once we have left school, there are no required health classes, no "empowerment" books to help us through the health challenges we may face after puberty. Whether we are 18 or 80, as adults we are expected to "just know" how to find a doctor or what our blood pressure should be, or how to eat healthy, and so on. It's overwhelming when we don't even know where to start.

We wrote this book to change that, to provide you with information from experts in medicine who are all women and who bring that perspective to the content of each chapter in the questions they suggest you ask your clinician and in their pearls of wisdom. Our goal is for you to be an empowered patient who positively impacts the trajectory of your own health, wellness and ultimately your life. Let's do this!

The term "woman" is frequently used in this book to refer to the target audience, although the material discussed applies to anyone with a uterus, cervix, or vagina. We recognize that not all people with these body parts identify as women and that not all people who identify as women have these body parts.

You can reach us at:
Mary I. O'Connor, M.D.:
mary.oconnor@vorihealth.com
Kanwal L. Haq, M.S.:
takingcareofyoubook@gmail.com

How to use this book

We are so glad you have picked up this book! It is not a book that you must read cover to cover (although we hope that you will), but rather an easy-to-use and practical resource that allows you to simply flip to the chapter you are interested in. You can read it in any order, and you can come back to different chapters at any time.

This is not a medical textbook, either. This is a book for women, written by women. The book's purpose is to be a resource for all of us. Our chapters are written in a direct and approachable style, keeping away from medical jargon as much as possible. However, because the language of medicine and health care is unique, we have inserted medical terms as definitions (often in parentheses) so that you can better recognize and understand the information that may be presented to you by your health care team.

We have divided the book into three sections:
- **Women and the current health landscape** These chapters focus on the ways in which women access and navigate health care in the United States, today.
- **Common clinical conditions** These chapters discuss common medical problems (clinical conditions), how they can be prevented, how they are treated and how they differ in women compared

with men. Each chapter also contains questions to ask your health care team and pearls of wisdom from women who are experts on each condition.
- **Taking care of you** These chapters discuss changes we can make, as individuals and as communities, to live our healthiest lives!

Some of the chapters refer to other chapters within the book. If you read the referenced chapters, you will have a more comprehensive understanding of the information presented in your chapter, but it is not required. If you'd like to learn more about a topic, you'll find select sources by chapter at the end of the book.

We are grateful to the amazing women who contributed to our book. They are smart, accomplished and leaders in their fields. You can learn a bit about their backgrounds at the end of each of their chapters. Each of these contributors is a champion for better health care for women, and we applaud our collective efforts.

We truly hope you find this first edition of our book helpful on your health care journey. We love feedback and would like to hear your thoughts on how we can make the next edition an even better resource to empower women!

The figures in this book are not anatomical drawings but rather fun illustrations to help with understanding and context. We hope you enjoy them as much as we do!

"Caring for myself is not self-indulgence, it is self-preservation, and that is an act of political warfare." – Audre Lorde

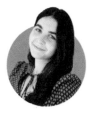

Margot Sarkozy - she/her
Margot created most of the illustrations in this book. She is an undergraduate at Yale University majoring in neuroscience. She aims to attend medical school and eventually become a neurosurgeon. Margot hopes to increase representation of all women in medical textbooks through her illustrations.

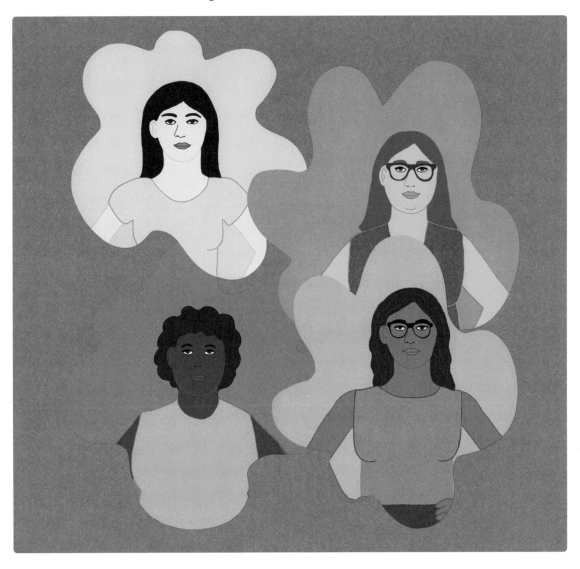

What is 'women's health'?

Stephanie S. Faubion, M.D., M.B.A.

If you're a woman who at some point has had less than satisfying health care interactions or outcomes, you can probably relate to why this book is important to you. Now, more than ever, it is critical that health care be individualized, and that means considering factors that might particularly influence *your* risk of disease and how it is treated.

Sex and gender are key components when considering how women experience disease, how diseases manifest in women, and even how treatment is approached. Our biological sex matters. Whether you are a woman and have XX chromosomes or a man with XY chromosomes, your genes determine many aspects of disease risk and expression. Gender — the social constructs under which we live, including cultural norms, roles and relationships — also matters.

As women, we tend to be caregivers. We often put our own health at the bottom of our to-do lists given all of the other things that take precedence in our lives, such as caring for children, parents and pets; maintaining careers; doing laundry, grocery shopping and cooking; you name it! Indeed, we are often more diligent about maintaining our cars than our own bodies!

Why is it that we need to be given permission to take care of ourselves? And when we finally do see our clinicians — medical professionals who provide health care and guidance to their patients — why does it often feel like no one is hearing what we are saying, or that a one-size-fits-all approach is being offered that doesn't take into account who you are as an individual?

Navigating the health care system brings another set of challenges — knowing what type of clinician to see, knowing when virtual health care is appropriate and when it might not be enough, and knowing when to seek help at an urgent care center or a hospital emergency department and when to wait for a regular appointment.

Let's face it. Women in general, and particularly women of color and sexual and gender minority women, have not always been factored into this whole health care schema. Medicine as we know it today has been based on the 70-kg (155-lb.) man in every aspect. Prior to the early 1990s, female animals or humans were not included in research studies. One reason for this was the historical misconception that women are just like men, and that there are no significant differences between the sexes outside of reproduction. Another was the belief that female animals might cause problems with studies because of cyclical hormonal variations.

These beliefs resulted in significant sex-biases in research that unfortunately continue to impact the care of women. Consider that the majority of medications on the market today were tested in male animals and male humans — which explains why most of the medications taken off the market in the last 20 years were due to harmful (adverse) effects in women. The National Institutes of Health (NIH) mandated inclusion of women and minorities in clinical research trials in its Revitalization Act of 1993. However, it wasn't until 2016 that investigators were required to include sex as a biological variable in the design, analysis and reporting of laboratory animal and human studies. Still, even today, the results of many studies are not reported by sex, leaving significant gaps in our understanding of sex differences in health and disease.

Why is all of this important to understand? In order to individualize care for women, we need to look through a sex-and-gender lens. For you to receive care that is specific to you, your clinicians need to take into account not only your genetic makeup, but also your life circumstances, the stressors you are under and your goals and preferences. No one has a better understanding of your body than you do, and you have the ultimate control over what happens to your body. Although your clinicians have certainly undergone many years of training and may have years of experience, you should feel empowered to get involved in making decisions about your health care. That means feeling comfortable speaking up, asking questions, communicating your concerns and desires about your health, and seeking a second opinion, if needed.

Remember, you are your own best advocate, and your voice is the most important in any discussion about your health. Therefore, arming yourself with the information you need about your health and how to navigate the health care system is key and will put you in a better position to be a proponent for your health. Advocating for your own health has numerous potential benefits, including increasing your health literacy, boosting your sense of control and confidence in your health care decisions, and even improving your adherence to treatments and your health outcomes.

Taking Care of You: The Empowered Woman's Guide to Better Health was written for women who want to better understand their health and become active advocates for their own well-being. In these pages, you will learn how to find the right medical professional to partner with and how to walk into your clinician's office feeling prepared and knowledgeable on how to collaborate with your clinician to make the best health care decisions.

This book is a much-needed "how-to" guide on women's health. Its chapters cover an A-Z list of common conditions and diseases in women. Each chapter includes information about prevention, treatment, why the condition matters to women, and questions to ask your health care team. From mental health issues such as anxiety and depression to common concerns such as breast cancer, heart disease and vaccinations, your questions on a wide variety of topics will be answered.

"Behind every healthy woman is herself."

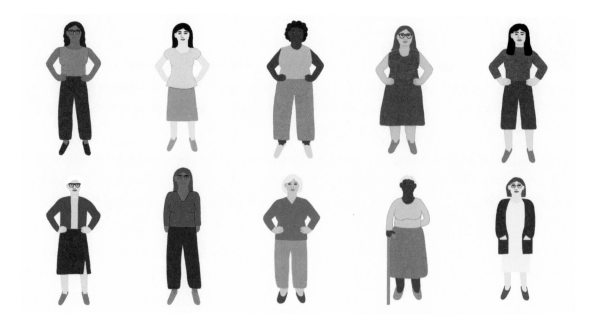

You will also discover a "Pearls of Wisdom" section for each topic, all curated by an impressive group of experts in the field. You will read about the importance of additional research to advance the health of women — a feat that is only possible with the representation and participation of underrepresented groups, including women of color and gender minorities.

Whether you have concerns about your health now or are hoping to be proactive and learn ways to live well in future years, you will find practical information here that you can use today. You play the most important role in determining your health and individualizing your care, and this book will empower you to be your own best advocate.

"Women need to be empowered to be their own best advocates for their health."

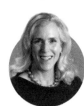

Stephanie S. Faubion, M.D., M.B.A. - she/her
Dr. Faubion is Chair of the Department of Medicine at Mayo Clinic in Jacksonville, Florida, and Director of Mayo Clinic Center for Women's Health. She specializes in the health of women with particular focus on menopause, women's sexual health and healthy aging.

Part 1

Women and the current health landscape

1
The role of social determinants in women's health

Sadiya Muqueeth, Dr.P.H., M.P.H.

WHAT ARE SOCIAL DETERMINANTS OF HEALTH?

What do you think of when you think of the word *health?*

Health, as defined by the World Health Organization, is "a state of complete physical, mental, and social well-being and not merely the absence of disease." Hospitals, doctors and nurses (clinicians), and the health insurance companies and agencies that pay for care (payers) are part of the system that provides health care services. Access, quality and affordability of these services are critical to health outcomes, including everything from mending fractured bones to providing life-saving chemotherapies. Health care services alone, however, do not determine health status.

For many conditions, a person's zip code better predicts health outcomes than other factors. The circumstances in which we live, learn, work and play influence a range of health outcomes and are called social determinants of health (SDOH). These circumstances range broadly, from deeply entrenched social norms and political structures such as economic status, racism or discrimination to more specific conditions of communities such as transportation systems, availability of greenspace, housing affordability, food quality and health care access. When factors impact the individual or a family in particular, they are often termed "social needs" and the person is supported with tailored resources.

WHY ARE SDOH IMPORTANT?

Social determinants of health impact everyone. For some people, access to high-quality living conditions can protect them from increased risk of illness or help them manage disease more easily. For others, lower-quality living conditions make them more vulnerable to poor health and create barriers to overall health. When large groups of people or a community lives in areas with negative SDOH, managing the health of this population can be significantly more difficult and create health inequities. Times of stress, including short- and long-term disasters, economic instability and prolonged events, such as the coronavirus pandemic, worsen poor health outcomes.

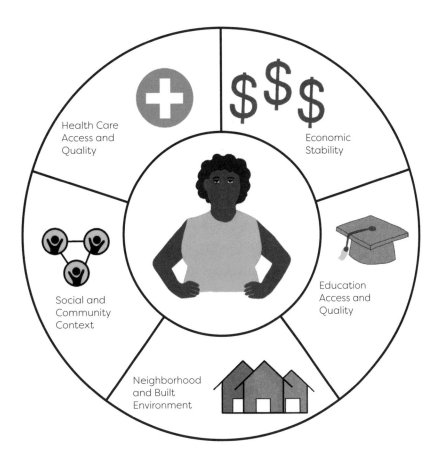

Health Care Access and Quality

Economic Stability

Social and Community Context

Education Access and Quality

Neighborhood and Built Environment

When these high-stress events interact with weak or negative SDOH, they can amplify the negative impact of SDOH on people's health status. In the midst of the coronavirus pandemic, many people in the United States experienced just that, creating further disparities in health outcomes.

WHY DO SDOH MATTER TO WOMEN?

Disparities and differences exist in women's SDOH and health outcomes compared with those of men. On average, women make $0.82 for every dollar that men make. During the pandemic, Black and Latinx women experienced the highest drops in job security. Job insecurity can lead to hardships, unstable housing and decreased ability to purchase nutritious food, all of which are factors connected to health. Women also experience a higher burden of intimate partner violence, which outside of physical injury, can lead to negative mental health outcomes across the lifespan.

Within the health care system, women may be less likely to be diagnosed properly and provided with lifesaving treatments, such as during heart attacks. Disparities between communities persist as Black women and American Indian/Alaskan Native women experience significantly worse pregnancy-related mortality outcomes than their white counterparts do.

These SDOH and health care inequities prevent women — especially women from communities that have been historically underserved and marginalized due to structural racism and lack of economic opportunity — from easily and efficiently managing their own and their families' health. In this context, in which women are more vulnerable to experiencing inequities and its ripple effects, services such as those described in this chapter may provide an opportunity to supplement and navigate barriers to health.

HOW DOES HEALTH CARE ADDRESS SDOH?

Knowing that community conditions impact an individual's health can seem, of course, quite obvious. But attempting to rectify the situation can be challenging in practice. If, for example, during a short 15-minute appointment your clinician encourages you to eat healthier, you may not have time to explain that you have limited resources to spend on food or that there are no grocery stores with healthy options in your neighborhood.

Increasingly, health care systems are realizing the impact of community conditions on health status and, additionally, are being held accountable for ensuring better health outcomes. As a result, they are beginning to engage in multiple approaches to better manage health outcomes and control preventable health care costs.

One approach is to screen people who come in for medical help to see who might have social needs and might benefit from non-

medical services that affect health. In fact, in 2017-2018, about one out of four hospitals screened for specific non-medical needs.

Social needs aren't the same as community conditions. Social needs refer to immediate barriers to health care that a person may face. One example might be transportation to and from frequent health care appointments, such as during prenatal care. Ideally, default community conditions would provide affordable, high-quality public transportation systems and a sense of safety, so that any woman could get to and from anywhere safely and easily. Each facet of this network is important to improving health: community conditions, social needs services, and assistance navigating health care inequities.

To find out about your unique social needs, health care systems may use a set of questions to identify your needs, provide you with appropriate information and connect you to relevant services. Different members of the health care team — for example, the front desk staff, medical assistant, community health worker, nurse or doctor — may ask you about challenges you might be experiencing. The questions may be asked directly, through paperwork completed during an appointment, or through care coordination services that provide outreach to you at your home after an event such as an unexpected hospitalization. Other health care systems may consider using publicly available information about neighborhood factors to identify opportunities to better connect their patients to services.

While the range of social needs and SDOH are vast and touch every aspect of daily life, the following are three common barriers and the respective services that a clinician or payer may support.

Example 1: Transportation security

The challenge Finding reliable transportation to and from regular health care visits can be difficult for some people. Whether due to high cost of transport, very long distances (as in rural areas) or limited public transportation options, transportation insecurity can cause missed appointments and delay medical care. Delays can lead to worsening health and increased health care costs, especially for those who have frequent appointments. Consistent and reliable transportation is important in managing medical care.

The services Both clinicians and payers may offer services to increase reliable access to health care through telehealth, ridesharing, vouchers and non-emergency medical transportation (NEMT). Telehealth, which increased in both demand and availability during the COVID-19 pandemic, allows people to meet with faraway clinicians from their home or a local clinic. For in-person appointments, some health care systems partner with ride-share apps or van programs that provide transportation to and from health care facilities. Others provide vouchers for buses, trains or taxis. Each state's Medicaid services also provide NEMT for pre-approved care, such as behavioral health services or preventive care, including prenatal appointments. Make sure to check the requirements around eligibility and services established by your state, insurance company and clinic.

Example 2: Food security and physical activity

The challenge Eating a healthy diet and engaging in regular exercises isn't always as simple as it sounds. With 6 out of 10 adults in the U.S. living with a chronic disease and 4 out of 10 living with two or more chronic illnesses, lifestyle changes are common recommendations from clinicians. Balanced nutrition and an active lifestyle can lower the risk of chronic illnesses such as diabetes, hypertension and high cholesterol. But eating a nutritious diet is significantly more challenging when a person is experiencing hunger, food insecurity or a tight budget. People experiencing food insecurity are more likely to have increased emergency department visits, hospitalizations and health care costs.

The services To address these problems, some clinics, hospitals and doctors' offices are screening their patients for food insecurity and offering connections to supplemental food and nutrition programs. Programs may be linked to local food banks, established by clinicians or insurance companies, managed by the health department, or independently delivered. Called "food as medicine," "food pharmacies," or "produce prescriptions," these programs are intended to support access to affordable, nutritious foods to manage health conditions. "Medically tailored meal programs" are especially designed by credentialed dietitians or nutritionists for people who require unique diets to meet complex dietary needs, such as renal disease.

Long-standing federal programs such as the Supplemental Nutrition Assistance Program (SNAP) provide benefits to supplement food budgets based on financial need. Realizing that women's health and young children's health are often uniquely vulnerable, the Special Supplemental Nutrition Program for Women, Infants and Children (WIC) offers women and children access to food, health care referrals and nutrition education. While each state's program differs, women who are pregnant, breastfeeding and non-breastfeeding postpartum are eligible for services. Infants and children up to age five who are found to be at nutritional risk are also eligible.

Like a nutritious diet, exercise is a necessary aspect of life and is linked to a range of health factors from weight management to stress relief to healthier aging. Your clinician might write you a "prescription" to get outside and get active through programs like NatureRx or ParkRx, or encourage you to enroll in a group fitness program hosted by the health system or your insurance company. These programs are intended to promote more physically active lifestyles, encouraging you and your family to get outside to your nearby park, public space or exercise facility.

Example 3: Housing security
The challenge Stable housing that you own, rent, or stay in as part of a household cannot be taken for granted. Housing insecurity has some of the deepest consequences on health and well-being. Whether the problems include homelessness, unstable housing options, having to move frequently, affordability or quality of housing, each challenge impacts health outcomes. Studies have shown that housing is linked with mental health, substance use, intimate-

partner violence, asthma-related emergency department visits and many other outcomes. Safe, affordable, consistent and quality housing protects health and well-being.

The services Both housing insecurity and housing environment are key social needs that impact health. Program models such as Housing First support people experiencing homelessness in choosing housing opportunities that do not have significant eligibility requirements, based on the value that housing is a basic need. Other initiatives focus on quality of housing. Asthma is one of the reasons people, especially children, visit the emergency departments often. Asthma can result from unhealthy residential environmental factors such as secondhand smoke, mold, mildew and substandard arrangements. These environmental factors increase the risk of asthma attacks.

Initiatives such as medical-legal partnerships place lawyers and paralegals in health care settings to help people address legal issues linked to health status. Other initiatives such as those focused on lead-paint exposure among pregnant women refers families to public health departments. Lead-based paint, commonly used to paint homes before 1978, is linked with significant health effects. Exposure to lead-based paint can lead to miscarriage, pre-term birth and low birth weight among pregnant women, developmental challenges and anemia among children, and cardiovascular effects and other health implications among older adults. Public health departments may provide direct testing and care coordination as well as prevention services to educate communities. Some public health departments issue legally binding abatement notices and conduct re-inspection.

QUESTIONS TO ASK YOUR HEALTH CARE TEAM ABOUT SDOH

Depending on the social barrier you're facing, ask your clinician or a member of your health care team what options are available that can help you overcome the barrier. In addition, find out:

- What specific services are available?
- Who is eligible for the specific services?
- How much does the service cost and who pays for the services?
- How do you connect to the services?
- How long are the services available?

PEARLS OF WISDOM

- Remember, doctors, nurses and other clinicians want to help. In addition to taking care of your medical needs, your health care team may serve as a bridge to resources that you may not be aware of. The team's main goal is to make sure you stay healthy, not simply use health care services.
- Share the barriers you're experiencing and be specific, whether it involves completing screening questionnaires or having a conversation with the health care team. Research shows that as doctors learn more about their patients' social needs, communication between doctors and patients improves.
- The health professionals who take care of you are a team. Doctors don't work alone. Your team may include physician assistants, nurses, social workers, community health workers, home health aides, medical assistants and others. Some members of the team may have more information about social resources than others.
- Don't forget your insurance company. Health care systems support many programs, but other initiatives may be available through your insurance provider, public or private. Get to know the resources they offer and find out which ones you might be eligible for.
- Ask questions! Services vary by clinic, hospital and insurance provider, and also by where you live. Ask questions to get clarity on what's available and for how long, and what is covered by your insurance.
- Provide feedback! If you can, follow up with your health care team to tell them how it went. Clinicians don't always hear back about whether people connected with services and whether those services were helpful. Providing feedback can help you and future patients.

"Connected health systems serve women more effectively."

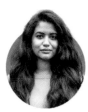

Sadiya Muqueeth, Dr.P.H., M.P.H. - she/her
Dr. Muqueeth is the Director of Community Health at Trust for Public Land and co-Founder/CEO of Hyphen Health, LLC in Baltimore, Maryland. She specializes in community health interventions and strengthening public health systems.

2
Challenges faced by women of color

Marshala Lee, M.D., M.P.H., and Nadiyah Fisher

HOW DO WOMEN OF COLOR NAVIGATE HEALTH CARE BARRIERS?

Prioritizing your health is crucial for determining your quality of life. Each of us has only one body and mind for our entire lives; we must take care of ourselves. A common goal for most women is to be in good health. Statistically, those who live healthier lives live longer. At first glance, the way to preserve health seems simple: visit the doctor regularly, exercise, eat a balanced diet and get enough sleep. But these common suggestions are often too simple and fail to address the complex nature of the health care system.

Navigating the health care system can be challenging for anyone, but women of color face unique barriers. Women of color often stand at the intersection of multiple obstacles, experiencing the combined effects of racial, gender, ethnic and other forms of discrimination while simultaneously navigating systemic racism, socioeconomic inequities, cultural and language differences, mistrust, stigma, and institutional structures in which disparities remain the status quo.

If you're a woman of color, you're likely aware of the multitude of ethnic and racial differences in health outcomes that exist. This can make applying the "simplest" of common health care solutions difficult and intimidating. These differences in health and health care between groups that stem from broader inequities are oftentimes preventable and are referred to as health disparities. For various reasons, many health outcomes, including maternal health outcomes, are worse for women of color than for those of white women.

WHAT ARE SOME HEALTH DISPARITIES THAT IMPACT WOMEN OF COLOR?

Research has shown that women of color sometimes receive poorer quality of care and are less likely than white women to have their pain treated appropriately due to historical misconceptions. For example, in a study including over 400 medical students and residents, some participants suggested "simpler" and "less severe" treatment options for Black women, even though they had the same diagnosis as women in different racial groups. This is unacceptable, and is an example of Black women receiving

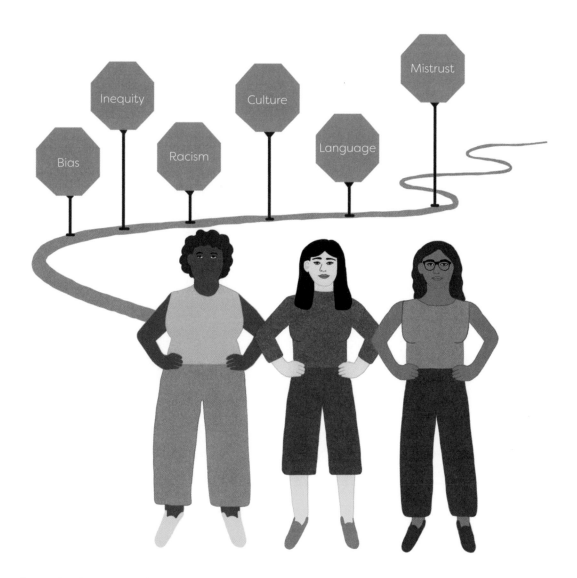

substandard care. The following are other examples of health disparities that exist for women of color:

- Heart disease is the leading cause of death for most women in the United States, but Black women have an even higher risk of dying from heart disease, at a younger age, than white women do. Approximately 60% of Black women have some form of heart disease.

- Whereas heart disease is the leading cause of death for most women in the U.S., cancer is the leading cause of death among American Indian and Alaska Native populations. More specifically, lung cancer is the most common cause of cancer death among American Indian and Alaska Native women.

- Black women are three to four times more likely to die from pregnancy-related complications than white women are. Black women are also three to four times more likely to experience a severe disability resulting from childbirth than white women are.

- American Indian and Alaska Native, Hispanic and Black women have higher rates of diabetes and resulting disability than white women do.
- American Indian and Alaska Native women have disproportionately higher rates of mental health problems than other women in the U.S. do.
- Hispanic, Black and some Asian women, when compared with white women, have lower levels of health insurance coverage, with Hispanic women facing the greatest barriers to health insurance. Hispanic women are three times as likely as white women and nearly twice as likely as Black women to be uninsured.
- Hispanic, Black and Asian women have around the same prevalence rates for mental illness, but Asian women are less likely to be treated for mental health concerns.
- Women of color are disproportionally affected by postpartum depression. They face postpartum depression at a greater rate — almost two to three times more — than all new mothers.

These statistics are alarming and can be overwhelming for women of color who may be personally affected by one or more of these conditions. Such statistics can instill additional mistrust in the health care system and prevent women from seeking help.

However, it's important to remember that these statistics represent symptoms of health inequity rather than the cause. The specific reasons for health disparities among women are multifactorial and emerge from a complex interplay of factors such as social determinants of health, clinician bias, access to health care and biological factors.

PEARLS OF WISDOM

While there's no simple solution to combating health disparities, we must work together to develop comprehensive strategies for improving the quality of care and social determinants of health for women of color. We must empower women of color to take an active role in their health and eliminate the factors that negatively impact their health care experiences. The following are a few recommendations for women of color as they navigate the health care system. Feel free to modify these recommendations so they are useful for you!

Do your research and choose wisely
Finding a doctor or other clinician who listens to you and is sensitive to your needs is important even if difficult at times. Word-of-mouth and online ratings can be useful tools when seeking a culturally competent clinician. Look at multiple resources and websites before scheduling an appointment. Websites such as healthgrades.com and vitals.com are great tools for reading patient reviews of clinicians.

Understand your risks
To get the most out of your visit, be open and honest with your clinician. It's important that you and your clinician are aware of your family medical history. Genetic risk factors can increase the chances of developing a disease. Ask your family members to share their medical history with you so that you can be mindful of possible risk factors. Discuss your personal and family medical history with your clinician to ensure that you're receiving the best care possible, including appropriate screenings to check for

diseases early on in the disease development process. Early detection helps foster early intervention.

Ask questions

Before your appointment, write down a list of questions to ask during your visit. We tend to remember things more clearly when we jot them down on paper. When talking with your clinician, ask for help understanding medical tests, prescribed treatments, medications and lab results. Feel free to research the side effects of different treatments on trusted websites.

Often, clinicians use medical jargon — scientific words, abbreviations and shorthand descriptions — when explaining diagnoses and treatments. Tell your clinician if you don't understand what's being said. No question is too simple. It's important that you fully understand what your clinician is telling you and that you understand the treatment plan that's being laid out for you. If you need a language interpreter, ask for one. There are people trained to interpret medical terms; use these services!

If you try all of these steps and you're still confused by what your clinician is saying, ask if someone else from the care team, such as a nurse or physician's assistant, can step in and explain it in a different way. If not, you may need to find a new clinician.

Be supported

Two minds are better than one! Consider bringing someone you trust to your next appointment or hospital stay. This person can bring up concerns that you may not have thought of, which in turn may help you speak up and remember important

details during and after your visit. Scientific jargon or language can make it hard for a patient to understand what is going on with their body. A second person can help explain the information in plain language.

Review your medical records

If something isn't documented in your medical record, it's like it didn't even happen! Your medical records must be accurate, complete, and clearly document your medical history and goals of care. As a patient, you have the right to access your medical records. Ask for and review documentation from your visit to ensure accuracy and gain clarity about next steps. This is a perfect opportunity to ask questions about what is in your care plan. Reviewing your medical records is also a way to see if there are patterns in your health that might need to be addressed. Consider storing an extra copy of your medical records in a secure location to ensure that it is easily accessible in an emergency.

Speak up

No one knows you better than you know yourself! A physician should always provide an open and honest environment for you. If you have a negative experience with a clinician, say something. Speak with a supervisor, patient relations specialist or someone on the hospital's medical ethics team. Contact information for the patient relations specialist and medical ethics team can be requested from the care team and is also typically accessible via the hospital's website or the information phone line. The patient relations team typically provides a centralized place where patients, family members and visitors can voice their concerns, grievances or complaints and have them reviewed. A medical ethics consultation may help whenever there is an unresolved ethical concern, offering recommendations that you (or your family) may use in health care decision making and providing reassurance of your grievances.

Consider a second opinion

A second opinion makes a difference if you're faced with a tough decision or dealing with a complex medical condition. You might want to consult a doctor with more experience in treating your condition, such as a specialist. A specialist is a physician who is trained in a specific area of practice (for example, a cardiologist specializes in the diagnosis and treatment of diseases of the heart). Or you might just be looking for a better doctor-patient relationship. Not every doctor will be the right fit for every patient. Getting a second opinion might provide you with more information regarding your condition, may confirm or question the first doctor's diagnosis and treatment plan and help you better determine next treatment steps.

Breathe

Your health can be uncertain sometimes. Even with proper care, results take time. If you're confident in the care you're receiving, take a moment to breathe. Avoid fixating on diagnoses. The best way to cure, fight or prevent a disease is to be consistent and confident.

"Eliminating health disparities must be a central tenet in the women's health movement."

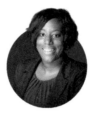

Marshala Lee, M.D., M.P.H. - she/her
Dr. Lee is a board-certified family medicine physician and the Director of the Harrington Community Partnership Fund at ChristianaCare's Institute for Research on Equity and Community Health in Wilmington, Delaware. Dr. Lee is committed to fostering a healthier world by empowering communities to live healthier lives, decreasing health workforce shortages, eliminating health disparities, and providing culturally appropriate care.

"Acknowledging the history of mental health and dismantling stigma in women of color is imperative to their health."

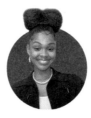

Nadiyah Fisher - she/her
Nadiyah Fisher is an undergraduate at the University of Pittsburgh studying Neuroscience and Psychology. After graduation, Nadiyah plans on pursuing a degree in medicine; more specifically, a Triple Board Program in Pediatrics and Psychiatry. In the future, Nadiyah hopes to provide affordable and culturally specific mental health care to underserved communities of color.

3

Special considerations: Sexual and gender minority women

Diane Bruessow, M.P.A.S., P.A.-C., DFAAPA

WHO ARE SEXUAL AND GENDER MINORITY (SGM) WOMEN?

Sexual minorities have a sexual orientation — that is, a sexual attraction, behavior or identity — that is same-gender-loving. Sexual minority women may be lesbians or bisexual women or may use other terms to describe their sexuality.

Gender minorities have a gender identity that is incongruent with assigned sex at birth — such as a person whose assigned sex was male, and whose gender identity is female or nonbinary. Gender minorities may use other terms, such as transgender, to describe their gender identity.

Lesbian, bisexual and transgender women represent only a portion of sexual and gender minority women.

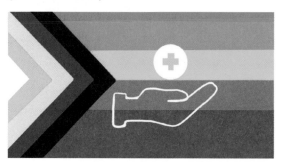

WHAT UNIQUE HEALTH CARE CHALLENGES DO SGM WOMEN EXPERIENCE?

SGM women generally face two primary health care challenges.

The first challenge is making sure that as an SGM woman you are heard and that your health concerns are being addressed. Doctors and other clinicians may assume that you are straight (heterosexual) and cisgender (when gender identity and sex at birth are congruent). Clarifying assumptions is especially important when:

- Completing paperwork when you are meeting with a new clinician or being admitted to a hospital
- Talking with your clinician
- Ensuring that a treatment plan will be effective for you
- Having a satisfying health care experience

Sharing your sexual orientation, gender identity and assigned sex at birth with your clinician makes a difference. Electronic health records have fields for sexual orientation and gender identity and assigned sex at birth because this important information helps your clinician give you the best health care.

The second challenge is that SGM women may experience additional health disparities (see Chapter 1). This means that your medical and mental health needs and experiences may be different from those of other women. SGM women are less likely to have health insurance coverage, access to quality health services, a stable source of health care, immunizations and inclusion in public health infrastructure.

CAN THESE CHALLENGES BE PREVENTED?

Yes! The higher rates of unhealthy behaviors and mental health issues including depression (see Chapter 24) and anxiety (see Chapter 12) are associated with a lack of affirmation. For example, compared to non-SGM women, SGM women who don't receive acceptance from their families experience up to eight times higher rates of suicidal behavior, substance use, and other unhealthy behaviors. SGM women who are affirmed in their sexual orientation and gender identity experience rates of depression and anxiety similar to those of most other women.

As a SGM woman, a key step toward receiving effective health care is finding a clinician you can trust and who can be an ally. Equally important is staying up to date on immunizations, such as getting vaccinated against the human papilloma virus, a virus that increases the likelihood of certain cancers, and following recommended schedules for cancer screenings. Medical professionals know that early detection of cancer saves lives, while being diagnosed later is often more deadly.

You're more likely to experience improved health care and health outcomes when your clinician is aware of your sexual orientation and gender identity and can provide culturally competent medical care (see Chapter 6).

WHY DO THESE CHALLENGES MATTER TO SGM WOMEN?

As a SGM woman, you may know someone who experienced bias and discrimination in health care. But don't let that stop you from seeking health care or disclosing key information to your clinician. Avoiding health care or not disclosing important information can result in poorer health care experiences and health outcomes for yourself and other SGM women.

Having strong social supports in place can help you build resilience, which is a positive factor necessary to counteract assumptions, bias and discriminatory practices.

QUESTIONS TO ASK YOUR HEALTH CARE TEAM ABOUT SGM HEALTH

For all SGM women
- Before making an appointment, ask if the practice has any LGBT patients. You don't have to give your name during that initial call.
- Let your clinician know up front how you describe yourself and your partner(s).
- Ask your clinician to use your chosen

name and pronouns, and to describe your partners in the manner you advise.

For gender minority women

- Ask your clinician to take an "organ inventory." This is an opportunity to discuss the body parts you have and the terms you use to describe them, as well as your medical and surgical transition-related history.

PEARLS OF WISDOM

SGM women have unique health needs and face unique challenges associated with experiences of bias and discrimination when accessing health care. Instead of avoiding health care, seek out affirming health care professionals and settings using online resources such as:

- GLMA (formerly the Gay and Lesbian Medical Association) Provider Directory **www.glma.org**
- World Professional Association for Transgender Health Member Directory (WPATH) **www.wpath.org**
- Healthcare Equality Index, an annual LGBT health benchmarking tool that evaluates health care facilities **www.hrc.org**

If you feel that a clinician discriminated against you because of your sexual orientation or gender identity, you can file a complaint with the U.S. Department of Human Services (**www.hhs.gov/ocr**).

Finding a clinician you are comfortable with is essential to your health!

"Health professionals have a broader understanding of women's health now that we know sex and gender are different concepts."

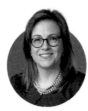

Diane Bruessow, M.P.A.S., P.A.-C., DFAAPA - she/her
PA Bruessow has an appointment to the Department of Internal Medicine and is faculty in the Yale School of Medicine Physician Assistant Online Program in New Haven, Connecticut. She specializes in transgender medicine and practices at Healthy Transitions, in Montclair, New Jersey.

4

Is Google your first responder?

Kanwal L. Haq, M.S., and Amy Bantham, Dr.P.H., M.S., M.P.P.

SEARCHING FOR HEALTH INFORMATION ONLINE

How many times have you found yourself with an unusual symptom or ailment and then quickly opened your phone to Google what it means? A lot of us do it! Whether we are searching for information for ourselves, or trying to help a family member or friend, many women search for health information online.

While the act of searching for health information online is not harmful in and of itself — it's good to be concerned about your health! — it is important to recognize that searching for health information online is only a starting point. Online searches are not the final answer, and certainly not a diagnosis. In the following sections, we discuss the process of seeking health information and how online searches can be used as steppingstones for seeking care safely and effectively.

EVALUATING THE RELIABILITY OF INFORMATION ONLINE

When searching for medical advice online you will likely find yourself sifting through an overwhelming amount of information, since there are websites covering almost every single health topic. While some of your search results may provide information from a reputable medical institution, your results can also produce social media posts, blogs, open forums, news articles, advertisements and so on. Search engines such as Google, Yahoo, or Bing do not verify the information they present.

To determine the reliability and accuracy of health information, focus on three main things:
- Who is providing the information?
- When was the information provided? How recent is it?
- What is the goal of the information? Why is the information being provided?

Who is providing the information?
Reliable websites will tell you where their health information came from; in fact, some websites will have teams of qualified individuals vetting the information found on their sites. Other sites may not have this level of vetting but will list the author's name and credentials at the top or bottom of the article or post.

When browsing a health site, make sure that the information was written or reviewed by a qualified medical professional and that their credentials align with the expertise they are providing (see Chapter 5). If an author isn't listed, you can determine whether the information you have found is credible and trustworthy by contacting the site owners. Reliable websites will have a separate "About Us" or "Contact Us" page or will have their contact information listed at the bottom of the page.

Sometimes, your online search may result in blog posts, chat rooms, discussion groups or social media posts, such as from Facebook, Twitter, Instagram, Whatsapp, TikTok or other sites. These platforms create online communities where people can connect with friends, family and strangers. If people you know post information on these types of websites, it does not mean that the information is necessarily true or false. But do your homework. Check the original sources of information and make sure the original source is not someone's opinion, but fact based upon scientific evidence.

In science and medicine, information (even if provided by a credentialed expert) is validated through a process called peer review. This is the gold standard of quality control. When new information is presented in the scientific community, other experts conduct a rigorous check, scrutinizing the new finding or discovery to determine if it is indeed true before it is widely shared with others.

For example, Wikipedia is one of the largest and most utilized websites in the world, but many of the health article contributors are not credentialed medical researchers or professionals. In fact, anyone can write and publish a Wikipedia article — you don't even have to provide your real name to contribute. While this is changing, with more medical professionals taking it upon themselves to update Wikipedia articles, Wikipedia does not currently provide the same rigorous quality control as peer-reviewed publications, such as journals and books.

Perhaps the quickest way to determine who is providing the information is by determining who is hosting the information online. You can do this by looking at the domain suffix — the last part of a domain name, such as ".com," ".net" or ".edu." A great place to start is by looking at websites that end in ".gov." Only federal, state, local and territorial government organizations are eligible to obtain a .gov domain. That means these websites are owned by the United States government, and the information provided is based upon peer-reviewed science. Some of the top sites include:

- Centers for Disease Control and Prevention (CDC) at **www.cdc.gov**
- Office on Women's Health (U.S. Department of Health & Human Services) at **www.womenshealth.gov**
- The .gov websites maintained by your state's Department of Public Health, for example, at **www.health.ny.gov**
- National Institutes of Health (NIH) and its 27 specialized institutes, at **www.nih.gov**
  › NIH's MedlinePlus at **www.medlineplus.gov**

The next option is to consider web addresses that end in ".edu." These websites are associated with educational institutions and must be accredited in order to have received the .edu domain name registration. The information you find on these sites will be vetted and regulated by qualified individuals. A few examples of regularly accessed .edu websites include:

- Harvard Health Publishing at **www.health.harvard.edu**. This is Harvard Medical School's consumer health education division, which draws upon the expertise of its faculty members and clinicians in order to provide easy-to-understand medical information for the general public.
- Go Ask Alice at **www.goaskalice.columbia.edu**. This is an online health "question and answer" resource that draws upon the expertise of health researchers and specialists at Columbia University. Initially, this website was developed to help students make informed health decisions, but it is now open to everyone and aims to provide "reliable, accurate, accessible, and culturally competent health information."

Another common domain, ".org," is often used by nonprofit organizations. Many top health care institutions are nonprofits. However, these domains can be a bit trickier to navigate in terms of reliability because, in contrast to .gov and .edu domains, which undergo a vetting process to receive the domain, .org is an unrestricted domain that can be used by anyone. Look for .org websites that belong to reputable nonprofit organizations and that explain how their information is reviewed. Some examples of nonprofits that offer reliable health information include:

- Mayo Clinic at **www.mayoclinic.org**

- Cleveland Clinic at **my.clevelandclinic.org/health**
- American Academy of Family Physicians' consumer website at **www.familydoctor.org**
- Johns Hopkins Medicine at **www.hopkinsmedicine.org/health**

Other websites, primarily .com and .net domains, are owned by businesses or individuals. With these websites you may need to further identify when the information was provided and for what purpose in order to determine reliability.

When was the information provided? How recent is it?

Science is constantly changing. Look for the most current information. You can often find out when a website was edited or reviewed by looking for a date at the bottom of the page. A good rule of thumb is that the information should be no older than three years (although with COVID-19 we have learned that even three months can bring about significant discovery and change!)

What is the goal of the information? Why is it being provided?

Even when websites provide accurate and current information, the site may not be providing the most relevant information for you. Thus, it is vital to know why the site was created, which can help you better assess the content provided.

Sometimes the primary purpose of the website is to inform or explain, but sometimes it is to advertise a product or a service. For example, if we do a search on the phrase, "Do I have COVID-19?" several sites come up, including commercial sites that aim to sell COVID-19 tests and tele-health subscriptions. While an at-home test or a doctor can help you determine if you have COVID-19, this website in and of itself does not help you address the question of whether you have COVID-19. In contrast, the CDC's website offers a self-checker tool that takes you through a series of questions to determine if you might have COVID-19, along with advice on how to proceed (search **www.cdc.gov** for "corona-virus self-checker"). In this case, the CDC's website is going to be more helpful.

However, just because a website is trying to advertise a service or product does not mean that it may not be helpful or reliable. Many websites offer a range of services from information and education to advertisement. One example is psychologytoday.com, which provides articles related to mental health but also advertises for many mental health professionals who are accepting new patients. This brings us to why you should see a clinician when you have a health concern.

SEEKING A CLINICIAN AFTER FINDING INFORMATION ONLINE

Finding information online helps us become more informed. But we can't rely on any single website to provide us with a diagnosis or treatment plan. It is always a good idea to seek care from a medical professional when you have a health concern.

One study found that out of the 72% of Americans who reported looking up health information, nearly 50% decided that their symptoms didn't need the attention of a clinician. This is an alarming statistic because relying solely on search engines for decision making can keep you from accessing and receiving proper care when you need it.

Even if you use a symptom-checker tool from a trustworthy source, such as the CDC, research shows that you will receive a correct diagnosis only 34% of the time, and that is only in relation to simple health concerns. Complex cases need a much more conscientious approach, which requires the support of a clinician.

Still, searching online can help us ask questions about our concerns, and asking questions helps us better communicate those concerns. When preparing to see a clinician, you can do your own homework by asking yourself:

- What symptoms am I specifically experiencing? (Try to describe your symptoms clearly.)
  › This could be anything such as headaches, dizziness, lightheadedness, pain, aches, fever, unexplained weight loss or weight gain, lumps, changes in appetite, difficulty sleeping, bone or joint stiffness, bladder or bowel concerns, changes in menstrual cycle, chest pain, shortness of breath, vision changes, hearing changes, skin changes, rashes, bumps, mood changes (for example, feeling sad, lonely or anxious), trouble with memory or thinking, changes in mobility, challenges with intimacy or sexual activity, and so forth.
- Where do I experience the symptoms?
  › Certain parts of your body? Everywhere?

› Is the pain sharp? Or dull?
- When do I experience these symptoms?
  › Do you experience the symptoms or pain suddenly?
  › Or do they occur constantly? Or only at a specific time of day or night? Do they recur at certain times? When doing certain activities?
  › When did the symptoms start?
  › How long do you experience these symptoms? Seconds? Minutes? Hours? Days?
  › How often do these symptoms occur? Daily? Every so often?
- Does anything make these symptoms better?
- Does anything make these symptoms worse?
- Do these symptoms keep me from going out or doing my usual activities?

Sometimes when we are feeling anxious we might be reading with a "glass-half-empty lens," and asking these specific questions can help us reevaluate what we found online in light of what we are actually experiencing.

SHARING THE INFORMATION YOU FOUND ONLINE WITH A CLINICIAN

It is beneficial for you to share your symptoms and what you found online with your clinician. Share what you searched for, why you searched for it, what you found and where you found it.

If you found some potentially frightening results online, your clinician may acknowledge your concerns but may start by asking you a list of questions about your background and well-being, instead of focusing on your search results. Your clinician is not being rude or dismissive of your concerns but seeking additional information in order to make an accurate diagnosis.

Your clinician may ask about major life changes or stressors — such as losing a job or a home, facing challenges within your family, dealing with the death of a loved one, coping with a global pandemic — because such factors can drastically impact your health and manifest as a number of different symptoms. Be open and honest with your clinician about any challenges you may be experiencing, as it will help them help you. Share your symptoms, what you found online and the following:
- Any allergies or drug reactions
- All medications you're taking, including prescription drugs, over-the-counter medicines (anything from pain relievers to eyedrops to laxatives), vitamins, supplements and herbal remedies
  › Name and dose of medication
  › Date you started taking a medication
  › When you take it
  › How often you take it
  › What you take it for (many medications can serve multiple purposes)
  › If it does (or doesn't) work for you
- Lifestyle
  › Any past hospitalizations or major accidents or injuries
  › Alcohol, tobacco and other drug usages
  › Your daily diet
  › Your daily activities
  › How much you exercise
  › Sexual activity
  › Sexuality

- Complete family medical history including information about your grandparents, parents, siblings, aunts, uncles and cousins and their experiences with:
  - Heart disease
  - High blood pressure
  - Stroke
  - Cancer (list which type)
  - Any other conditions you may be concerned about

Sharing all of this information will hopefully help you avoid invasive and unnecessary testing, but if testing is needed, you can ask your clinician:

- What type of testing is needed to confirm my symptoms?
- Why is the specific test being done? Is it the only one?
- Are there any harmful or uncomfortable side effects of the testing?
- How many steps are involved in the testing? What is required of me?
- When will the test results be provided? How?
- What information will testing provide?
- Who can be called if there are further questions about the testing?

USING INFORMATION PROVIDED BY A CLINICIAN

Hopefully the end process of your online search leads you to a clinician who can provide you with the right diagnosis and treatment. You should always feel empowered to ask:

- What is the name of my condition?
- How long will this condition last?

- How will this condition be treated or managed?
- How will this condition affect me? In the short term? Long term?
- What are the treatment options? Which treatment is recommended for me? When do I need to start treatment?
- What medications will I need, if any? For how long? Will these medications interact with anything I am currently taking? How will I know if the medication is or is not working? Are there any side effects I should be prepared for? Will my insurance cover it? How much will it cost me?
- Why do I have this condition?
- How can I learn more about this condition? How can I learn more about the treatment?

If you do not understand your clinician's response to any of these questions, or if your clinician uses medical terms you are not familiar with, always ask them to clarify! The Medical Library Association (**www.mlanet.org**) has an online tool called "What did my doctor say" that can help you learn about different medical terms, but a good clinician should always explain!

Unfortunately, not even the best clinicians can answer every question every time. However, good clinicians will tell you when they don't have answers and will help you find someone who does. If you don't feel listened to, or something in your gut tells you that you didn't arrive at the right diagnosis and treatment, your journey does not need to end there. Keep in mind that not all clinicians offer the same medical advice. You may need to find the right clinician for you (see Chapter 6).

PEARLS OF WISDOM

Women rely on the internet more heavily than men do to understand health concerns, engage with others about health, and use technology to support health goals for themselves and their families. This is not surprising considering that women have more health needs, are more often caregivers, and make 80% of health care decisions for their families. Searching for health information online can make women more informed health care consumers and better self-advocates, if they use credible health information to ask questions.

However, women should not rely on the internet to self-diagnose and then delay or skip clinical care. No website is a substitute for a qualified clinician. Remember, when your health concerns are urgent, you should immediately seek professional medical care, not Google!

"I'm sick and tired of being sick and tired."
– Fannie Lou Hamer

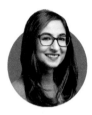

Kanwal L. Haq, M.S. - she/her
Kanwal is a medical anthropologist passionate about creating more connected, more informed, and more equitable systems of care. She specializes in community-based participatory research and builds accessible tools, resources, and programs for women around the globe. Kanwal currently leads the NYC women's health programs at the Arnhold Institute for Global Health at Mount Sinai's Icahn School of Medicine.

"Women can use health information from trusted sources to be powerful and informed advocates for their health."

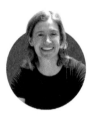

Amy Bantham, Dr.P.H., M.S., M.P.P. - she/her
Dr. Bantham is the CEO/Founder of Move to Live® More with a mission to help people live healthier, longer, more active lives. She focuses on addressing physical inactivity, chronic disease and social determinants of health through cross-sector collaboration and innovation.

5
Who are clinicians?
They're not just physicians

Fatma Haiderzad, D.N.P., M.S., C.R.N.A.

WHO ARE CLINICIANS?

You may think that a clinician is a physician. If you do, you're only partially correct. Doctors make up a percentage of well-trained and effective medical professionals who provide patient care, also called health care clinicians or clinicians. Many clinicians are doctors, but not all of them are. Nonphysician clinicians can also diagnose, treat and provide ongoing management of common illnesses and even some complex ones as part of a health care team. Often these clinicians are referred to as advanced practice providers (APPs).

Legally, a health care provider can be defined as any clinician who is authorized to operate within their scope of practice as defined by state law, from whom your health insurance will accept medical certification to verify the existence of a health condition or authenticate a claim for benefits. Scope of practice describes the procedures, actions, and processes that health care providers are allowed to perform in keeping with the terms of their licenses. This chapter describes the various categories of allied health professionals and how they might fit into your health care.

WHAT IS THE ROLE OF AN ADVANCED PRACTICE PROVIDER?

Advanced practice providers are certified and trained clinicians who provide medical care. They work one-on-one with their patients and often become the person you interact with the most when accessing health care. You need to know who they are and what they do, as it is highly likely that they may care for you.

The most common advanced practice providers who may take care of you in a clinic or hospital include the following:

Advanced practice registered nurses (APRNs)
APRNs are registered nurses who hold a master's degree and an APRN license. APRNs are educated, trained, certified and licensed in one of four roles:

Certified nurse practitioners (NPs) Nurse practitioners (NPs) are the majority of the APRN workforce. NPs provide comprehensive primary, acute, and specialty care. They also focus on health promotion, disease prevention, health education, counseling, and disease management.

Clinical nurse specialists (CNS) CNS practitioners focus on community health, managing the complex care of vulnerable populations, educating and supporting staff on best clinical practices, and advancing safety within health care systems.

Certified registered nurse anesthetists (CRNAs) CRNAs, also known as nurse anesthesiologists, are qualified to deliver the full spectrum of anesthesia care for people undergoing surgery or having a baby. They provide more than 50 million anesthetics in the United States annually and offer anesthesia in more than 80% of rural hospitals in the U.S. Half of these rural hospitals use a CRNA-only model for obstetric care.

Certified nurse-midwives (CNMs) CNMs deliver a range of primary health care services, including gynecologic care, childbirth, and newborn care. CNMs provide primary and preventive care for reproductive and sexual health.

Doctor of nursing practice (DNP)

Many APRNs go on to pursue a doctoral degree (DNP) to expand their clinical roles to include more administrative, leadership, and teaching roles.

Physician associate or assistant (PA)

A PA holds a master's degree. Like NPs, PAs can diagnose illness, develop and manage treatment plans, and prescribe medications. PAs can also serve as critical members of a surgical team and work with surgeons to support the care of patients before and after surgery.

Despite the difference in titles, all advanced practice providers have a lot in common with physicians, including the ability to serve as primary care providers and become board-certified in a specialty. So the next time you have an appointment with an advanced practice provider, go with the confidence that they are well-qualified to meet your health needs.

WHERE DO ADVANCED PRACTICE PROVIDERS WORK?

Advanced practice providers can work in many different health care settings, including various types of clinics and hospitals. Their scope of practice varies depending on their education and the state where they practice.

For example, in many states, NPs can have a fully independent practice, without physician collaboration, supervision, or oversight. In other states, NPs practice either under the supervision of a physician or with a collaborative agreement with a physician. In such cases, the physician regularly reviews the care the NP is providing to a percentage of patients in the NP's practice.

As a patient, you can always ask your advanced practice providers what type of practice they have, what conditions they are comfortable treating, and for which instances you would need to be referred to a physician. If your advanced care provider has a supervising or collaborative physician, know who that physician is and be sure you are comfortable with the training and credentials of that physician. Remember that you are always in charge of your health care and the clinicians you see.

WHY SHOULD WOMEN KNOW ABOUT ADVANCED PRACTICE PROVIDERS?

As a patient, you should know the different members of your health care team and the advanced practice providers who are vital members of this team. In addition to diagnosing and treating different health conditions, advanced practice providers are also frequently involved in health promotion and education, preventive health care and screening, and patient advocacy. These activities position them well to play an active role in caring for your health.

You may sometimes find it difficult to get a prompt appointment with a physician. An advanced practice provider may be able to address your health care needs more quickly than a physician. APPs are often able to spend more time with you than a physician might be when explaining a condition, and can explain it in plain language instead of using complex medical terminology. For example, if you are diagnosed with prediabetes, an APP can explain the

journey ahead, including who will be a part of your diabetes care team — such as a physician, APP, dietitian, and other medical professionals — treatment plans and options, and warning signs to watch out for. Knowing what to expect can help you feel less anxious about a diagnosis and more hopeful, knowledgeable, and empowered to make changes. Ultimately, these factors can lead to better health outcomes.

Some APPs have additional training and expertise in providing primary care services specifically to women and are known as women's health nurse practitioners (WHNPs). WHNPs receive specialized training that includes:
- Care related to common and complex gynecologic, sexual and reproductive health concerns, the menopausal transition, and postmenopause health care
- Uncomplicated and high-risk pregnancies and postpartum care after labor and delivery

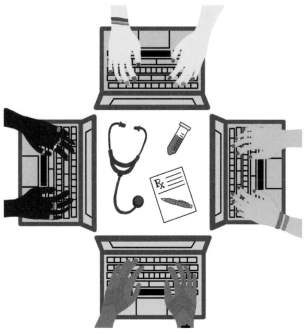

- Sexual and reproductive health care for women and their partners
- Care for uncomplicated nongynecologic health problems
- Care that is inclusive of all gender identities and respectful and responsive to each person's needs and preferences

QUESTIONS TO ASK YOUR ADVANCED PRACTICE PROVIDER

When you first contact an APP, find out what type of practice the APP has.

If you're seeing an APP who has an independent practice:
- What conditions are you comfortable treating?
- When would you refer me to a physician?

If you're seeing an APP who practices with a supervising or collaborative physician:
- Who is your supervising or collaborative physician? (This will allow you to know who the physician is and check out the credentials and background of the physician.)
- How regularly do you interact with the physician?
- Will you be discussing your evaluation of me and your recommended treatment plan with the physician?
- How will you communicate the outcome of this discussion with me?

PEARLS OF WISDOM

Advanced practice providers are well-trained medical professionals who deliver outstanding care for many conditions. Most routine medical conditions can be treated by an APP. While complex medical conditions may be best evaluated by a physician, APPs may be able to see you for an appointment more promptly, spend more time with you, and better coordinate referral to a physician for complex conditions. Remember that you are in charge of your health care. Leveraging the strengths of the diverse members of your health care team can help you achieve better health outcomes.

"We, as a nation, must make women-centered health care a priority, via education and advocacy, as the wellness of individuals, families, and communities depends on it."

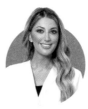

Fatma Haiderzad, D.N.P., M.S., C.R.N.A. - she/her Dr. Haiderzad is self-employed in Miami, Florida, and Chicago, Illinois. Dr. Haiderzad is a health care entrepreneur and board-certified anesthetist. She leads health care venture capital at Lurra Capital and has interests in health equity and digital health solutions including telehealth, artificial intelligence and machine learning.

6
Finding the right clinician

Mara Gordon, M.D., and Kanwal L. Haq, M.S.

WHEN SHOULD I LOOK FOR A CLINICIAN?

The short answer is right now. Don't wait for a problem to establish care with a primary care clinician, since they will work with you to prevent health concerns from becoming full-blown crises. Developing a relationship with a good primary care clinician will help you be your healthiest self, rather than just "slapping bandages" on issues as they arise.

Having a primary care clinician can help with logistical issues such as getting vaccines or filling out paperwork you need for school or work. A primary care clinician can also order referrals, which are sometimes required by your insurance, for health services such as seeing a dietitian, a physical therapist or specialists. Your primary care clinician may also help coordinate care between different specialists, which can sometimes be confusing to understand and navigate.

Establishing care with a primary care clinician is a good time to take stock of your overall health. In the United States, physical health is often considered legally and financially separate from mental health, oral health, and overall wellness. For example, your health insurance probably won't cover dental visits or veggies from the farmers' market. However, a good primary care clinician will still want to hear that you're getting to the dentist, exercising regularly, eating healthy foods, finding positive ways to cope with stress and engaging in a social community. Your primary care clinician can help you see the big picture of your health and stay on top of preventive care. Think of your primary care clinician as the quarterback of your health care team.

WHO IS THE RIGHT CLINICIAN FOR ME?

Before you start looking for a primary care clinician, take some time to reflect on what you need from her. This can help you put together a list of practices to consider. Here are some important considerations as you're thinking about where you'll establish care.

Insurance
Call your insurance provider and find out which primary care practices are considered in-network. Seeing a clinician who accepts your insurance can save you a lot of money in the long run, so it's worth investigating

fully from the start. If you're considering a clinician who isn't in-network, call to ask what kinds of bills you might expect for co-pays or procedures. Also ask if you'll be charged for phone calls, email messages, forms you need to fill out, and telehealth visits.

Location

How far are you willing to travel to see your clinician? If you anticipate needing regular visits, it might be convenient to be able to walk, bike or take public transportation.

Hours

If your schedule makes it difficult to get to appointments during normal business hours, you may want to go to a practice with evening or weekend hours. You may also consider a group practice, with lots of clinicians that may make it easier to squeeze you in for appointments at odd hours.

Telehealth

The ability to get medical care via video and phone has exploded during the COVID-19 pandemic. Ask any clinician you're considering if it's something they offer, and under what circumstances.

Electronic health records

What kind of electronic health record (EHR) does the practice use? Is there a patient portal you can access? A patient portal is a secure app or website where you can access your records, contact your clinician, schedule appointments, pay your bills and update your health information. There's some research that shows using a patient portal may help you monitor chronic conditions and stay up to date with preventive care.

Affiliated hospitals and specialists

Despite technological advances in medical record keeping, many hospital systems don't share records. That means unless your primary care clinician works for the same hospital system as your specialists, your primary care clinician won't be able to read what your specialists write about you. It can also make it difficult for your primary care clinician and specialists to communicate easily. If you anticipate needing specialty care, a procedure, or if you've been hospitalized in the past, you may want to choose a primary care clinician who works in the same hospital system as the specialists.

Languages

If English isn't your first language, it's a great idea to look for a primary care clinician who speaks your native language. Ask friends and family for their recommendations or do a quick Google search. If you can't find a clinician who is fluent in your preferred language, ask about interpretation services that may be offered by your clinician. Find out if these services would be in-person, virtual, or over a telephone. Also ask if services are available 24/7.

Demographics

The research is mixed on whether having a clinician who matches your demographics improves your health. Different cultural groups have different perspectives, ideas, customs, and stigmas around health care services, so it is perfectly acceptable to seek a clinician who is aware of, understands, and respects your cultural, religious, and other personal beliefs and traditions. Some studies suggest that Black patients may have better experiences with Black clinicians. Other studies show that women patients don't need to see women clinicians to feel satisfied with their care. However, if you prefer a female clinician, you should feel comfortable seeking one out.

On-call services

Find out what happens if you have an urgent after-hours question. Is there an on-call service where your concerns can be addressed by a clinician? Who staffs it? Will you be charged?

Pediatrics and geriatrics

Many family medicine clinicians and physicians certified in both internal medicine and pediatrics see both adults and kids. If you care for young children or older adults, you may find it helpful to take them to the same clinician you see.

Procedures and scope of care

Many primary care clinicians offer a host of common services. These include:

- Routine gynecologic care, such as pap smears or long-acting reversible contraception (for example, intrauterine devices)
- Joint injections
- Mental health care, such as treatment for depression, anxiety, or addiction

Many practices also offer what's called integrated mental health care, which means that your primary care clinician works with a therapist in the same office to coordinate therapy and medicines for mental health concerns. Some family physicians also provide prenatal and abortion care. You should feel empowered to ask about all of these services when you're establishing care. A one-stop shop for your health

can make it much easier to get the care you need.

HOW TO CONDUCT A QUALITY CHECK WHEN LOOKING FOR A CLINICIAN

There are a lot of great clinicians out there. The next step is finding the one who is perfect for you.

Ask around

We recommend starting with recommendations from family, friends and colleagues you trust. Nothing beats a personal suggestion.

Search online . . . to a point

Most clinicians assume that their patients are Googling them! Take a look at their professional profiles and see what they choose to highlight — it can give you valuable information about them. Online reviews may or may not be helpful because they're often unregulated and tend to attract either really happy or really unhappy patients. We also suggest prioritizing factors other than a clinician's pedigree. It's easy to look up their credentials if you want to, but communication style is probably more important than where they went to medical school.

Shop around

We encourage you to make "getting to know you" appointments with multiple clinicians. As you're preparing to invest in a relationship with a new clinician, make sure you find one that is right for you.

Staying up to date

It's imperative that your clinician stays up to date with medical research. When you make those first appointments, you should feel empowered to ask how the clinician continues their own education. Do they read medical journals, attend conferences, or teach students themselves? Academic practices — where clinicians teach trainees such as students or medical residents — are often a great place to find those who love to follow medical research, although being a patient at an academic practice may mean you'll also be seen by students and trainees in addition to your own clinician.

It's not just about the clinician

You'll also be interacting with nurses, medical and nursing assistants, and front desk staff. Make sure they treat you with respect, too, since you'll inevitably be interacting with them in addition to your clinician.

Trust your gut

When you meet your potential clinician, how do you feel? Do they actively listen, making eye contact with you, not the computer? Do you have a chance to ask questions? Do you feel rushed? Do they ask what the matter is, along with what matters to you? How do you feel disclosing personal information? Does your clinician explain their thinking and decision making in a way you understand?

Speak up

If you have a specific complaint that's easy to fix, it might be helpful to give your clinician feedback. Clinicians are used to it,

Evaluating

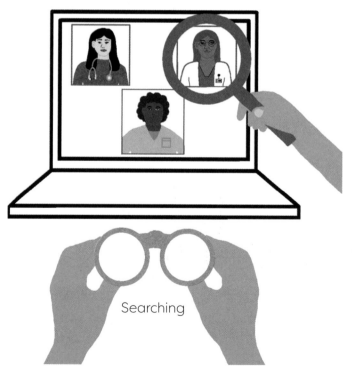

Searching

so feel free to share suggestions such as "I need time to ask questions during each visit," or "Please summarize your recommendations in writing."

It's OK to break up

If you don't feel comfortable with your clinician after that first appointment — or after the first 10 — it's OK to seek care elsewhere. For example, if you feel like your clinician doesn't listen well or you feel dismissed, it's well within your rights to find somebody new.

PEARLS OF WISDOM

As you embark on your search for a primary care clinician, it's important to understand some basics about health care in the United States and equip yourself with strategies to get the best out of the relationship.

Visits are short and sweet

Short appointments are the unfortunate reality of modern medical care. Most primary care practices offer visits that are between 10 and 20 minutes long. (The exception to this is concierge medicine, sometimes known as direct primary care, where you pay a fee in addition to your insurance costs for greater access to your clinician.) Make sure you have realistic expectations for what you can accomplish during this period of time. You can always make a follow-up appointment.

You and your clinician are on the same team

Sometimes, it can feel like your clinician doesn't share your priorities. You want to talk about your back pain, for example, and she wants to talk about your blood pressure. Remember that your clinician is trained to prioritize emergencies, so if she's worried about something, it's likely a health problem that needs to be addressed urgently. However, it should still feel like you're on the same team. Your clinician should be asking both "What is the matter?" and "What matters to you?" By bringing up what is perhaps most important to you, both you and your clinician can have a focused agenda during the visit. For example, if your clinician tries to redirect the agenda for a visit, discuss it directly: "It seems like you want to talk about my blood pressure, but today, I want to work on my back pain." You may not be able to fix everything in one visit, but a good clinician will make room to address what matters to you. This is part of shared decision making (see Chapter 7) and leads to better health care and experiences.

Stick to one or two challenges

Since primary care appointments are so short, you'll be better served if you thoroughly address one or two issues that matter to you in your time with your clinician rather than trying to tackle too many at once and failing.

Write it down

Bringing a list of questions with you can help you stick to those one or two problems and make sure you get every last concern about those specific problems addressed. Keep track of your symptoms in a simple diary in your smartphone or take pictures of a rash; this can help you make sure you're giving your clinician an accurate portrait of your symptoms.

A good plan can take time

Despite the impression you might get from watching a show like *Grey's Anatomy*, sometimes the right diagnosis and the right plan can take time. A good clinician will never blow off your symptoms or make you feel dismissed, but it can take multiple visits for even the best experts to arrive at a diagnosis. And when you get the right diagnosis, finding an effective treatment plan can take time and hard work. Sometimes the best treatment is no treatment at all, or involves a holistic approach like focusing on exercise, stress management, and healthy eating. Don't be too quick to jump ship for a clinician who offers a fast fix, since sometimes the most effective remedies require patience.

You're entitled to a second opinion

Clinicians expect that you'll seek out second opinions, especially for serious conditions or before a procedure. You should feel empowered to hear from other clinicians regarding a diagnosis or a plan of action. Do be up front when you're seeking a second opinion — that will help both your original clinician and the new one, whom you're seeing for that additional opinion, tailor the visits to your needs.

Don't settle

You're investing in a long-term relationship, so connecting with the right person may take a while. That's OK. Be honest with yourself and your clinician about what you need.

"Liberation and justice for women will always be bound up with women's access to health care."

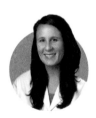

Mara Gordon, M.D. - she/her
Dr. Gordon is an assistant professor of Family Medicine at Cooper Medical School of Rowan University in Camden, New Jersey. She serves as a primary care physician for patients of all ages and has a special interest in reproductive health and mental health in the primary care setting.

"Selfish prudence is too often allowed to come between duty and human life."
– Dr. Rebecca Lee Crumpler

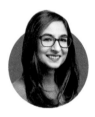

Kanwal L. Haq, M.S. - she/her
Kanwal is a medical anthropologist passionate about creating more connected, more informed, and more equitable systems of care. She specializes in community-based participatory research and builds accessible tools, resources, and programs for women around the globe. Kanwal currently leads the NYC women's health programs at the Arnhold Institute for Global Health at Mount Sinai's Icahn School of Medicine.

7
Shared decision making and you

Mary I. O'Connor, M.D., and Kanwal L. Haq, M.S.

WHAT IS SHARED DECISION MAKING?

Making decisions regarding medical treatment can be difficult and have a great impact on you and your family. Is that surgery right for you? Should you take this medication, which has potential side effects? Should you get a vaccine?

Medicine has traditionally been very paternalistic. This means that the person in authority (the doctor) makes decisions for you based on what that person believes is in your best interest. Often such "decisions" are recommendations for you to have certain tests or procedures, without a more comprehensive discussion about the potential advantages and disadvantages of these recommendations. Say, for example, you develop back or knee pain and are referred to a surgeon. The surgeon evaluates you and recommends a magnetic resonance imaging scan (MRI) in an attempt to identify what is wrong. Was there any discussion with you regarding the potential option of not getting an MRI at that moment and instead starting with, for example, physical therapy for your pain?

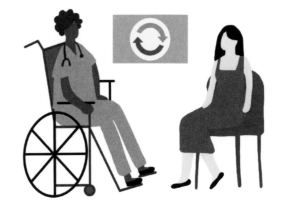

This is an important conversation because inappropriate MRIs may lead to inappropriate surgery. The result is that 17% to 50% of spine surgeries and 20% to 34% of knee replacement procedures may be unwarranted. But you may not be comfortable questioning the physician, who after all did go through medical school and several years of training to help guide you. However, that does not mean that the physician should be dictating certain tests or treatments without first ensuring that you understand the options and potential outcomes and agree to proceed. What should happen is a process called "shared decision making" (SDM).

MAKE THE BEST DECISION FOR YOU

Shared decision making is defined as "a process in which both the patient and health care professional work together to decide the best plan of care for the patient." Taking into account your values, goals and concerns, your clinician helps you learn more about your health condition, as well as the testing and treatment options available to you and their potential risks and benefits. What is critically important to understand is that SDM is not simply information your clinician gives you about your options. It's a conversation between you and your clinician to help you make the best decision for you.

WHY DOES SDM MATTER TO WOMEN?

For women, SDM is especially important. The gender gap in medicine is real and complex. For example, research shows that older women tend to receive fewer physician services than men with similar health needs do. One study showed that women with significant knee arthritis receive less medical information and less encouragement to participate in the decision to undergo knee replacement surgery than do men with the same condition. Many physicians — especially surgeons — are men, and may project an authoritarian presence. As a result, women may be afraid to ask questions for fear of being labeled "difficult." If you feel uncomfortable asking your clinician questions, please find another clinician who creates a safe and welcoming atmosphere for you.

ASK ABOUT SDM TOOLS

SDM is supported by patient decision aids (PDA), which are tools that help people become involved in decision making by making clear what the decision is, providing information on options and outcomes, and clarifying personal values. To understand how PDAs work, let's look at one example — the Movement is Life Shared Decision Making tool. This tool is designed for people with knee pain, with the goal of empowering them to take an active role in their health care journey. It is also designed to help address health disparities in knee pain between genders, races and ethnicities. It projects a likely outcome of treatment based on age, gender, race and ethnicity, education level, severity of knee pain, level of physical function and potential impact on lost work productivity.

The image on the next page shows how the Movement is Life Shared Decision Making tool works. It features a 67-year-old African American woman with obesity and hypertension who is on Medicare and has a high school education. She has moderate knee pain (5 out of 10 on the pain scale) that limits her ability to function fully in daily life.

The PDA tool shows that if she does nothing, her knee pain and physical limitations will increase with time and negatively impact her productivity if she is working outside the home. It also shows that if she increases her level of physical activity, loses some weight and uses nonprescription medications for her pain, she can significantly improve her symptoms and decrease their impact on her productivity. Her symptoms would also improve with

Shared decision making

The following chart demonstrates how shared decision making works with the Movement is Life tool for knee pain. The chart shows how an older woman with knee pain, high blood pressure and obesity might work through different scenarios with her clinician.

Arrows below show changes relative to today

Knee pain	What would happen if you:	YEAR 1	YEAR 3	YEAR 6
1 — No Pain 10 — Extreme Pain	Do nothing	5	6 ⬆	7 ⬆
TODAY: 5 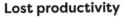	Increase activity, lose weight and take nonprescription medications	0 ⬇	2 ⬇	5
	Do physical therapy, receive corticosteroid injections and take prescription medications	2 ⬇	2 ⬇	5

Activity level	What would happen if you:	YEAR 1	YEAR 3	YEAR 6
1 — No Limitation 10 — Extreme Limitation	Do nothing	5	6 ⬆	7 ⬆
TODAY: 5	Increase activity, lose weight and take nonprescription medications	0 ⬇	2 ⬇	5
	Do physical therapy, receive corticosteroid injections and take prescription medications	0 ⬇	2 ⬇	5

Lost productivity

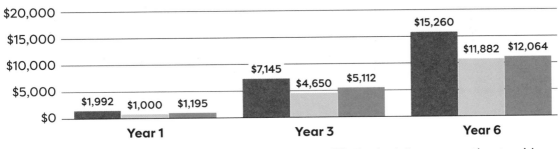

	Year 1	Year 3	Year 6
No Treatment	$1,992	$7,145	$15,260
Increased activity, weight loss, nonprescription medications	$1,000	$4,650	$11,882
Physical therapy, corticosteroid injections, prescription medications	$1,195	$5,112	$12,064

 No Treatment

Increased activity, weight loss, nonprescription medications

Physical therapy, corticosteroid injections, prescription medications physical therapy, cortisone injections into her knee joint and prescription medications.

PDA tools exist for a variety of conditions. The next time you have an important medical decision to make with your clinician, ask if there are decision support tools to help the two of you make a shared decision.

PEARLS OF WISDOM

Almost all treatments in medicine have both benefits and risks — some with greater risks than others. Your clinician brings valuable knowledge and experience to your decision making, but you are the most important person in the conversation, because this decision is about your health. Aim to make the health care decisions that are best for you, guided and supported by your trusted clinician through shared decision making.

"Women need to have their voices heard by their doctors and other members of their health care team."

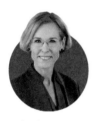

Mary I. O'Connor, M.D. - she/her
Dr. O'Connor is co-founder and Chief Medical Officer at Vori Health, an innovative health care enterprise with a mission to empower all people to lead their healthiest lives. She serves as Chair of Movement is Life, a national nonprofit coalition committed to health equity. Dr. O'Connor is a past chair of the Department of Orthopedic Surgery at Mayo Clinic in Jacksonville, Florida, and Emerita Professor of Orthopedics at Mayo Clinic. She specialized in bone and soft tissue tumor surgery and hip and knee replacement surgery.

"If society will not admit of women's free development, then society must be remodeled." – Elizabeth Blackwell

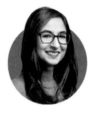

Kanwal L. Haq, M.S. - she/her
Kanwal is a medical anthropologist passionate about creating more connected, more informed, and more equitable systems of care. She specializes in community-based participatory research and builds accessible tools, resources, and programs for women around the globe. Kanwal currently leads the NYC women's health programs at the Arnhold Institute for Global Health at Mount Sinai's Icahn School of Medicine.

8
Telemedicine: Getting the most out of your care

Erkeda DeRouen, M.D.

WHAT IS TELEMEDICINE?

There are many names for telemedicine. Telehealth, digital medicine, virtual health, and remote monitoring are just a few. Telemedicine visits can be via telephone, video, email, and even text.

In traditional care, office visits consist of obtaining a history of the present illness (learning the "story" of what is causing concern), performing a physical checkup during which you are evaluated via visual examination and physical touch, and discussing the diagnosis and plan for treatment.

With telehealth, a major component of the physical examination is missing — the ability of your doctor or other clinician to touch you! However, this sort of disadvantage can be offset by having you do certain movements that your clinician can see, such as lifting your arms over your head or walking. Telehealth can also be supplemented with a variety of growing technological aids. Since most diagnoses can be made by your clinician by obtaining the

history or "story" of what happened, telemedicine is a great place to start care.

The delivery of telehealth care comes in many shapes and sizes. For instance, some forms are affiliated with your primary care office, while others are delivered by privately owned companies with little or no connection to your primary care home. Still others are connected to large hospital systems. Knowing which type of telehealth visit you are having may help you know what to expect in terms of the personal information that you may need to share. In this chapter, we're primarily talking about a telemedicine encounter, which involves the ability to obtain an evaluation, diagnosis, and recommendation for treatment by using internet-connected devices in a location that is separate from your physician or another clinician.

WHEN SHOULD TELEMEDICINE BE USED?

The following are a few examples of situations in which telemedicine can be used.

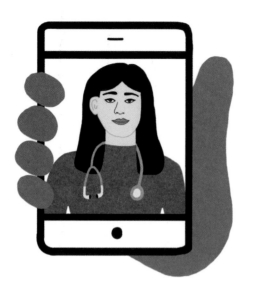

Preventive care

Individuals can obtain some preventive health screenings and education remotely. This also applies to follow-ups after hospitalizations to help prevent hospital readmission. Telehealth is revolutionary, but it has boundaries. You still need in-person care for "hands-on" procedures, such as Pap smears. Or you may need a higher level of evaluation, depending on the information you provided. When a clinician tells you that she needs to see you in person to get more clarity, it means that she is giving you comprehensive care!

Straightforward concerns

Imagine developing an itchy rash after a hike outdoors. With telemedicine you can phone a doctor, share an image, and obtain a diagnosis and proposed treatment right from your living room sofa!

Chronic care

Telemedicine can be very helpful for individuals with chronic medical conditions that require regular medical visits. For many people, managing diabetes, high blood pressure and heart disease can be safely and effectively done with telemedicine.

Mental health care

Mental health care can be provided through telemedicine. A little-known fact is that the first cases of telehealth in the U.S. were in the mental health field in the 1960s. During the COVID-19 pandemic, virtual mental health visits have exponentially increased.

HOW SHOULD YOU PREPARE FOR A TELEMEDICINE VISIT?

To get the most benefit from a telemedicine visit, it is important to be prepared. Provide as much information to your clinician as possible. Much of your diagnosis and treatment plan depends on the story that you tell your clinician about what's been happening to you. This is not the time to be shy or vague. Pretend that you're talking to your best friend and tell your clinician everything!

What's happening?

At the very minimum, you will need to communicate:

- What is concerning you?
- When did your concern start?
- How much is your concern affecting your daily life?
- What makes it better or worse?
- Is your concern constant or intermittent?
- What have you tried to make it better?
- How is it impacting your life?

Additionally, you should be prepared to provide:

Medical history

No one knows your medical history better than you. Depending on where your clinician is working, much of your health record may not be available to her. If you are using a telehealth company that is not affiliated with your primary care office, let them know all of the things that you have been diagnosed with, as they could be related to your current diagnosis and treatment.

List of medications

Medication lists are super important. Provide your clinician with a list of everything that you are taking, including supplements or vitamins. Some of what you're taking may be contributing to your symptoms, and some may interact with potential medications that you may need.

List of allergies

Always share your allergies to medications with your clinician, to avoid allergic reactions. Never assume that this information is recorded in the system!

Vital signs

Vital signs are very, very, very important! They give your clinician the inside scoop as to how your body is responding to stress or infection. Do not guess about certain values, such as body temperature, as these values are used to determine the treatment of a condition. It is better to say "I do not know" than to say that you have a fever without measuring your temperature. A fever is defined by specific body temperatures — 100.4 degrees Fahrenheit or higher. Also, providing information, such as telling your clinician that you have a cough in addition to a fever, could be the deciding factor (among a few other things) in your diagnosis. For example, providing all the information that you're able to could make the difference between a diagnosis of a viral infection and a diagnosis of pneumonia.

HOW CAN TELEMEDICINE DECREASE HEALTH CARE DISPARITIES?

The American health care system is full of health care disparities. Much of this is due to the infrastructure of our society, in which socioeconomic factors create large gaps in resources. There are many social determinants of health (see Chapter 1) that affect people in all aspects of life. In particular, access to health care is influenced by interconnected factors such as educational access and quality; economic stability; neighborhood environment; and community. Biases run rampant. Telemedicine can help bridge some of these gaps since it's not tied to location.

Telemedicine can also provide a great opportunity to expand access to care in rural areas, where 9% of U.S. physicians care for 20% of the country's population. Additionally, it can provide opportunities for people to engage with medical care by decreasing some physical barriers to attending office visits, such as lack of transportation or decreased availability of medical caregivers in an area.

WHY DOES TELEHEALTH MATTER TO WOMEN?

Telemedicine has reimagined women's health. Now you can obtain medication refills, such as birth control, using digital care. You may have the option of obtaining close follow-up care during pregnancy without needing to go in person for each of those closely scheduled visits. The flexibility of telehealth can also help women who may otherwise avoid health care because of time or schedule constraints. Digital health can provide a way for women to access care that fits into their life structure while avoiding the hustle and bustle of an office visit. For example, you may not need to take off work for a checkup visit if you're using more-flex-ible telehealth hours. And if you have children, you won't need to find a babysitter to attend a virtual follow-up visit.

PEARLS OF WISDOM

Although there are limitations in performing the physical exam, telemedicine is a fantas-tic option for many medical concerns. It is often used as an adjunct to in-person care. Sometimes, it can provide access to those who may not have sought care without it. It is important to appear at a virtual visit with as much information about your medical history, medications, allergies and current symptoms as possible.

For telemedicine to work well and be effective in today's society, women need access to technology, including the internet. State medical licensing agencies must support health care workers performing telemedicine. Trust between women and their clinicians should be established to promote the best outcomes and experience. This may be more challenging in the virtual environment when a woman hasn't met the clinician before. We must keep working to improve telemedicine technology in order to meet the goal of decreasing bias and disparities.

"Visualize your highest self and start showing up as her!"

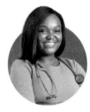

Erkeda DeRouen, M.D. - she/ her
Dr. DeRouen is a Medical Consultant who practices telemedicine and is triple board certified in Family, Diversity, & Lifestyle Medicine with a focus on Telehealth.

9

Urgent care versus the emergency department

Tehreem Rehman, M.D., M.P.H.

WHAT ARE URGENT CARE CENTERS?

Urgent care centers are places where you can get quick and convenient basic health care. Typically, urgent care centers offer extended night and weekend hours, walk-in appointments and a limited number of higher-level services. The vast majority of urgent care centers can process lab tests, perform X-ray imaging and provide stitches. Most centers can deliver routine immunizations and administer fluids through an IV if necessary. Over 80% of urgent care centers can provide orthopedic-related care, such as splinting and casting.

While the demand for emergency department (ED) services has grown significantly in the past few years, the number of urgent care centers also has grown tremendously, surpassing the growth of hospital emergency departments in the U.S. Currently, there are about 9,200 urgent care centers in the U.S. collectively seeing 122 million people each year. This comes out to an average of 36 people seen each day per facility. In comparison, there are only 4,200 EDs, which provide services to 137 million

patients each year. On average, 89 people are seen each day at every ED.

Most urgent care centers operate independently of hospitals. However, an increasing number of hospital systems are opening their own urgent care centers for people needing help with common clinical conditions. When an urgent care center is available in a neighborhood, residents are almost four times less likely to go to the ED. This is a good thing, because a visit to the urgent care center for a common health concern can help you avoid crowding, longer wait times and overstretched resources. It will likely cost you less, too. Common procedures and diagnostics cost about 11 times more when administered at an ED versus an urgent care center.

Incidentally, telemedicine (see Chapter 8) can also be used for many common conditions that might be evaluated at an urgent care center. Virtual visits are even more convenient than using an urgent care center because they can be scheduled at a time that's convenient for you and can take place in your own home. Basic lab tests and X-rays cannot be performed with a telemedicine visit, although your telemedicine clinician can order those tests and you can go to a test center to have them done.

HOW ARE URGENT CARE CENTERS DIFFERENT FROM EMERGENCY DEPARTMENTS?

Urgent care centers are not obligated to provide services to those who cannot pay, and unfortunately urgent care services are not always available for publicly insured or uninsured women. However, a hospital emergency department must see everyone regardless of their health insurance status.

In some situations, going to a hospital ED is more appropriate than going to an urgent care center. If there is any concern about a life-threatening illness such as a heart attack or stroke, for example, an urgent care center will immediately refer you to a hospital ED.

Common triggers for an ED referral include abnormal vital signs, such as an irregular heart rate or high blood pressure. You might also be referred to an ED if you appear confused and are behaving unusually.

If you are older or taking medicines for multiple conditions, your condition may be more complex and require more testing than an urgent care center can provide. If you require advanced imaging tests, such as ultrasound or a CT scan, you'll likely be referred to an ED, since less than one-fifth of urgent care centers are equipped to offer these advanced services.

WHY SHOULD YOU CARE ABOUT THE DIFFERENCE?

Urgent care centers can provide access to care when you are unable to get an appointment with a primary care clinician. Often, people who have public health insurance are disproportionately harmed by this inability to get help from a primary care clinician. One study showed that only 1 out of 4 people with Medicaid was able to obtain a primary care appointment within seven days after discharge from an ED, and the overall appointment rate was a little over 50%. In comparison, over one-third of people with commercial insurance were able to get an appointment within seven days and their overall appointment rate was almost 80%. As a result, urgent care centers are often a more feasible option for people who have public insurance, but they may not accept people with public health insurance or those without insurance.

For common conditions, regular use of urgent care centers rather than a primary care setting can result in increased cost, redundant testing and fragmented care.

Similar to the way that urgent care centers provide easy access to primary care, EDs can more easily provide access to specialty care. For instance, if you had a procedure performed recently and the surgeon is a member of the ED health care system, the ED care team is more likely to actively involve the specialist in your care in a timely fashion. Additionally, the type of health insurance you have may affect your access to a particular specialist. Some research suggests that specialists are more likely to see a publicly insured or uninsured patient if the patient was referred from the ED. For example, if you have been suffering from migraines without relief at home and your neurology appointment is not for another six months, a visit to the ED can treat your symptoms and may help you see that neurologist sooner. However, a visit to the ED does not mean that you will be able to get an elective surgery, such as removal of your gallbladder, any faster.

In other situations, urgent care centers can stabilize a person who is in critical condition and expedite that person's transfer to an ED without having to rely on emergency medical services (EMS), which traditionally facilitate access to EDs for critically ill people as appropriate. Some urgent care centers have privileges to directly admit people to certain hospitals without having to go through the ED. However, urgent care centers are usually staffed by nurse practitioners, physician assistants, and internal medicine or family medicine doctors. These clinicians are trained to care for children and adults, including pregnant women, as well as to perform common procedures. However, they do not undergo the same degree of training in resuscitation and stabilization of critically ill people that is required of emergency doctors, which is why urgent care centers refer appropriate transfers to the ED.

There is a risk of over-transferring people from urgent care centers to EDs. Approximately one of every four people transferred to EDs from urgent care centers is ultimately discharged directly from the ED and does not stay in the hospital. Some experts have proposed that EMS clinicians redirect people from the ED to an urgent care center

when appropriate. Yet, 1 person out of 10 was inappropriately diverted to an urgent care center. This can cause delay in your access to high-level care and potentially result in poor health outcomes.

As someone who may not be in medicine, you may find it difficult to know when to go to the ED and when to go to an urgent care center. That is why it is important to educate yourself on the differences between the ED and an urgent care center.

The most common reasons urgent care centers transfer people to an ED include deep or jagged wounds (lacerations), broken bones (fractures), skin infection (cellulitis), pneumonia, and nonspecific abdominal or chest pain. Some lacerations require more complex repair and, depending on the location of the laceration, may even require the involvement of a specialist such as a plastic surgeon. If a fracture is unstable or bone is exposed, an ED referral will prompt a consultation with an orthopedic surgeon. Cellulitis or other skin infections sometimes require IV antibiotics and possibly even hospital admission for close monitoring. For older adults or people who need oxygen, the ED referral helps with admission to the hospital for further care. Nonspecific abdominal pain, especially in older adults, usually requires more specific imaging such as a CT scan, which can be performed in an ED. Although urgent care centers can perform electrocardiograms — a heart test that looks for abnormal electrical signals — and other basic labs, urgent care staff will likely refer someone with chest pain and any abnormal test results to the ED for further observation or evaluation by a specialist.

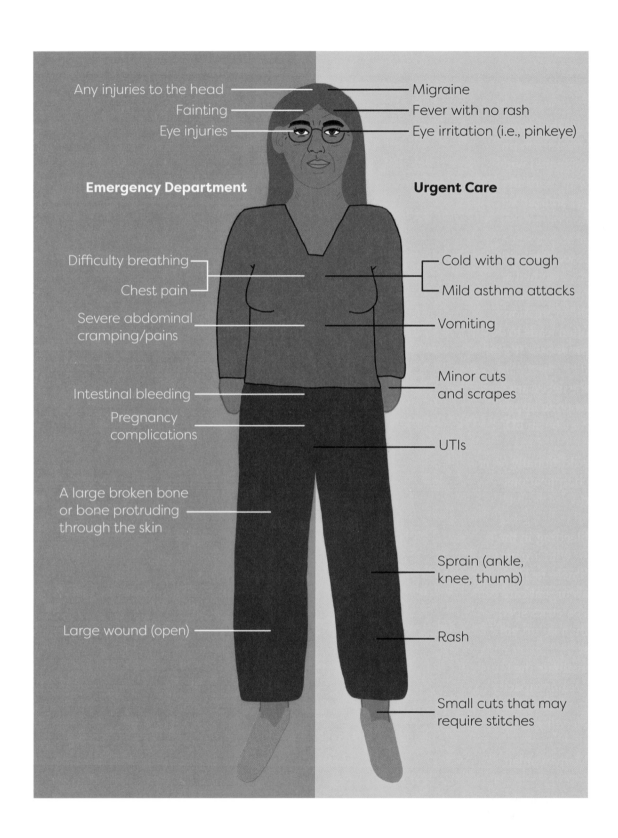

Any injuries to the head

Fainting

Eye injuries

Migraine

Fever with no rash

Eye irritation (i.e., pinkeye)

Emergency Department

Urgent Care

Difficulty breathing

Chest pain

Cold with a cough

Mild asthma attacks

Severe abdominal cramping/pains

Vomiting

Intestinal bleeding

Pregnancy complications

Minor cuts and scrapes

UTIs

A large broken bone or bone protruding through the skin

Sprain (ankle, knee, thumb)

Large wound (open)

Rash

Small cuts that may require stitches

WHY DO THESE DIFFERENCES MATTER TO WOMEN?

Life-threatening emergencies, such as heart attacks, can present differently in women compared with men. Women often present with more atypical symptoms, such as generalized weakness or feelings of indigestion rather than the crushing "elephant-sitting-on-the-chest" pain that is typically associated with a heart attack. Because of this, women are at risk of being misdiagnosed. In fact, there is documented bias in the evaluation of chest pain in women that often leads to delayed care and worse prognosis. It's important for women to have their chest pain evaluated in a place that has the necessary resources and expertise to respond appropriately, which in many cases may be an ED.

Additionally, women with pregnancy complications — such as leaking fluid, decreased fetal movement at greater than 20 weeks gestational age, and vaginal bleeding in the second or third trimester — who are unable to see their OB-GYN in a timely fashion should go to an ED and not an urgent care center. An ED has access to obstetrics specialists and is more likely than an urgent care center to have ultrasound imaging available to immediately evaluate the fetus. Additionally, an ED has greater capacity to initiate life-saving treatment, such as blood transfusions, if bleeding is significant.

Many women, not just those of reproductive age, are disproportionately affected by structural determinants of health inequity. These include housing instability, food insecurity and caregiver burden. Women are also more likely to suffer from certain mental health concerns, such as anxiety, depression and post-traumatic stress disorder (PTSD). The impact of psychosocial factors on a woman's health and symptoms is more likely to be addressed appropriately in an ED rather than in an urgent care center. Health care teams in EDs have access to greater resources and interdisciplinary partners such as community health workers, social workers, and care managers. For mental health concerns, women can be connected to crisis counselors, psychiatrists and other mental health specialists.

QUESTIONS TO ASK YOUR HEALTH CARE TEAM

At the urgent care center:
- Do I need to be transferred to an ED?
- If I am being transferred to an ED, why?
- Is there any chance that my symptoms could be related to a life-threatening illness that you can't test for here?
- What additional testing do I need to get for this condition that you cannot test for here?
- When should I follow up with my primary care clinician?
- Are you a doctor?

(Not all clinicians have the same level of training. Urgent care centers are often staffed by nurse practitioners and physician assistants.)

At the emergency department:
- Why are these tests being ordered?
- What are we waiting for?
- Are you a doctor?

› If yes, are you the attending or resident doctor?

(Residents are appropriately supervised and trained to treat you and often can help expedite your workup in the ED. However, the final decision about your care lies with the attending physician.)

- How can I get hold of my nurse if I need something addressed urgently (for example, using the bathroom, or feeling pain or worsening of symptoms)?
- Is my condition managed by a specific specialist at your hospital?
    › Who is that specialist?
    › Is that specialist on call today?
    › Has the specialist been notified that I am in the ED?

PEARLS OF WISDOM

Women are experts on their own bodies. Even if your symptoms do not follow a traditional pattern, you could still be at risk of a life-threatening illness. Urgent care centers can sometimes be more accessible when you do not have access to a primary care clinician. However, urgent care centers are not just smaller emergency departments. Advocate for yourself by knowing what urgent care centers can and cannot provide for you, and when obtaining care is crucial, that you receive the higher level of care that an ED is likely to provide.

"Women are the experts on their own bodies."

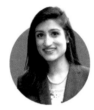

Tehreem Rehman, M.D., M.P.H. - she/her
Dr. Rehman is an emergency physician and an Administration, Operations, and Quality Fellow at the University of Colorado School of Medicine. She specializes in population health management, value-based care and health equity.

Part 2

Common conditions impacting women

10
ACL tears

Monique S. Haynes, M.D., M.P.H., M.B.A., and Elizabeth C. Gardner, M.D.

WHAT IS AN ACL TEAR?

The anterior cruciate ligament (ACL) is a rubber band-like structure in the knee that connects the femur (thigh bone) with the tibia (lower leg bone). It holds these bones in proper position during motion, preventing the tibia from rotating too much or moving too far in front of the femur. Unfortunately, you probably know someone who has injured their ACL, or at least heard of someone who has. Most often the ACL is injured when someone is running and changes their speed of movement abruptly or pivots to a new direction. It can also be injured when a force is applied directly to the knee — for example, during a sports game or a motor vehicle accident. Many people who experience ACL tears describe hearing a loud popping sound and then having significant swelling of the knee shortly after. They might also describe a sensation of the knee "giving out" when pressure is applied to the joint, or when they move quickly in a different direction.

CAN ACL TEARS BE PREVENTED?

While ACL tears cannot be completely prevented, there are ways to reduce the risk of injury. These methods aim to optimize proper nerve and muscle control of the knee, increase power and balance, and improve core strength and stability.

Bracing
A supportive brace is often used both to prevent injury and to stabilize the knee when returning to a sport after ACL surgery. While there is no strong evidence that wearing a brace can prevent injury to the ACL, braces do prevent injuries to the medial collateral ligament (MCL), another important ligament on the inside of the knee. When deciding whether a brace might be beneficial, it's important for you and your clinician to consider your specific activities and individual risk factors.

Injury prevention programs
Multiple ACL prevention programs have been developed to try to improve certain modifiable risk factors for ACL injury, such as abnormal movement patterns and faulty nerve-muscle communication patterns. Most of these neuromuscular programs are successful in reducing injury rates, typically by using prescribed exercises performed consistently over a specific time frame. While the specifics of each program vary, here are some common features.

Front view of the knee

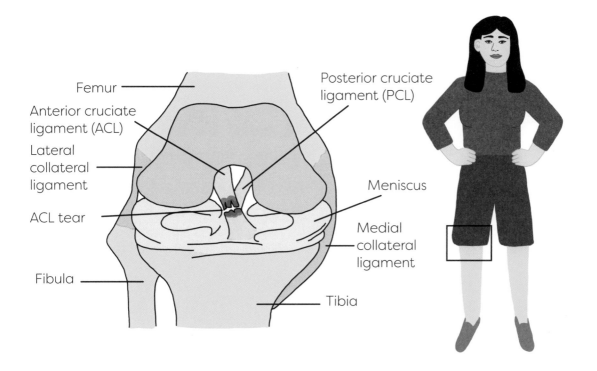

Femur
Anterior cruciate ligament (ACL)
Lateral collateral ligament
ACL tear
Fibula
Posterior cruciate ligament (PCL)
Meniscus
Medial collateral ligament
Tibia

Balance training This type of training focuses on improving stability. Participants practice exercises in unstable positions, such as catching a ball while balancing on one leg or while standing on an uneven or wobbly surface. The goal is to improve the body's ability to stabilize itself.

Strength training Focusing on core and hamstring muscles, these exercises use resistance bands, body weight, free weights or machines to strengthen the muscles that stabilize the body and the knee.

Agility training Agility refers to the ability to change body position or direction quickly and effectively. Agility training focuses on controlled change of direction. Participants practice foot placement and body alignment techniques at fast speeds. These exercises aim to improve the body's control while pivoting or cutting, which are particularly high-risk activities for ACL tears.

Jump training These exercises have two purposes. The first is to develop power during agility exercises, such as bounding. The second, which is even more important, is the focus on proper landing mechanics, which are commonly faulty in those who have experienced an ACL tear.

Stretching These exercises involve using classic static stretches (holding stretches for a period) to address problematic muscle imbalance or tightness and improve the flexibility of nearby tendons.

HOW ARE ACL TEARS TREATED?

A medical professional can usually detect an ACL injury by doing a series of physical exam maneuvers. The maneuvers put stress on the ACL and test its ability to keep the knee stable. An account of how the injury happened, as well as details about subsequent sensations of instability, are often very helpful in making a diagnosis. In many cases, an MRI is done to confirm suspicion of an ACL tear.

If an ACL tear is detected, the next step is to decide whether to treat the injury with surgery or with nonsurgical therapy. This decision depends on several factors, including the severity of injury to the ACL, whether other injuries are also present, your own personal circumstances and what you anticipate your physical demands will be in the future.

Nonoperative treatment of ACL tears

For some women, the best treatment for an ACL tear is non-surgical. Typically, successful nonoperative treatment includes a course of physical therapy to recover from the injury that caused the tear and to optimize movement patterns and strength, such as described in the neuromuscular prevention programs in the previous section. Consistent low-risk exercises allow many women to continue to lead active lives. Some women may decide, with their clinician, to wear a brace for some activities and may modify their activities to avoid particularly high-risk sports.

Operative treatment of ACL tears

Surgery is often the preferred option for younger athletes — particularly those involved in high-risk pivoting sports — and for people who experience ongoing instability despite appropriate non-surgical treatment. The surgery is typically performed as an outpatient procedure — meaning you don't stay overnight in the hospital — using a minimally invasive approach with a camera (arthroscopic procedure).

ACL reconstruction The current gold standard for treating ACL tears is ACL reconstruction. During reconstruction, the injured ACL tissue is removed from the knee joint and replaced by other tendons, taken either from another location in the body (autograft) or from a cadaver donor (allograft). There are pros and cons to each graft choice — review them carefully with your surgeon. The most common grafts are from the patella tendon, hamstring tendons, quadriceps tendon or multiple different allograft options. The graft is shaped to mimic and ideally function like the original ACL. Reconstruction is usually effective in restoring knee stability and allowing people to return to physical activity. As with any procedure, however, it is not without risk. It has been associated with decreased thigh muscle strength, pain in the front of the knee, and potential development of osteoarthritis.

ACL repair ACL repair is another procedure that can treat ACL tears. During ACL repair, the original ligament is kept in place and fixed, so there is no need for a graft. Unfortunately, most ACL tears don't heal well even after the torn ends are surgically reconnected. For this reason, repair procedures have historically been associated with less favorable outcomes, which is why reconstruction has become the recommended method of surgical treatment.

However, newer imaging techniques make it possible to identify tears that may be more suitable for repair, resulting in a renewed interest in ACL repair. Recent studies have shown that ACL repair can be effective depending on the location of the tear and the techniques used by the surgeon.

Postsurgical rehabilitation No matter which treatment technique is chosen, consistent rehabilitation, often supervised by a physical therapist, is key to maximizing the outcome after surgery.

Initially, rehabilitation is aimed at recovery from the surgery itself. Physical therapy helps to decrease swelling and helps you regain motion and muscle strength. However, in the months after surgery, rehab exercises are focused on the same neuromuscular training patterns that are emphasized in the ACL injury prevention programs mentioned earlier.

The pace of rehab is governed by your progress and by the healing process following the ACL surgery (ligamentization). The current recommendation is to wait at least nine months after surgery to return to high-risk sports. This is because your strength, balance and movement patterns typically are still improving during this time. There are physical and psychological assessments that can be helpful in guiding a safe return to high-risk activities. In the years and decades following treatment of an ACL injury, it is important to remain active and maintain a healthy weight to counteract the potential development of osteoarthritis.

WHY DO ACL TEARS MATTER TO WOMEN?

Young age and high-level participation in sports increase the risk of an ACL tear. Unfortunately, so does being female. It is estimated that female athletes are at least three times as likely to have an ACL injury as male athletes are. The theory is that this increased risk is due to both physical and movement technique differences between women and men. Physically, women's bodies are more commonly in a "knock-kneed" alignment, also known as valgus. This position puts extra strain on the ACL, particularly when landing from a jump or when changing direction. Additionally, the size of the intercondylar notch, the area of the knee where the ACL sits, is smaller in women than in men, increasing the predisposition to injury.

During activity, there are several differences in the way that many women move compared with men. For example, many women will land from a jump in a more upright position, knock-kneed and often flat-footed, rather than on the balls of their feet. This puts more strain on the ACL. Women also tend to have "quadriceps dominance," which means the strength of their quadriceps overpowers the strength of their hamstrings. This becomes problematic when decelerating or changing speed.

Beyond identifying factors that put you at risk of experiencing an ACL tear, it is also important to understand what factors affect your outcome if you sustain an ACL injury — specifically your ability to regain function and return to your preferred sports and activities after a tear. Studies have shown

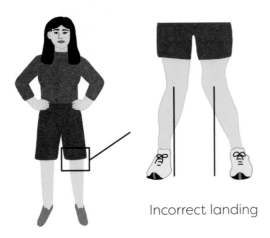

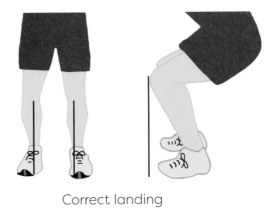

Incorrect landing   Correct landing

that while men tend to express more positive expectations about their recovery, women are unfortunately less likely to return to playing sports after an ACL tear. Factors that make it more likely that a person will return to play include engagement in care, a strong relationship with the operating surgeon and health care team, comprehensive education about the procedure and the recovery, and a strong social support system. This shows how important it is for you to be active and informed in your health care journey. Educate yourself as much as possible about your injury and treatment options so that you can make informed treatment decisions and feel empowered in your recovery.

QUESTIONS TO ASK YOUR HEALTH CARE TEAM ABOUT ACL TEARS

- How can I become involved in a training program to prevent an ACL injury?
- Are there specific factors about the way I am built or what I do that put me at risk for tearing my ACL?
  › Are there specific activities that put me at risk for tearing my ACL?
- How will I decide if ACL surgery is right for me?
  › Are there specific physical or lifestyle factors that might help me decide whether surgery is the best option for me?
- What is the recovery period like after ACL reconstruction?
  › How long will it take for me to heal enough to go back to work?
  › How long will it take for me to heal enough to go back to playing sports?
- If I decide to treat my ACL tear nonoperatively, what are the risks that I will face?
  › What is the likelihood that I will need surgery in the future?
- How likely is it that the ACL reconstruction could fail?
  › If it does fail, would I need another surgery?
- How concerned should I be about developing osteoarthritis in the future?

PEARLS OF WISDOM

ACL tears are common injuries that disproportionately affect women. As with all medical conditions, the best treatment is prevention. Fortunately, there are many prevention programs that have been shown to significantly decrease the risk of ACL injury. If an ACL injury does occur, education about the treatment options, both surgical and non-surgical, and collaboration with the entire treatment team — including your surgeon and physical therapist — are important to achieving the best outcome.

"Women should feel empowered, informed, and supported when making decisions about their health."

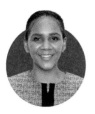

Monique S. Haynes, M.D., M.P.H., M.B.A. - she/her
Monique Haynes is a current resident with the Rush University Orthopedic Surgery Residency Program.

"Women empowered by knowledge are equipped to be an advocate for their own health and wellness."

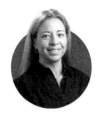

Elizabeth C. Gardner, M.D. - she/her
Dr. Gardner is the Head Team Orthopaedic Surgeon for Yale University Athletics and Associate Professor of Orthopaedic Surgery at Yale University School of Medicine. She specializes in orthopedic sports medicine surgery, primarily of the shoulder and knee.

11

Anemia

Miriam Kwarteng-Siaw, M.D., and Maureen O. Achebe, M.D., M.P.H.

WHAT IS ANEMIA?

Anemia is a condition of low hemoglobin in the body. Hemoglobin is the protein in red blood cells (RBCs) that helps carry oxygen from the lungs to all parts of the body including the brain, heart and lungs. Oxygen is essential for the body to function normally. When there are not enough RBCs, the level of hemoglobin is low, and this means that the blood cannot carry the needed supply of oxygen. This low supply of oxygen in the tissues causes the symptoms of anemia, which include fatigue, headaches, chest pain, shortness of breath, and depression.

CAN ANEMIA BE PREVENTED?

Sometimes anemia can be prevented. It depends on the cause of anemia. Prevention of anemia is more complicated if it has a genetic or hereditary cause, or if it is due to other illnesses. In these cases, it's important to seek help from a hematologist, a doctor who specializes in blood conditions such as anemia.

The most common reason for anemia is that bone marrow is not making enough blood because it does not have enough iron. Avoiding blood loss and getting enough iron in your diet can help prevent this type of anemia. Low levels of nutrients such as vitamin B12 and folate also can lead to anemia. Eating a healthy and varied diet, rich in foods with multiple nutrients, is another important way to prevent nutritional anemia.

While there are many causes of anemia, all can be grouped into two broad categories:
- Bone marrow is not making enough blood (decreased red blood cell production)
- The body is losing too much blood (excessive loss of red blood cells)

HOW IS ANEMIA TREATED?

Treatment depends on what is causing the anemia, so the first step is figuring out the cause.

Iron deficiency anemia
To treat the most common anemia, iron deficiency anemia, eat foods rich in iron such as spinach, collard greens, beans, beef, many grains and liver. However, dietary iron may not be enough to supply all of

Impact of anemia

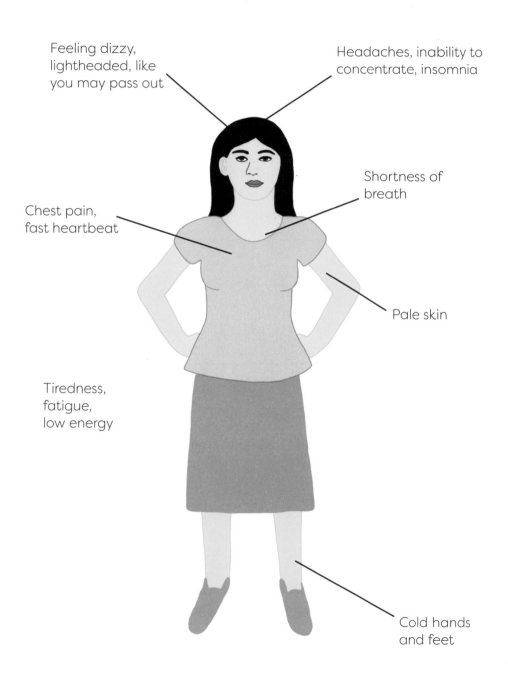

Feeling dizzy, lightheaded, like you may pass out

Headaches, inability to concentrate, insomnia

Shortness of breath

Chest pain, fast heartbeat

Pale skin

Tiredness, fatigue, low energy

Cold hands and feet

Causes of anemia

Bone marrow not making enough blood	Body losing too much blood or red blood cells
Not enough nutrients for bone marrow blood production Iron deficiency Vitamin B12 and folate deficiency Erythropoietin deficiency (due to kidney disease)	**Blood loss** Excessive menstrual bleeding GI blood loss (blood in stool or black stool, caused by colon cancer, for example) Trauma bleeding (such as from a motor vehicle accident)
Suppression of bone marrow production Inflammatory conditions Autoimmune diseases (such as rheumatoid arthritis or lupus) Cancer	**Shortened RBC lifespan** Hereditary anemias (such as sickle cell disease or thalassemia) Infections (such as babesiosis or malaria) Acquired hemolytic anemias
Diseases of the bone marrow Aplastic anemia Leukemia Myelodysplasia	

your iron needs, so you may need to take over-the-counter iron supplements. Iron tablets are easily accessible and inexpensive but can cause side effects such as constipation and black stools in some people. One tablet of iron a day or every other day is usually enough. Your body can absorb iron more easily if you take it with vitamin C or orange juice.

When dietary and supplemental iron are not enough to improve iron deficiency, iron given intravenously, through your veins, can be an effective solution. Very severe anemia requires a blood transfusion. Blood transfusions are reserved for severe cases of anemia or for anemia that occurs rapidly. For instance, blood transfusions may be needed when a large volume of blood is lost due to a traumatic injury, such as a severe automobile crash. When you lose blood quickly, the only way to replace it in time to prevent serious complications is through a blood transfusion.

Anemia caused by other nutrient deficiencies

Other common causes of anemia are deficiencies of nutrients such as vitamin B12 and folate. Vitamin B12 is found exclusively in animal proteins, so vitamin B12 deficiency is more common if you follow a strict vegan or vegetarian diet. If you have Crohn's disease, or you have had gastric bypass surgery, in which part of the stomach or intestines is removed, your risk of vitamin B12 deficiency anemia is increased. Folate deficiency, on the other hand, is rare in the United States because of federally mandated folic acid fortification of food.

If your body lacks vitamin B12 or folic acid, taking vitamin B12 and folic acid supplements can help treat the anemia associated with these deficiencies.

Pregnancy-related anemia

Pregnancy is another cause of anemia. As a fetus grows, it needs iron, which is drawn from the mother's iron stores. If mothers don't have enough iron stores, mothers and babies are at higher risk of poor outcomes such as preterm births, low birth weights and small-for-gestational-age newborns. Thus, treating iron deficiency anemia early in pregnancy is essential to a healthy pregnancy and a healthy baby. If you develop iron deficiency anemia during pregnancy, work closely with your obstetrician and a hematologist to treat it.

WHY DOES ANEMIA MATTER TO WOMEN?

Anemia is one of the most common medical problems in the world and extremely common in women. It can cause women to experience fatigue, headaches, shortness of breath or depression. According to the World Health Organization (WHO), anemia affects one in four individuals in the world — in other words, around 1.62 billion people. Yet, if anemia is so common, why don't we know more about it? The reason is that it affects mostly preschool-aged children and women of reproductive age (15-49 years). Due to monthly menstrual blood loss, women are at particularly high risk of developing anemia. Pre-menopausal women, women with heavy menses and pregnant women are at greatest risk of getting anemia. In our research looking at

individuals with anemia, approximately 90% of participants were women. Anemia causes dizziness, headaches, chest pain, shortness of breath, a racing heartbeat, fatigue, pale skin and cold hands and feet. Anemia has a significant impact on well-being and daily functioning of women.

QUESTIONS TO ASK YOUR HEALTH CARE TEAM ABOUT ANEMIA

For all women

- How low is my blood level? Or how bad is my anemia?
- What is the cause of my anemia? Is there more than one cause?
  › Can the cause of my anemia be prevented? Can it be treated? If so, how?
- What can I do to help myself?
- Do I need to see a hematologist for my anemia?

For women with anemia caused by nutritional deficiencies

- What are the causes of my nutritional deficiency?
- What foods should I eat to increase my iron, vitamin B12 and folate levels?
- Do I need to take additional supplements?
  › What are the next steps if oral supplements do not help?
- Will you check for bleeding in my stomach and intestines if I have iron deficiency anemia?

For women with severe anemia

- Is my anemia bad enough that I may need a blood transfusion?
  › If so, will I need blood transfusions often?

> What are the risks of getting a blood transfusion?

- Can I have a referral to a hematologist for my anemia?

PEARLS OF WISDOM

Anemia has a significant impact on well-being and daily functioning. Always ask your doctor to check for anemia if you suffer fatigue. Anemia can develop very gradually, so you may be anemic before you realize it.

Also keep in mind that anemia itself can be a sign of another serious medical condition, so it is always important to investigate and determine the cause of the anemia. When anemia goes unnoticed or unrecognized, it can have a negative impact on your quality of life. If you don't know to ask your doctor to check for anemia and insist on it being investigated and treated, you may suffer needless fatigue, depression, poor pregnancy outcomes and decreased work capacity.

Having anemia is not normal and it should be addressed by your primary care clinician or a hematologist.

"A woman's health is her capital."
– Harriet Beecher Stowe

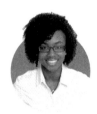

Miriam Kwarteng-Siaw, M.D. - she/her
Dr. Kwarteng-Siaw is a Clinical Fellow specializing in Internal Medicine at Brigham and Women's Hospital in Boston, Massachusetts.

"The health of the nation depends on the health of women."

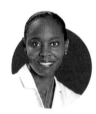

Maureen O. Achebe, M.D., M.P.H. - she/her

Dr. Achebe specializes in the study of blood disorders (hematology). She is the Clinical Director of the Non-Malignant Hematology Clinic at the Dana Farber Cancer Institute, Medical Director of the Brigham and Women's Hospital Ambulatory Infusion Center, and Director of Brigham and Women's Hospital Sickle Cell Center. She is an Assistant Professor of Medicine at Harvard Medical School.

12
Anxiety

Caitlin L. McLean, Ph.D., and Michelle A. Silva, Psy.D.

WHAT IS ANXIETY?

Anxiety is a common and often healthy emotional response that occurs when what's demanded of you feels like more than you can effectively manage. It is a general feeling of unease or apprehension about what is to come. Anxiety occurs on a continuum and all people experience it from time to time. In fact, anxiety can sometimes be beneficial because it activates the body to respond more quickly. In some cases, it may even optimize physical performance. This can be helpful in certain situations, such as being aware of your surroundings when you're somewhere new or preparing for a job interview.

When you perceive an event to be overwhelming or frightening, your body has an automatic physiological reaction called the "fight-or-flight" response. The perception of threat activates your body's sympathetic nervous system and triggers an acute stress response. This includes the release of adrenaline and the stress hormone cortisol. These substances prepare the body for activation so you can either fight the threat or flee to safety. For some people, nonthreatening situations, such as challenges at work, can trigger this response. Repeated activation

of this biological alarm system over time can harm the body and contribute to a heightened perception of threat and anxiety even in the absence of an actual threat.

Although anxiety is similar to stress, they are not the same. Stress is generally understood as a time-limited response to an external trigger, whereas anxiety is often persistent and does not go away even in the absence of a stressor. Exposure to excessive and chronic stressors can increase the risk of developing an anxiety disorder. When feelings of stress or anxiety become so persistent and intense that they begin to interfere with daily life — such as your ability to meet home or work responsibilities or get along with others — or cause other changes in behavior, it may be time to seek professional attention.

The COVID-19 pandemic serves as an example of how a sense of uncertainty and unpredictability can trigger universal feelings of anxiety, regardless of age, gender and cultural background. Stressful and challenging situations — such as work or school demands, intimate relationships, pregnancy and parenthood, medical procedures or the death of a loved one — can increase the intensity and frequency of

Anxiety disorders risk factors

- Brain structure
- Genetics
- Parenting style
- Societal pressure and expectations
- Social learning
- Socioeconomic status
- Trauma exposure

experiencing anxiety. Additionally, experiences with racism and discrimination can prompt and maintain anxiety.

How common are anxiety disorders?

Anxiety disorders are the most common mental health concern in the United States. They affect approximately 1 in 5 adults each year and nearly 1 in 3 adults over a lifetime. How anxiety disorders affect people can vary across different cultural groups, as can the signs and symptoms. For example, some studies suggest that white Americans are more likely to have certain types of anxiety disorders than are Black Americans, Latinxs (the term "Latinxs" is used as an inclusive description for people with Latin American or Hispanic heritage), and Asian Americans. However, Black Americans are more frequently diagnosed with post-traumatic stress disorder (PTSD).

What causes an anxiety disorder?

The causes of an anxiety disorder are not perfectly defined. Research indicates that anxiety disorders are likely influenced by a combination of genetic and environmental factors. Anxiety disorders tend to run in families, and people who have a parent with an anxiety disorder are at especially high risk. This familial link may be due both to biology and personality type.

Social influences also may be associated with the development of an anxiety disorder. For example, most children look to a caregiver for cues in ambiguous situations. If the caregiver is demonstrating fear, the child may be more likely to interpret the situation as unsafe and learn to model the caregiver's behavior. Experiencing negative or traumatic events, such as abuse or neglect, can increase a person's likelihood of developing an anxiety disorder.

Types of anxiety disorders

There are different types of anxiety disorders*. The most common ones, and their main characteristics, are:

Generalized anxiety disorder	Pervasive worry about a range of topics (both major life events and minor daily stresses) or fear of something bad happening
Panic disorder	Unexpected and repeated episodes of intense fear accompanied by physical symptoms that may include chest pain, heart palpitations, shortness of breath, dizziness, or abdominal distress and the fear of having another episode
Specific phobias	Intense, persistent, irrational fear of a specific object, situation or activity that poses little or no actual danger
Agoraphobia	Extreme or irrational fear of entering open or crowded places, of leaving one's own home, or of being in places from which escape is difficult
Social anxiety disorder	Fear of evaluation, meeting people, being observed or performing in front of others
Separation anxiety disorder	Recurrent and excessive distress about being away or anticipating being away from home or loved ones, or about losing a parent or other loved one to an illness or a disaster
Post-traumatic stress disorder*	Unwanted memories (like flashbacks or nightmares), avoidance of reminders, negative changes in thinking or mood, and increased arousal (being on guard, irritable) in response to experiencing or witnessing a traumatic event
Obsessive-compulsive disorder*	Repeated thoughts, urges, or mental images that cause intense anxiety (obsession) accompanied by urges to do something in response to the obsession (compulsion)

*Post-traumatic stress disorder and obsessive-compulsive disorder, while not currently categorized as anxiety disorders, have many similarities to anxiety disorders.

What are the signs and symptoms of an anxiety disorder?

People experience anxiety disorders in different ways, but some common signs and symptoms of anxiety include:

- Feeling nervous, restless or tense
- Experiencing a persistent sense of impending danger, panic or doom
- Having an increased heart rate
- Breathing rapidly (hyperventilation)
- Sweating
- Trembling
- Feeling weak or tired
- Being afraid of losing control or going crazy
- Having trouble concentrating or thinking about anything other than what's causing you to worry
- Having trouble sleeping
- Experiencing gastrointestinal (GI) problems (such as stomach pains, nausea or diarrhea)
- Avoiding specific situations that make you feel afraid or anxious (such as social events or interactions, being on airplanes or elevators, contact with animals, exposure to heights or storms, medical procedures, or injury)

CAN ANXIETY BE PREVENTED?

Yes and no. Since anxiety is a common emotion that can be helpful at times, you can't necessarily prevent anxiety from ever occurring. However, the following are things that you can do to help reduce anxiety and keep it from taking over your life and developing into a disorder.

Become aware of life stressors

Take some time to reflect on what is currently going on in your life, to recognize stressors that are affecting you, to consider a lifestyle change or to think of ways that you can cope with those stressors. This type of self-reflection can be helpful in managing anxiety.

Avoid alcohol, nicotine and caffeine

Often people will use substances such as alcohol or nicotine to create an immediate sense of relaxation. But these substances can increase anxiety and tension in the long run. Caffeine stimulates your fight-or-flight response. Studies show that caffeine can make anxiety worse, even triggering an anxiety attack. For some, it may be helpful to entirely avoid alcohol, nicotine and caffeine.

Set yourself up for a good night's rest

Sleep difficulties can cause anxiety, and anxiety in turn can disrupt your sleep, creating a vicious cycle. Excessive worry also makes it harder to fall asleep and stay asleep through the night. To get quality rest:
- Try to keep a regular sleep schedule.
- Make your bedroom comfortable and free of disruptions.
- Avoid electronic screens and blue light an hour before bed.
- Follow a relaxing bedtime routine, such as journaling or taking a warm bath or shower.

Engage in physical activity

Physical activity can help ease symptoms of anxiety and make you feel better. It may also help keep anxiety from coming back once you're feeling better. Some research indicates that more exercise is better for anxiety, but the key is to do what you can! Save strenuous activity for earlier in the day,

Anxiety: Head, heart and gut-related symptoms

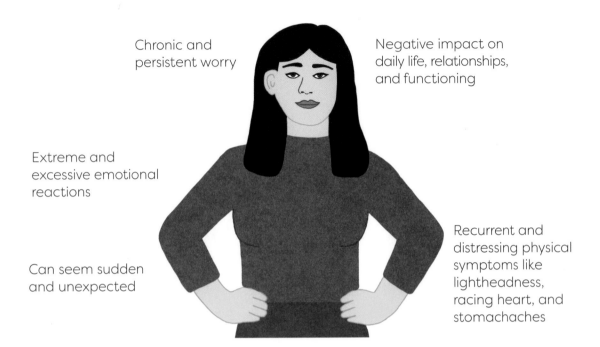

Chronic and persistent worry

Negative impact on daily life, relationships, and functioning

Extreme and excessive emotional reactions

Can seem sudden and unexpected

Recurrent and distressing physical symptoms like lightheadness, racing heart, and stomachaches

though, as intense exercise too close to bedtime can activate your body at a time when you are trying to relax.

Write your thoughts down

Writing down your thoughts is a way of slowing your thinking and allowing yourself to work through your thoughts, one at a time. Doing this can help you identify ongoing worries, problems and concerns you may have. Over time, your log can help you learn to recognize patterns, and ultimately how to cope. Also, listing current worries or tasks for the next day can help you feel less consumed by worry. Just be careful not to get stuck reading over your list for too long. Instead, make your list and then release it. Setting a timer can be helpful.

Practice self-care

Self-care is taking time to do something just for yourself. This might be having a cup of tea with minimal distractions, taking a walk or a bath, practicing some breathing techniques or reading a book or magazine. For some people, taking care of themselves may mean scheduling time to see friends or family, or participating in other kinds of social activity. For others, scheduling self-care can increase feelings of anxiety, since it may be seen as adding "one more thing" to their day. Self-care is individualized and, in some cases, it might mean paring down activities that are no longer necessary, useful or meaningful to you. It can take time to create your own toolbox of effective strategies — be alert to what works for you!

HOW ARE ANXIETY DISORDERS TREATED?

Before beginning treatment, it is important to rule out any underlying physical problems that may explain your symptoms. Your clinician may ask you about any physical symptoms you're experiencing and suggest a blood test to check for signs of an underlying disease or condition.

Since there are different anxiety disorders, you'll want to receive a thorough evaluation by a mental health specialist, as well. This is someone trained to diagnose and treat mental health conditions. This person may be a psychiatrist, psychologist, psychiatric nurse practitioner or other licensed mental health provider.

Undoubtedly, anxiety can be debilitating and interfere with your ability to live a satisfying life.

In these cases, your mental health provider may recommend an initial combination of medication and psychotherapy.

Psychotherapy

Psychotherapy, also referred to as counseling or talk therapy, is often recommended to treat anxiety and can be very effective. The most common approaches are cognitive behavioral therapy and exposure therapy.

- **Cognitive behavioral therapy (CBT)** explores how negative thoughts and ways of looking at the world influence your behavior and trigger feelings of anxiety. The goal is to change your thoughts and thought patterns so that you can decrease negative and unpleasant emotions, and ultimately change your behavior.
- **Exposure therapy** involves reducing avoidance to the situations that trigger fear and anxiety. Most people try to avoid things, situations or people that cause them anxiety or discomfort. During exposure therapy, the goal is to gradually expose you to your fear so that you can learn to build control over the experience and reduce your feelings of anxiety.

Medication

Your clinician can help you determine the best option for you in terms of medications. Common medications for anxiety include selective serotonin reuptake inhibitors (SSRIs) and serotonin and norepinephrine reuptake inhibitors (SNRIs). These medications are classified as antidepressants and tend to have a lower risk of serious side effects in comparison to other medications used for managing anxiety.

Benzodiazepines are a type of sedative that decrease the physical symptoms of anxiety but are recommended only on a short-term basis because they can be habit-forming. Because of the possibility of dependence, benzodiazepines are not recommended for people with alcohol or drug misuse.

It is important to remember that medication will not be a miracle cure. Make sure you understand the side effects, withdrawal patterns and risk factors of each medication so that you can make an informed decision.

Mind-body approaches

These approaches focus on the connection between your mind, body and behavior that affects your overall health. Mind-body approaches can be helpful in managing and preventing anxiety and may include:

- Acupuncture
- Massage
- Meditation and mindfulness
- Relaxation (such as breathing exercises, guided imagery and progressive muscle relaxation)
- Tai chi
- Qigong
- Yoga
- Hypnotherapy

Research results vary on how effective these different approaches are for anxiety disorders. Mind-body approaches may be used in addition to psychotherapy and medication, and consultation with your primary care clinician is recommended.

WHY DOES ANXIETY MATTER TO WOMEN?

Women are almost twice as likely as men to have an anxiety disorder. Women are more likely to be diagnosed with each of the various anxiety disorders, with the exception of social anxiety disorder, which affects women and men equally.

Some research suggests that differences between men and women may be, in part, due to women's fluctuating levels of sex hormones, particularly estradiol and progesterone, during the reproductive cycle. Research suggests that women experience worsening anxiety symptoms during phases of the reproductive cycle that are marked by reduced hormone levels — particularly the premenstrual phase, which can occur up to two weeks before menstrual bleeding occurs.

Anxiety may also affect women more than men due to socialization processes. For example, society may place different gendered expectations on the expression of anxiety and on acceptable coping styles.

Available evidence indicates that women tend to experience more severe symptoms of anxiety than men do. They are also more likely to seek and engage in treatment for anxiety disorders than are men. Whether there are differences in treatment response by gender remains inconclusive.

QUESTIONS TO ASK YOUR HEALTH CARE TEAM ABOUT ANXIETY

- Do I have any underlying medical problems that might be causing my symptoms of anxiety?
- Am I on any medications or using other drugs that might be causing my anxiety?
  › *This includes nonprescription medications, herbal remedies and teas.*
- What type of anxiety disorder do I have?
  › What are my treatment options for this particular anxiety disorder?
- Will I need to take medication for anxiety?
  › Is it OK to take this medication with other medications I may be taking?
  › Will I take it every day, or as needed?
  › How long will I need to take it?
  › What side effects can I expect from the medication?
  › Is there a way to minimize or prevent side effects?

"Health care providers must appreciate the fullness of women's lives and recognize individual beliefs and needs to provide the best possible care."

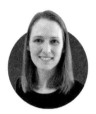

Caitlin L. McLean, Ph.D. - she/her
Dr. McLean is a fellow in Women's Health at the VA San Diego Healthcare System and the University of California San Diego in San Diego, CA. Her clinical and research interests focus on the impact of trauma on women's health and on psychological interventions for the treatment of trauma-related problems.

"Women deserve the right to health care that is accessible, holistic, and sensitive to their unique needs and preferences."

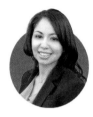

Michelle A. Silva, Psy.D. - she/her
Dr. Silva is a clinical psychologist at the Connecticut Mental Health Center and Assistant Professor in the Department of Psychiatry at the Yale School of Medicine. Her professional interests include the assessment and treatment of immigration-related trauma among Latinx communities and the role of social justice and advocacy in professional training and practice.

13
Asthma

Megan Conroy, M.D., M.A.Ed., and Jennifer McCallister, M.D.

WHAT IS ASTHMA?

Asthma is a disease of inflammation in the airways of the lungs. This inflammation causes:

- Swelling in the lining of the airways
- More mucus production in the airways
- Overgrowth of the muscles that surround each airway, making the airways prone to tightening (bronchoconstriction)
- Narrowing of the airways, reducing airflow when breathing out or exhaling (obstruction)

The inflammation caused by asthma makes it difficult to breathe. Without asthma, the airway tube is wide open, the muscle around the tube is relaxed and there is no inflammation or mucus. With asthma, the muscles around the airway tubes become thicker and tighter, and the tubes become inflamed and filled with mucus, resulting in less airflow.

This narrowing of the airways causes the characteristic signs and symptoms of asthma, such as wheezing, shortness of breath, chest tightness and cough. Symptoms may vary in frequency and in intensity: on some days, breathing will feel good; on other days, asthma symptoms may flare (asthma attack).

A diagnosis of asthma is based on a couple of factors. One is that you have the typical symptoms of asthma. The other is the results of your lung function tests. These are tests that measure how much air moves in and out of your lungs as you breathe. If these tests show that your lung function varies over time and that there's limited and variable air flow out of your lungs when you exhale, you may have asthma.

Asthma is a common disease. About 1 out of 13 people living in the U.S. have asthma. At the same time, many other diseases produce signs and symptoms that are similar to those of asthma. Up to 30% of people who have been told by a doctor that they have asthma may have symptoms caused by something else entirely.

CAN ASTHMA BE PREVENTED?

You can't prevent asthma altogether, but there are ways to reduce your risk of asthma.

There isn't one singular cause of asthma, and there are many different factors that combine to put a person at risk of asthma. The condition results from a complex

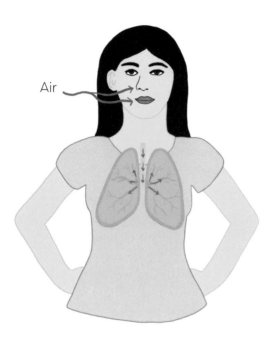

The relaxed muscles of the tubes allow air to flow through easily

The thick muscles of the mucus-filled tubes prevent air from flowing

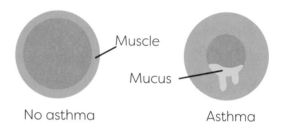

Muscle

Mucus

No asthma

Asthma

interaction between genetics and the environment, in ways that aren't completely understood. Risk factors for asthma are quite diverse, and many are not changeable.

Maintaining a healthy weight, not smoking and avoiding exposure to secondhand smoke are ways that you can reduce your risk or your children's risk of asthma. Tobacco exposure — both from active smoking and from secondhand smoke — is associated with a greater risk of asthma. Children born to mothers who smoke are twice as likely to develop asthma, but smoke exposure during childhood from other sources also increases the risk of asthma.

Avoid triggers

Symptoms of asthma typically vary over time and may flare up during an asthma attack. Certain factors may trigger symptoms in a person with asthma, such as

breathing in smoke, air pollution, high pollen seasons for people with seasonal allergies, vigorous exercise, breathing very cold or very humid air, or upper respiratory infections, among others.

Each person's triggers vary. But you may be able to prevent flaring asthma symptoms by avoiding known triggers, such as smoke, or making certain changes to your environment, such as keeping windows closed during high pollen seasons. Talk with your doctor about what triggers your asthma and how you can prevent asthma attacks.

HOW IS ASTHMA TREATED?

Asthma is commonly treated with inhaled medications. After confirming your diagnosis of asthma, your physician can select the right treatment for you based on how frequently you have symptoms. People who have symptoms every day typically require scheduled inhalers. Others who might only have symptoms of asthma a few times a month may need a different treatment strategy.

The treatment your doctor recommends may change over time as your symptoms change — adjusting medications as necessary to improve quality of life and lung function while minimizing side effects and the risks some medications can bring. Know that you can manage your own asthma using an asthma action plan that you create with your doctor.

Maintenance inhalers

Most, but not all, people with asthma benefit from a maintenance inhaler that is taken daily. Maintenance inhalers contain a steroid medication and are taken once or twice daily as prescribed. Maintenance steroid inhalers target and treat the cause of asthma by reducing inflammation in the lungs. Some maintenance inhalers also include a second medication that is a long-acting version of albuterol, a medication that relaxes the muscles of the airways to allow better airflow.

Reliever inhalers

Everyone with asthma should have a reliever inhaler. Reliever inhalers act quickly to open up constricted airways. They provide quick but temporary relief. Albuterol is the most common reliever medication. It can be administered by an inhaler or delivered by a nebulizer — a machine that turns the medication into a mist, which is easier for some people to breathe in. Reliever inhalers are important to have in a crisis, since asthma

symptoms can flare up at unpredictable times. Reliever medications alone are only appropriate for very mild asthma, in which symptoms occur less than twice a month.

Regular assessments

It's important that you and your doctor regularly evaluate how well your asthma treatment plan is working. Discuss with your doctor how frequently you have symptoms, how often you require quick relief medications, whether you wake up at night with symptoms of asthma, whether you are limited in your activities because of asthma, whether your asthma flares up and whether you have side effects from your medications. Your doctor will also likely monitor your lung function with lung function tests.

If your asthma has been well controlled for several months or more, discuss with your doctor a trial of reducing the amount of medication you use to control your asthma. Alternatively, if you continue to have asthma symptoms twice a week or more, or if symptoms wake you from sleep, limit your activities, or result in reduced lung function, there may be a need to increase your asthma therapies.

If you're using your reliever medication more than twice a month and don't have a maintenance inhaler, ask your doctor about increasing therapies for your asthma. Likewise, talk to your doctor about increasing asthma therapies if you have a maintenance inhaler but are using your reliever medication more than twice a week. Inhaler technique is key to taking your medication correctly but is neither self-explanatory nor easy. Ask your doctor or pharmacist to show you the proper technique or visit the manufacturer's website for your prescribed medication to find videos on how to take your medication correctly. Ask your doctor to assess whether you are using your inhaler correctly.

Additional factors

Asthma and the inflammation it causes in the lungs can be worsened by other factors such as allergies, postnasal drip, acid reflux, nasal polyps, sleep apnea or repeated swallowing into the airway (aspiration). Other prescription or over-the-counter medications can impact how well asthma is controlled. Improving asthma control often requires addressing these other co-factors in addition to inhaler medications.

Biologic injectable medications

Sometimes asthma remains uncontrolled despite treatment with high-dose maintenance inhalers and appropriate management of other co-factors that impact asthma. If this happens, your doctor may recommend injectable medications that target the specific type of inflammation contributing to your asthma. These medications are typically managed by a lung or allergy specialist and may be administered in your doctor's office. You can even learn to give some of these at home.

WHY DOES ASTHMA MATTER IN WOMEN?

Women are more likely than men to develop asthma as an adult. After age 40, asthma is predominantly a disease seen in women, whereas in childhood, boys develop asthma more frequently than girls. Hormone changes occurring around menopause appear to put women at risk for the development of asthma around or after menopause.

Pregnancy also can impact asthma control or the frequency of asthma symptoms. Among women with asthma who become pregnant, one-third experience a worsening in asthma control, one-third have similar control and one-third see improved control. For women whose symptoms worsen during pregnancy, it's crucial to have effective proactive asthma care, as this can have implications for both mother and baby.

Poorly controlled asthma changes the structure of your lungs. This can result in reduced lung function as you age. Poor control of asthma can limit your daily activities and prevent you from fulfilling your responsibilities at home or at work.

Exposure to substances in your workplace may contribute to the worsening of your asthma. While it's possible to develop asthma in almost any environment, certain occupations, such as health care workers, custodians and hair stylists, may be at higher risk of asthma due to exposure to latex, chemicals and dyes. The best way to prevent your asthma from worsening in the workplace is to minimize your exposure to substances that trigger your symptoms. Wear masks and other protective equipment as needed.

QUESTIONS TO ASK YOUR HEALTH CARE TEAM ABOUT ASTHMA

For all women with asthma
• Is the diagnosis certain to be asthma,

or could my symptoms be caused by something else?

- What would be considered "good control" of my asthma?
    › Am I reaching the goals for control and lung function that you have for me?
- Am I using my inhalers correctly?
- Are there specific environmental or lifestyle changes I can make to improve the control of my asthma?
- How can I avoid or minimize triggers of my asthma symptoms?
- Are there other diseases, such as allergy, sinus disease or acid reflux, that impact my asthma?
- How can I take charge of monitoring and managing my own asthma?
- Would it be OK for me to monitor my asthma with a peak flow meter at home?
- Can we make an asthma action plan?

For those with moderate to severe asthma

- Should I see a lung specialist?
- What type of inflammation drives my asthma?
- Is my lung function impaired because of my asthma?
- Could allergy testing be helpful to understand triggers for my asthma and inform how I can reduce allergen exposures in my home or workplace?
- Would biologic injectable medications be appropriate to help control my asthma?

For pregnant women with asthma

- Should I continue my current inhalers?
- Should I have more frequent health care visits for my asthma during pregnancy?
- If I decide to breastfeed, how will my asthma regimen impact breastfeeding?

PEARLS OF WISDOM

Asthma has the potential to impact many realms of your life, but with the right management plan it shouldn't limit your life. Achieving good asthma control will help to preserve lung function. You can be empowered to monitor and manage your asthma by working with your doctor to make a personalized plan for your asthma.

"Personalized, whole person care should be the standard."

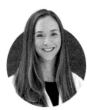

Megan Conroy, M.D., M.A.Ed. - she/her
Dr. Conroy is an Assistant Professor of Medicine in the Division of Pulmonary, Critical Care, and Sleep Medicine at The Ohio State University Wexner Medical Center in Columbus, Ohio. She practices critical care medicine as well as pulmonary medicine with a specialization in difficult-to-treat and severe asthma.

"Gender-specific care for women ensures the best care possible."

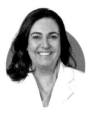

Jennifer McCallister, M.D. - she/her
Dr. McCallister is the Associate Dean of Medical Education at The Ohio State University College of Medicine and a Professor of Medicine in the Division of Pulmonary, Critical Care, and Sleep Medicine at The Ohio State University Wexner Medical Center in Columbus, Ohio. She specializes in the care of patients with severe asthma and asthma in pregnancy.

14
Blood clots

Tiffany M. Cochran, M.D., M.H.A., and Holly L. Thacker, M.D., FACP

WHAT IS A BLOOD CLOT?

A blood clot occurs when blood has changed from a liquid to a thickened gel-like or semisolid state — from liquid to a clump. Blood clotting is a natural process. When there is bleeding from an injury, such as a cut, the clotting process stops the bleeding. Through a cascade of events, different blood components come together to create the clot, overlying the injured blood vessel. Clot formation (thrombosis) helps seal off the wound, prevents further bleeding and reduces the risk of infection to the body. After the injury heals, the body naturally dissolves the clot.

At times, a clot may not naturally dissolve, or a clot may occur in a blood vessel, such as an artery or a vein, where there is no injury. This type of blood clotting tends to happen when the blood has an increased tendency to clot (hypercoagulable blood) and when the blood flows too slowly through the veins (venous stasis).

Veins carry deoxygenated blood back to the heart, so a clot formed in a vein hinders the return of blood to the heart (see illustration on next page). These vein clots tend to cause swelling and pain because they are like a traffic jam, holding up the blood that is trying to go back to the heart. When a blood clot forms in a vein close to the skin, it's called superficial venous thrombosis. When a blood clot forms deep in the veins, it's called deep vein thrombosis (DVT). These clots develop most often in leg veins but also can occur in veins in the arms, neck and pelvis, and in other large blood vessels.

Sometimes a clot in a vein may detach from its point of origin and travel all the way up to the lungs, where it gets stuck and obstructs blood flow. A clot that lodges in a lung is called a pulmonary embolism (PE) and can be extremely dangerous. Venous thromboembolism (VTE) is a broader term used to define both DVT and PE.

Blood clotting can also occur in the arteries, which are vessels that transport oxygenated and nutrient-filled blood away from the heart to the rest of the body. Compared to veins, blood pressure in the arteries is much higher. Clotting in arteries usually occurs when there is a buildup of fat and cholesterol deposits (plaques) within the artery. This buildup decreases the width of the artery. The blood still needs to get through, so it forces itself through the narrow opening. This elevates pressure in the artery

What a blood clot looks like in your veins

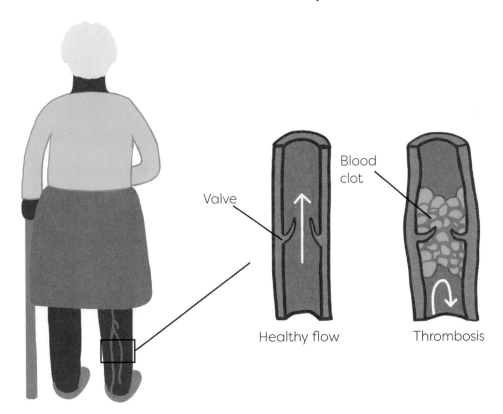

Valve

Blood clot

Healthy flow

Thrombosis

further, which can cause plaques to rupture. When this happens, the molecules that are released in the rupture cause the body to overreact and form an unnecessary clot in the artery. Plaques also can become dislodged and block blood flow through the artery, leading to a potential heart attack (Chapter 32) or stroke (Chapter 58).

CAN BLOOD CLOTS BE PREVENTED?

You can decrease the risk of blood clots by taking these simple steps.

Know if you're at higher risk
This step is essential if you're being admitted to the hospital or undergoing surgery.

Your health care team can review your medical history and the medications you take to identify if you are at higher risk for blood clots. You may receive a preventive blood thinner to help decrease the chance of DVT or PE.

Know your family history
Specific genetic mutations can increase the likelihood of blood to clot. Examples of such gene mutations include:
- Factor V Leiden
- Protein C and S deficiency
- Antithrombin
- Antiphospholipid syndrome
- Methylenetetrahydrofolate reductase (MTHFR) mutations

For people who experience recurring blood clots or unexplained (unprovoked) blood clots, it's important to uncover the reasons for their hypercoagulable blood.

Become more physically active

Immobility dramatically increases the risk of a blood clot, particularly a DVT in the lower leg. Less calf muscle activity decreases blood flow in the lower legs. This decreased blood flow increases the likelihood of a clot forming. If you have been physically inactive for a long time — for example, on a long airplane flight — find an opportunity to get up and move around. Walk the aisle, if permitted, or move your feet up and down (calf pumps) to increase blood flow in your legs.

Maintain a healthy weight

A greater than average body mass index (BMI) increases the chance that a blood clot will develop, especially when accompanied by other chronic medical conditions. Losing excess body weight is one way to reduce the risk of clots.

Adopt a healthy and nutrient-rich diet

Nutrition has an integral role in both triggering and preventing blood clots. High-fat and processed foods increase the risk of obesity, diabetes and high cholesterol levels, which could promote formation of blood clots. A heart-healthy diet can reduce your risk of thrombosis by decreasing not only the buildup of plaques in your arteries (atherosclerosis) but also by creating an environment that decreases the risk of blood clot formation. Certain nutrients can act to prevent clots and can be part of VTE treatment. For example, vitamin E is known to cause blood thinning. If you have

a history of VTE, talk to your clinician about taking 600 IU of vitamin E daily to thin your blood and make it less prone to clotting. Also, avoid oral menopausal hormone therapy and oral estrogen agonists/estrogen antagonists if you've had blood clots in the past.

Stay hydrated

Dehydration can increase the risk of VTE. Drinking plenty of fluids positively impacts overall health and can decrease the risk of thrombosis.

Be aware of the effects of medications

Certain medications may promote clotting, such as:

- Oral hormonal contraceptive pills
- Selective chemotherapy drugs, such as tamoxifen
- Estrogen agonists/estrogen antagonists (formerly referred to as selective estrogen receptor modulators or SERMs) used to prevent osteoporosis and reduce estrogen-positive breast cancer, such as raloxifene
- Oral medications for genitourinary syndrome of menopause (GSM), such as ospemifene
- Oral menopausal hormone therapy (OMHT)

HOW ARE BLOOD CLOTS TREATED?

The standard treatment for a blood clot is anticoagulant therapy — medications that stop the blood-clotting process. Anticoagulants, known as blood thinners, prevent the blood from further clotting. As a result, the blood clot cannot increase in size, allowing the body to start the breakdown of the blood clot (fibrinolysis). People with certain conditions — such as active cancer, genetic mutations for thrombosis or a high risk of VTE — often need anticoagulant therapy. Types of anticoagulants include:

Low molecular weight heparin (LMWH)

This is a blood thinner medication that is injected under the skin. It is often used in lower doses to help prevent blood clots after certain types of surgery, during a hospital stay or in some people with cancer who are at higher risk of blood clots. Heparin can also be used in higher doses to treat a blood clot.

Warfarin

This anticoagulant is taken orally. It requires dietary modifications — vitamin K-rich foods such as green, leafy vegetables make warfarin less effective — and frequent blood test monitoring to ensure appropriate blood thickness.

Direct oral anticoagulants (DOACs)

These newer anticoagulants offer some advantages over established blood thinners such as warfarin. DOACs do not require weekly monitoring as warfarin does, for example. However, blood test monitoring of kidney and liver function is still necessary. Examples of DOACs are apixaban, betrixaban, dabigatran, edoxaban and rivaroxaban. These DOACs are frequently prescribed to people with atrial fibrillation who are at increased risk of stroke.

Other treatments

In life-threatening situations or when a large clot is present, other forms of treatment may be used, including the following.

Catheter-based thrombolytic therapy During this surgical procedure, a long tube (catheter) is inserted into a blood vessel and directed at the blood clot. The tube delivers medication to dissolve the targeted blood clot.

Thrombolytics These are emergency drugs given to dissolve clots.

Thrombectomy This is a procedure in which the blood clot is surgically removed.

WHY DO BLOOD CLOTS MATTER TO WOMEN?

Women are at greater risk of developing blood clots, both PE and DVT. Contributing to this risk are pregnancy, hormonal contraceptive use and oral menopausal hormone therapy.

Pregnancy

Women have a higher risk of developing a blood clot during their childbearing years. VTE is one of two leading causes of maternal death worldwide, and it can be prevented. The highest chance for these clots to occur is right before delivery and right after childbirth. Advanced age at the time of pregnancy increases the risk of developing a blood clot during pregnancy. Being aware of these risk factors and following preventive strategies established by your clinician can decrease VTE risk during pregnancy.

Hormonal contraceptive use

Many women use hormonal birth control pills as their preferred method for preventing an unwanted pregnancy. Taking hormonal birth control pills increases the risk of a potential blood clot. However, this increased risk rarely results in the actual development of a clot. Based on available studies, only one woman out of every thousand women who are taking birth control pills will develop a blood clot. This data emphasizes how infrequently VTE happens with birth control pills.

Hormonal birth control patches and vaginal rings also increase VTE risk. Hormonal birth control delivered through a patch (transdermal birth control) may increase DVT risk more than is the case with oral or vaginal hormonal birth control because it can lead to higher hormone levels in the bloodstream. By contrast, transdermal and vaginal menopausal therapy are generally associated with a lower risk of VTE than oral menopausal hormone therapy, since the transdermal and vaginal approaches have less impact on liver proteins involved in blood clot formation.

Menopausal hormone therapy

Postmenopausal hormonal therapy also increases the risk of VTE, but not as much as hormonal birth control pills. This is because postmenopausal hormone therapy involves doses that are several times lower than hormone doses found in birth control pills. Nonetheless, the risk of VTE is still present. Oral estrogen alone has a lower VTE risk than oral estrogen-progestin. However, estrogen alone carries other risks. When not balanced by progesterone, estrogen can stimulate growth of the lining of the uterus, increasing the risk of endometrial cancer.

Bijuva, which contains bioidentical estradiol and natural progesterone, has not been shown to increase VTE. It can be an option if you are concerned about developing a blood clot but do not want to use estradiol patches, gels or sprays along with separate progesterone pills. However, if you've had a blood clot in the past or you have a known genetic mutation that increases your risk of a blood clot, generally avoid oral menopausal hormone therapy. Talk to your clinician about transdermal menopausal hormone therapy. Data from various studies indicate a lower risk of VTE with transdermal menopausal hormone therapy compared to oral menopausal hormone therapy.

Other factors play a role in blood clot development, such as obesity, immobility, advanced age, and long-distance traveling. The risk of a blot clot also increases in the time right after surgery. Before starting hormonal therapy, discuss with your clinician what other factors might affect your risk of blood clot development. Also ask about alternative options for hormone therapy if you have a family history of VTE due to a genetic disorder — such as factor V Leiden, protein C and S deficiency, antithrombin deficiency, MTHFR mutation or anticardiolipin antibodies.

QUESTIONS TO ASK YOUR HEALTH CARE TEAM ABOUT BLOOD CLOTS

- What are the next steps if I have a family history of VTE?
- How are blood clots diagnosed?
- If I develop a blood clot, how long will I have to take a blood thinner?
  › Is there a better anticoagulant to treat my blood clot?
  › Are there lasting complications from a blood clot?

- Can I still exercise while being treated for a blood clot?
  › Does moving around increase my risk of stroke or heart attack?
- If I'm traveling for a long time, how often should I move around to lower my risk of VTE?
- Am I on medications that increase my chances for VTE?
  › Can my medications be adjusted to lower my risk?

PEARLS OF WISDOM

Venous thromboembolism (VTE) remains a significant public health concern and can be avoided with appropriate preventive strategies. Being aware of your risk of VTE empowers you to have a conversation with your health care team to explore ways to reduce VTE risk. If you need hormone therapy, ask your health care team for a careful and individual risk assessment before you start treatment. If you have had a pregnancy or a delivery, with or without C-section, or if you have taken hormonal contraception and haven't ever developed a blood clot, your risk of VTE is likely low. Your risk of VTE is less certain if you have not had any conditions or gone through any therapies that increase the risk of VTE.

Adopting a healthy, active lifestyle is the best prevention for many medical conditions, including VTE. Taking charge of your health by being proactive, increasing physical activity and avoiding immobility is key. Understanding the risk-benefit equation for menopausal hormone therapy is fundamental as well. Most women under age 65 who are within 10 years of menopause and take hormone therapy, including oral menopausal hormonal therapy, have far more benefits from this therapy than risks. This includes improved quality of life and reduction of chronic diseases, along with increased longevity.

"We must empower the voices of all women to be heard within the health care system."

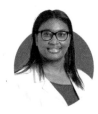

Tiffany M. Cochran, M.D., M.H.A. - she/her
Dr. Cochran is currently a second-year fellow in the Specialized Women's Health Fellowship at Cleveland Clinic Center for Specialized Women's Health. She specialized in menopause, hormonal therapy, menstrual disorders, female sexual dysfunction, and osteoporosis.

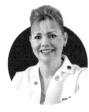

Holly L. Thacker, M.D., FACP - she/her
Dr. Thacker is director of the Cleveland Clinic Center for Specialized Women's Health and Professor, Cleveland Clinic Lerner College of Medicine of Case Western Reserve University.
She is a national expert in Specialized Women's Health with a focus on menopause, hormone therapy, and osteoporosis. Dr. Thacker's motto is the mission of the nonprofit she leads, Speaking of Women's Health: "Be Strong. Be Healthy. And Be in Charge."

15
Breast lump

Stacy Ugras, M.D., FACS

WHAT IS A BREAST LUMP?

Finding a breast lump is a common experience for women; many women feel at least one breast lump in their lifetimes. Breasts are not always smooth and homogeneous in texture. They can be nodular at their baseline, where the breast meets the chest wall, and they can fluctuate in texture and size over time. Breasts are sensitive to estrogen and progesterone, hormones that are at different levels during the menstrual cycle and over the lifespan of a woman. Lumps that may be prominent at one point in time may disappear or be difficult to find at another. The majority of breast lumps are benign, meaning they are not cancerous (malignant). Breast lumps may indicate a variety of conditions ranging from benign to potentially malignant.

Common causes of benign lumps
Common causes of benign breast lumps include the following:

Fibrocystic changes
This is a common condition affecting premenopausal women. It occurs when fibrous tissue and fluid-filled cysts develop in the breast. The condition causes painful breast lumps that come and go throughout the menstrual cycle. Most of the time, a fibrocystic lump is diagnosed with a combination of medical history, physical examination and imaging. Treatment is aimed at easing symptoms and can include reduction of caffeine intake, anti-inflammatory medication and sometimes oral contraceptive medications to help control hormone fluctuation.

Cysts: Simple and complex
Cysts cause 25% of masses in women 40 and older. More than half of women who have one cyst will experience additional cysts in their lifetime. Cysts are often hormonally sensitive, mobile, changeable in size throughout the menstrual cycle, and potentially painful. Ultrasound is the best way to characterize a cyst as either simple or complex.

Simple cysts Simple means the cyst is filled with benign-appearing fluid. Simple cysts can usually be left in place, but they are drained if they are causing excessive pain or if there is any question regarding the diagnosis. Often, they recur, as the wall of the cyst remains in place.

Complex cysts Complex means there is debris or bumpiness within the cyst. Complex

Breast lump characteristics

Benign breast lump	Concerning breast lump
Soft or rubbery	Hard
Painful	Painless
Regular or smooth shape	Irregular shape
Not fixed; mobile, moves around	Fixed to the skin or chest wall
No skin dimpling	Skin dimpling
Discharge is green or yellow	Discharge is bloody
No nipple retraction	Nipple retraction

cysts are sometimes drained or left in place and monitored, depending on the level of suspicion by the radiologist.

Fibroadenomas

These are some of the most frequent culprits behind the appearance of a solid mass on exam. Fibroadenomas are typically firm or rubbery, mobile, and usually not tender. Ultrasound imaging is often used to identify a fibroadenoma. If a fibroadenoma is small and has no concerning features on imaging, it is usually left alone. But if it looks like it might be worrisome, then your clinician will likely recommend a biopsy. If the biopsy confirms that the lump is a fibroadenoma, your clinician is likely to follow up with periodic physical exams and ultrasounds to monitor for any changes. If there is a concern that the fibroadenoma will continue to grow, even though it is benign, your clinician may recommend removing it.

Infections and skin conditions

In some cases, infections can present as fluid-filled pockets of pus, in which case they are drained. Some very small collections can be monitored, depending on how suspicious they look to the radiologist. Other infections can include skin infections, which are managed with antibiotics.

Breast lumps, while mostly benign, should not be ignored, as they may represent breast cancer. The above table compares the characteristics of a benign lump versus one that might be malignant.

Assessing a breast lump

To help you distinguish between a "normal" lump and a concerning one, it is important for you to perform a monthly breast self-examination.

If you notice a lump, try to assess the following characteristics.

Location Take note of where the lump is in your breast. Looking at the breast like a clock, at which hour is it located? How far from the nipple is it? Knowing this will help you find it again and help you show your clinician.

Breast self-examination

 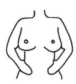 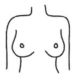

Stand in front of a mirror and visually examine your breasts from various angles.

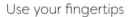

Use your fingertips   Clockwise   Side to side   Up and down

Features Determine the size and shape of the lump.

- Is it firm or soft?
- Is there one lump, or are there multiple similar ones?
- Does it move freely, or is it stuck to the surrounding breast?
- Are the edges smooth or irregular?
- Are there skin changes in the area? For example, is the skin red or thickened?
- Is there spontaneous or bloody nipple discharge?

Timing Where are you in your menstrual cycle?

As a rule of thumb, bring any new lumps to your clinician's attention for a thorough evaluation, which might include imaging and biopsy, if necessary. If there are any suspicious findings, your clinician can refer you to a breast surgeon. You may need to monitor the lump while waiting for an appointment. In this case, knowing the location and size will help. A lump that grows prior to your menstrual period but disappears afterward only to reappear again before your next period is likely benign. In general, malignancies don't change with your cycle and don't fluctuate in size over the course of a month or two.

CAN BREAST LUMPS BE PREVENTED?

Unfortunately, no. Breast lumps cannot be prevented. However, often what we perceive as a breast lump is just typical breast tissue or a benign fibrocystic change. One study demonstrated that only 27% of breast lumps had an identifiable cause other than fibrocystic change in women under age 40.

HOW ARE BREAST LUMPS TREATED?

If you note a lump, and it doesn't disappear over the course of a couple of months, bring it to the attention of your clinician, who will most likely perform a physical examination. The clinician will examine both breasts, looking at the skin of the breasts, palpating the entire breast area including the underarm (axillary) regions, which contain breast tissue and lymph nodes, and take note of the location, size, and characteristics of the lump. The clinician will also assess whether the lump adheres to surrounding tissue and note any skin changes.

After a thorough physical examination, your clinician may conclude:

- The lump is not a true mass. (However, your clinician will want to see if you've had a screening mammogram within the past year if you're 40 or older. If the screening mammogram was normal, the clinician will probably ask you to monitor the lump and return for a follow-up visit if it persists or worsens.)
- The lump is a mass and has benign characteristics on palpation (touch).
- The lump is a mass and has malignant characteristics on palpation.
- The lump is a mass with indeterminate characteristics on exam, meaning it could be benign or malignant.

Using imaging tests
If the doctor does find a discrete mass, imaging is typically used to better characterize the mass. Breast imaging techniques include mammography, ultrasound and MRI.

Mammography The standard for evaluation of a breast mass in any woman over 30 includes a mammogram. It is important to note that the imaging done to evaluate a mass is slightly different from routine screening mammography. When a particular lump is being assessed, the mammogram is a diagnostic mammogram. During a diagnostic mammogram, additional images are taken and the images are targeted at the mass.

Ultrasound Next, ultrasound is used to further evaluate the mass. In women younger than 30, ultrasound is often the only imaging technique used to evaluate palpable masses. This is because there is higher breast density in this younger age group that makes mammography less sensitive for detecting a mass. There is also a lower chance of malignancy in women under 30.

MRIs If the mass is not visible on a mammogram or ultrasound image, or if there is anything that is unclear, MRIs are conducted to help the radiologist or doctor clarify the diagnosis.

Classifying the results
Once imaging is complete, the radiologist characterizes the likelihood of malignancy based on imaging features. Using a numbers system called the Breast Imaging-Reporting and Data System (BIRADS), the radiologist classifies the mass (lesion) based on the odds that the mass is malignant. Use of this system provides a common way for doctors to describe what they see and helps define the need for follow-up imaging and tissue diagnosis. The BIRADS is divided into several categories, including:

- BIRADS-1 (normal)
- BIRADS-2 (benign)
- BIRADS-3 (probably benign, with a 2% or less chance of malignancy and follow-up imaging recommended)
- BIRADS-4 (greater than 2% chance of malignancy and a biopsy recommended)
- BIRADS-5 (highly suggestive of malignancy; followed by biopsy and breast surgery referral)

Importantly, just because a mass isn't seen on imaging doesn't mean the concern of a mass noted on a physical exam can be dismissed. Mammograms miss approximately 10% to 25% of cancers detectable by physical exam regardless of tumor size. Physical examination for palpable masses improves cancer detection over imaging alone. When combined, physical exam, mammogram and ultrasound have a sensitivity for cancer detection of 97%. If there is concern that the mass may be cancerous, a minimally invasive biopsy will likely be recommended. Once the biopsy is complete, it will take several days for a tissue specialist (pathologist) to evaluate the tissue sample and provide a diagnosis.

If the mass is cystic, the fluid within the cystic mass may be drained with a needle. If there is no concern for malignancy and the fluid from the cyst appears benign, further microscopic analysis may not be necessary. If there are any concerns, a pathologist can evaluate the fluid for malignancy.

Benign masses are often followed for one to two years after the initial assessment, with follow-up imaging at six-month intervals to check for any changes. If the mass grows, the recommendation will likely be to have the mass surgically removed (excised). If the mass hasn't changed after two years, the recommendation will most likely be for you to continue to monitor it on your own. Self-monitoring is important, as some benign lesions can change and become cancerous.

WHY DO BREAST LUMPS MATTER TO WOMEN?

Most women will experience a breast lump in their lifetime. It's important to monitor any breast lumps because they can be a sign of breast cancer. The average woman has a 12% lifetime risk of breast cancer. Early diagnosis of breast cancer improves the outcome (prognosis). In an analysis of data from the 2003 National Health Interview Survey, which included 361 women with breast cancer between 1980 and 2003, 25% of breast cancers were detected by self-examination. That number is high enough that every lump should be taken seriously and evaluated for underlying malignancy.

Sometimes, benign masses grow and cause pain, anxiety or cosmetic issues. Early removal of a mass that is growing reduces the risk of surgical complications and leads to a better cosmetic outcome. If a breast lump is causing anxiety, removing it, even if it is benign, is appropriate for some women under certain circumstances. Painful breast lumps — such as cysts, for example — can be managed with non-surgical measures such as medication and sometimes aspiration, which can help to alleviate pain.

While breast lumps occur more commonly in women, men should not ignore breast lumps, as men do have breast tissue and are susceptible to breast cancer. Male breast cancer accounts for approximately 1% of all breast cancers, with less than 0.5% of male cancer deaths being caused by breast cancer in the United States. Nevertheless, due to decreased awareness and screening, men who do have breast cancer are often diagnosed at a more advanced stage of disease and have a poorer prognosis.

QUESTIONS TO ASK YOUR HEALTH CARE TEAM ABOUT A BREAST LUMP

- Does the lump have suspicious features on my exam?
- Should I undergo breast imaging or have a biopsy?
- How should this lump be monitored?
- Am I at high risk for breast cancer based on my personal history and my family history?
- Should I see a breast surgeon?

PEARLS OF WISDOM

Check your breasts once a month after your period. Palpate the breast tissue and assess any skin changes. Use the "ugly duckling" rule — any lump that stands out and feels or looks different from the rest of your breast tissue warrants your attention and follow-up, as does any change in the appearance and feel of your breasts. Consider yearly screening mammography beginning at age 40. If you have dense breasts, talk to your clinician about more diligent examination.

"Women's health is complex but vital. We need to care for ourselves so that we can care for others."

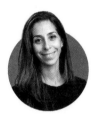

Stacy Ugras, M.D., FACS
Dr. Ugras is an attending surgeon at New York-Presbyterian Medical Center and Assistant Professor of Surgery at Columbia University Medical Center. She is a board certified general surgeon and fellowship trained breast surgeon specializing in all aspects of malignant and benign breast disease.

16

Breast cancer

Aixa E. Soyano Müller, M.D.

WHAT IS BREAST CANCER?

Cancer is a disease in which abnormal cells (cancer cells) grow and divide in an uncontrolled manner and are capable of invading nearby tissue and spreading to distant tissues. The type of cancer is determined by the tissue or organ where it started.

If cancer starts in the breast, it is called breast cancer. It begins when healthy breast cells change and proliferate without control into cancerous (malignant) cells, forming a mass called a tumor. Most of the time, what makes cells change and become malignant is unknown. Breast cancer cells can travel through the lymph nodes or the bloodstream and invade other organs, such as the bones, liver and lungs.

Types of breast cancer
There are different ways of classifying breast cancer. The three main subtypes of breast cancer are hormone positive, HER2 positive and triple negative.

Hormone positive This is the most common subtype of breast cancer and represents about two-thirds of breast cancers. These tumor cells have receptors for estrogen, progesterone or both and use these hormones as fuel to grow. Hormone positive breast cancer is more commonly seen after menopause.

HER2 positive About 20% of women with breast cancer have this subtype. It relies on the activation of a gene called human epidermal growth factor receptor 2 (HER2), which helps breast cancer cells grow. This type of tumor can grow quickly, but there are specific targeted treatments for this breast cancer subtype.

Triple negative This type represents up to 15% of breast cancers. When a tumor does not have estrogen, progesterone or HER2 receptors, it is called "triple negative." It is more common in younger women, women of African American or Hispanic descent, and women with a higher-risk breast cancer gene (BRCA1).

Subtypes are determined by doing specific tests on a sample of the tumor. These tests look for distinct receptors (biomarkers) on the surface of the cancer cells. Receptors are proteins that make the cell respond to certain substances, such as hormones or antibodies.

CAN BREAST CANCER BE PREVENTED?

There is no proven way to completely prevent breast cancer. There are some risk factors that cannot be controlled, such as age, race, ethnicity, the density of breast tissue, age at first menstrual period, age at the onset of menopause, personal history and family history of breast cancer. However, there are things you can do to decrease the risk of developing breast cancer.

Maintain a healthy weight

Obesity can increase body inflammation and hormone production. Studies suggest that being overweight or obese, especially after menopause, increases the risk of breast cancer. It also increases the risk of having the cancer come back after treatment. Participating in moderate to high-intensity regular physical activity for 30 to 60 minutes daily has been associated with lowering breast cancer risk.

Avoid long-term use of hormone replacement

Hormone replacement therapy is used to ease the symptoms of menopause, such as hot flashes, fatigue and bone loss. However, it also increases the likelihood of developing breast cancer and of finding it at a more advanced stage. Breast cancer risk increases the most during the first two to three years of taking hormone replacement therapy. There are many different types of hormone replacement therapy. If you take hormone therapy to relieve menopausal symptoms, talk to your clinician about using the lowest-dose formula for the shortest time possible. If you've been diagnosed with breast cancer or have a gene associated with a higher risk of breast cancer, such as the BRCA gene, don't use hormone replacement therapy.

Eat a healthy diet

The science isn't clear about which specific foods can help prevent cancer, but a balanced diet high in fruits and vegetables — and low in fat, processed meats and sugary drinks — can help you maintain a healthy body weight and lower the risk of cancer.

Avoid alcohol

Alcohol, even in small quantities, can increase breast cancer risk. It is best to not drink alcohol at all. At most, limit consumption to no more than one drink a day.

Get screened

Finding breast cancer early and getting prompt, adequate treatment are the most important factors in preventing death from breast cancer. Treating breast cancer when the tumor is small and cancer cells have not spread leads to better outcomes. Screening recommendations can change depending on whether your risk of developing breast cancer is average or high. Talk to your clinician about when and how often to get screened for breast cancer.

Current screening recommendations include:
- An annual screening mammogram, starting at age 40, for women with average risk of developing breast cancer
- Earlier mammographic screening for higher-risk women who may benefit from supplemental screening measures
- Supplemental screening with contrast-enhanced breast MRI for women with certain genetic mutations, a family

history of breast cancer or a personal history of radiation to the chest

- Breast MRI is also recommended for women who have dense breast tissue and a personal history of breast cancer or for women who were diagnosed with breast cancer by age 50

Stay vigilant if breast cancer runs in your family

If you have a strong family history of cancer, being vigilant about your breast health is extremely important. This includes getting to know your breasts by performing self-breast exams (see Chapter 15). If there are any changes in the appearance or feel of your breasts, report these changes immediately to your clinician. Stay up to date with your routine screening mammograms and talk to your clinician about what your personal risk is for developing breast cancer. If your risk is high, you may benefit from genetic testing and genetic counseling.

Preventive surgery

A very few women are at very high risk of developing breast cancer because of alterations in certain genes, such as BRCA, PALB2, TP53 or others. For these women, surgery to remove the breasts before cancer occurs (prophylactic mastectomy) can be an option.

Preventive medications

For some women with a high risk of developing breast cancer, prescription medications such as tamoxifen, raloxifene or aromatase inhibitors can be considered. This approach is also called endocrine prevention, chemoprevention or chemoprophylaxis.

HOW IS BREAST CANCER TREATED?

The treatment for breast cancer can be complex. Every person's cancer is different and unique. Before considering a treatment plan, members of your health care team think about many different factors, including the stage and subtype of your breast cancer, your age and health status, and whether or not you have reached menopause. Early breast cancer is treated in a multidisciplinary manner, meaning that different specialists participate in your care, including:

- A surgeon (surgical oncologist), who takes care of removing the breast tissue and lymph nodes that may be involved with breast cancer.
- A medical oncologist, who prescribes medications to help treat the cancer systemically, meaning everywhere in the body. Medications can include antihormonal therapies, chemotherapy and immunotherapy.
- A radiation oncologist, who uses radiation to treat the areas where the breast cancer was removed, to prevent the cancer from coming back (recurring).
- A plastic surgeon, who is often involved when the entire breast is removed and reconstruction is planned or desired.

Treatments include the following.

Systemic therapies

Systemic therapies use medications that circulate throughout the body to kill cancer cells and prevent recurrences. They can be prescribed one at a time or in combination.

Antihormonal therapies These therapies, also called hormone blockers or endocrine

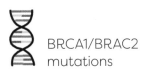

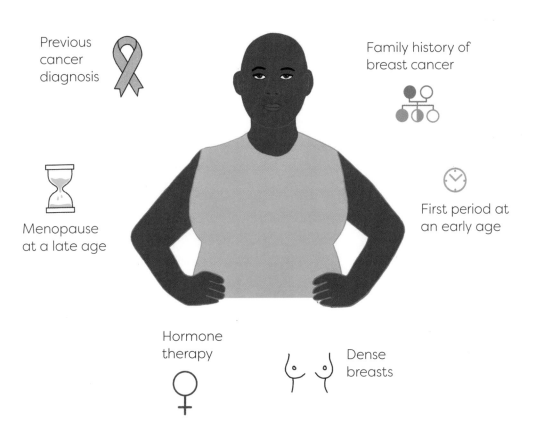

BRCA1/BRAC2 mutations

50 years and older

Previous cancer diagnosis

Family history of breast cancer

Menopause at a late age

First period at an early age

Hormone therapy

Dense breasts

therapy, include medications for hormone positive breast cancers. They are taken by mouth daily for 5 to 10 years. The most common drugs are tamoxifen, which is generally prescribed for pre- or perimenopausal women, and aromatase inhibitors (anastrozole, letrozole, exemestane) for postmenopausal women.

Chemotherapy Chemotherapy uses medications that kill rapidly growing cells. There are many different types of chemotherapy, and each one has a unique mechanism of action and possible side effects. Chemotherapy drugs can be administered orally or through a vein (intravenously).

Targeted treatments These are medications that work on a specific target. The most common treatments are antibodies against HER2. Antibodies are immune proteins that help identify specific cells that have receptors for that antibody. Targeted treatments used for HER2 positive breast cancers are usually given for one year. Antibody treatments also exist for triple negative cancers.

Immunotherapy Immunotherapy uses medications to help activate the immune system so that it can fight back against the cancer. Immunotherapy drugs can be given alone or in combination with chemotherapy. Their use is limited to certain subtypes of breast cancer.

Radiation

This treatment involves the use of high energy X-rays or other particles to destroy cancer cells. Radiation helps lower the risk of cancer recurrence in the breast. It is usually directed toward the breast, the chest wall or the underarm (axillary) lymph nodes. Many types of radiation therapy are available, along with many different schedules.

Surgery

Surgical procedures include the removal of the tumor and examination of the nearby lymph nodes. The type of surgery recommended depends on several factors, such as the size of the tumor, the presence or absence of lymph node involvement, the size of the breast, possible cosmetic outcomes and the overall treatment plan. The surgery performed will be one of two types:

- Lumpectomy, in which the tumor is removed but most of the healthy breast tissue remains.
- Mastectomy, in which the whole breast is removed, although the skin and nipple may be spared.

WHY DOES BREAST CANCER MATTER TO WOMEN?

Breast cancer is the most common cancer in women in the U.S. and worldwide, after some types of skin cancer. Following lung cancer (Chapter 42), it is the second leading cause of cancer-related deaths in women in the U.S. Approximately 1 in 8 women will develop breast cancer in their lifetimes making this cancer extremely common. Chances are that you or your family and friends already have been touched by breast cancer. Rarely, breast cancer can occur in men, too.

Breast cancer is more common in white women, but some of the more aggressive types of breast cancer are seen in Black women and Hispanic women. As such, outcomes vary among different races and ethnicities. In general, younger women — those younger than 40 years old — with breast cancer have worse outcomes than do older women.

Outcomes of breast cancer are partly related to how advanced the cancer is at diagnosis. This makes early detection a key part of improving outcomes for breast cancer. When breast cancer is detected early, treatment is highly successful.

QUESTIONS TO ASK YOUR HEALTH CARE TEAM ABOUT BREAST CANCER

- Who will be part of my health care team, and what does each member do?
- Am I a candidate for a lumpectomy?
  › Do I need a mastectomy?
  › Will I need lymph node surgery?
- What is the grade and stage of this disease?
- What are the biomarkers of my tumor?
  › What do these mean?

- What is the goal of each treatment?
- What are my treatment options?
  - › Are there clinical trials available for me to participate in?
- What are the possible side effects of treatments, and what can be done to ease them?
- What is my prognosis?

PEARLS OF WISDOM

Breast cancer is a diverse disease, and each person who has breast cancer experiences it in a unique way. As a result, many variables are involved in its treatment, and the way treatment affects each person is different. If you have breast cancer, try not to compare yourself and your progress to others with breast cancer. If you have a friend or relative with breast cancer, be supportive and engaged, but don't compare your friend or relative to others with breast cancer, either.

Communication is key to coping and understanding the expectations of breast cancer treatment. Make sure that you have a good system of communication in place with your health care team and that all of your questions are being addressed.

Early detection is key to success in the treatment and management of breast cancer. Be diligent and timely with your breast cancer screening schedule. Mammograms help save lives.

"The key to a healthy life is in prevention and screening."

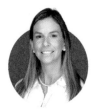

Aixa E. Soyano Müller, M.D. - she/her
Dr. Soyano is an Assistant Member in the Department of Breast Oncology at H. Lee Moffitt Cancer Center and Assistant Professor in the Department of Oncologic Sciences at the University of South Florida in Tampa. She is a medical oncologist and specializes in the multidisciplinary care of patients with breast cancer of any age, race, stage and subtype.

17

Carpal tunnel syndrome

Alana M. Munger, M.D., and Andrea Halim, M.D.

WHAT IS CARPAL TUNNEL SYNDROME?

The body's large, complex system of nerves is what enables a person to sense pressure, vibration and light touch. Nerves carry information from every part of the skin in the form of electrical signals, and those signals eventually reach the spinal cord and then the brain. Carpal tunnel syndrome (CTS) is caused by compression of one of the major nerves — the median nerve — that runs the length of the arm, goes through a passage in the wrist called the carpal tunnel and ends in the hand. The carpal tunnel itself is a channel that connects the hand to the forearm and contains the median nerve as well as nine flexor tendons.

The carpal tunnel's roof is made up of a fibrous ligament called the transverse carpal ligament. Because this ligament is less elastic than skin or muscle, any extra fluid or inflammation in the tunnel increases pressure within this space and on the median nerve. Pressure on the median nerve can lead to carpal tunnel syndrome. Many things can cause this to happen, including

overuse, tendonitis, pregnancy and infection. For many people, however, there is no clearly recognizable cause for the increased pressure within the space.

The median nerve controls the movement of all fingers except the pinky. If your median nerve is impaired or pinched, you might have a feeling of numbness and tingling in your thumb, index finger, middle finger or several fingers. People with longstanding nerve compression may experience nighttime pain. They often describe waking up at night with a painful numbness that can be alleviated by shaking the hands or running them under warm water.

There are some people, however, who do not demonstrate these "classic" symptoms of carpal tunnel syndrome and may experience numbness or pain in the index or middle finger that moves up into the forearm, or decreased sensation in the ring finger or small finger. If you have had this compression for a long time, you may experience a decreased ability to feel objects at your fingertips, decreased ability to grip objects tightly, or a tendency to drop things.

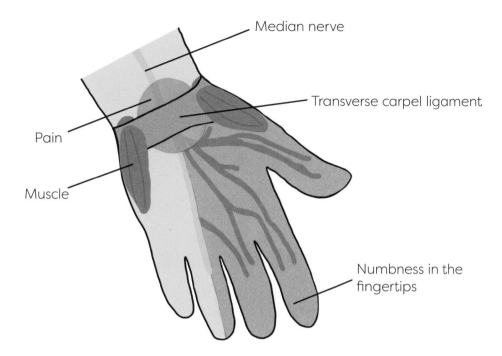

Median nerve

Transverse carpel ligament

Pain

Muscle

Numbness in the fingertips

CAN CARPAL TUNNEL SYNDROME BE PREVENTED?

Most cases of CTS develop gradually and do not have an identifiable cause. Some studies, although inconclusive, suggest that repetitive use of the wrist and fingers or repeated impact on the palm can increase the risk of CTS. While repetitive typing has not been shown to increase the risk of CTS, people who work with their hands are at higher risk of developing CTS. Specifically, large studies have shown that manual labor is a risk factor for carpal tunnel, likely due to heavy repetitive activity and constant wrist flexion. If you are in a profession that requires repetitive motions throughout the workday, try to take breaks in between these repetitive actions to relieve the pressure within your carpal tunnel.

HOW IS CARPAL TUNNEL SYNDROME TREATED?

Since other causes besides carpal tunnel syndrome may create numbness and pain in the hand and fingers, the first step is to have special tests done to rule out other problems:
- A nerve conduction study, which assesses how well the median nerve carries sensory signals across the carpal tunnel
- Electromyography, which looks for changes in the muscles that are innervated by the median nerve

Other causes of numbness and pain in the hand and fingers include:
- Cubital tunnel syndrome, or compression of the ulnar nerve
- Cervical spine disease, or compression of the spinal nerves as they leave the spine in the neck
- Neuropathy, or nerve problems caused by other conditions, such as diabetes, or by certain medications

Once other problems are ruled out and CTS is confirmed, treatment options include both nonoperative measures and surgery.

Nonoperative measures

Nonoperative measures are considered before surgery and include:

Wearing a wrist brace at night The use of a wrist splint is noninvasive and low risk and is the recommended first-line treatment for most women who are diagnosed with carpal tunnel syndrome.

Injection of a corticosteroid medication The corticosteroid medication is injected into the space around the nerve, the carpal tunnel itself. Reports show that more than 50% of people who receive corticosteroid injections experience continued relief of symptoms more than 6 months after the injection.

Surgery

Surgery is considered when symptoms cause significant sleep disruption, constant numbness or muscle weakness, and interference with work or day-to-day activities. A surgical release of the carpal tunnel involves cutting the fibrous tissue that creates the roof of the tunnel. This procedure does not require general anesthesia and can be performed by injected numbing medication into the skin and carpal tunnel. The procedure can be done in two ways:

Open carpal tunnel release This procedure involves an inch-long incision at the base of the palm, opening the roof of the carpal tunnel and allowing the surgeon to directly see the fibrous tissue.

Endoscopic carpal tunnel release During this procedure, the surgeon makes a smaller incision — about a quarter of an inch — through which a small camera is inserted into the carpal tunnel. The camera allows the surgeon to see the contents of the tunnel and see the incision in the roof of the carpal tunnel.

Although there are no differences in the long-term outcomes of either approach, endoscopic carpal tunnel release has been shown to allow an earlier return to work but an increased risk of temporary nerve injury. Talk to your surgeon about which option — an open or endoscopic release— is best for you.

WHY DOES CARPAL TUNNEL SYNDROME MATTER TO WOMEN?

Carpal tunnel syndrome is more common in women than in men. In addition, there are numerous female-predominant conditions that are risk factors for developing carpal tunnel syndrome. These include pregnancy and multiple inflammatory conditions, including rheumatoid arthritis and lupus.

Between 30% and 60% of women are diagnosed with pregnancy-related carpal tunnel syndrome. Women who develop carpal tunnel syndrome during pregnancy are more likely to develop symptoms in both hands and to experience less severe symptoms. Approximately 80% of these women experience symptom relief with nighttime wrist splinting. Thus, women with pregnancy-related carpal tunnel syndrome are less likely to require surgical release. However, if you experience severe symptoms during pregnancy, know that a surgical release of the carpal tunnel can be done without general anesthesia and will not place your baby at risk.

For more than 50% of women, CTS persists one year after childbirth, and in about 30% of women, CTS is still present three years after childbirth. If you continue to experience symptoms of CTS, see your clinician to find relief for your symptoms and to be evaluated for possible treatment.

QUESTIONS TO ASK YOUR HEALTH CARE TEAM ABOUT CARPAL TUNNEL SYNDROME

For anyone who develops symptoms of carpal tunnel syndrome, regardless of severity

- What treatment options do you recommend, given my specific symptoms?
- Is there anything I can do to prevent progression of my symptoms?
- Do I need electrodiagnostic testing in order to confirm the diagnosis of carpal tunnel syndrome?

For those who experience carpal tunnel syndrome in both the right and left wrist

- Can you inject both my left and right carpal tunnels at the same time?
- Can you perform a surgical release of both the right and left carpal tunnels in the same operation?

For those who wish to undergo a corticosteroid injection into the carpal tunnel

- What medication(s) will you be injecting?
- What are the potential side effects, both at the carpal tunnel as well as throughout my body, with this injection?
- How long will it take for me to experience relief of my symptoms?
- How long should I expect to experience relief of my symptoms?
- How many corticosteroid injections can I have before you would recommend surgery to release the carpal tunnel?

For those who wish to undergo a surgical release of the carpal tunnel

- Do you recommend an open or endoscopic carpal tunnel release?
- What are the risks associated with open versus endoscopic carpal tunnel release?
- How long will I be out of work?
- How long will I need to wear a bandage over the incision?
- What is the risk that my symptoms will not improve with the carpal tunnel release?

For pregnant and postpartum women who experience carpal tunnel syndrome

- I am in my first/second/third trimester. Is it safe for me to receive a corticosteroid injection into my carpal tunnel?
- I am lactating. Is it safe for me to receive a corticosteroid injection into my carpal tunnel?
- I am still experiencing carpal tunnel symptoms. When would you recommend surgical release of my carpal tunnel?

PEARLS OF WISDOM

Although nighttime pain and numbness affecting the thumb, index finger or middle finger are common signs and symptoms of CTS, some women may experience forearm numbness or numbness in the ring finger or little finger. If you think you have carpal tunnel syndrome, talk about it with your clinician and ask to have an electromyography done. Waiting to address carpal tunnel syndrome can lead to worsening symptoms and irreversible changes to your nerve.

If you have signs or symptoms of CTS, take them seriously. It is appropriate to see a hand surgeon if your electromyography confirms carpal tunnel syndrome or if you have persistent symptoms despite a negative electromyography. A hand surgeon should advise you on nonoperative treatment options and discuss surgical management depending on the severity of your symptoms.

"I learned a long time ago the wisest thing I can do is be on my own side, be an advocate for myself and others like me." – Maya Angelou

"It is the responsibility and privilege of surgeons to provide a thoughtful medical conversation to every patient, regardless of gender."

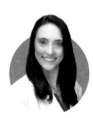

Alana M. Munger, M.D. - she/her
Dr. Munger is an orthopedic surgery resident physician at Yale-New Haven Hospital. She is also the creator, co-producer, co-editor, and host of the She Can Fix It Podcast, a podcast that involves interviews with female surgeons to highlight and empower the women of orthopedic surgery. Dr. Munger will specialize in bone and soft tissue tumor surgery.

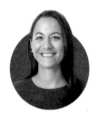

Andrea Halim, M.D. - she/her
Dr. Halim is an Assistant Professor of Hand surgery at the Department of Orthopaedics and Rehabilitation at Yale University. She serves as associate program director for the orthopedic program, as well as associate fellowship director for Yale's Combined Hand Fellowship.

18
Cervical cancer

Heidi J. Gray, M.D.

WHAT IS CERVICAL CANCER?

Cervical cancer is the third most common gynecologic cancer affecting women in the U.S., with approximately 10,000 to 12,000 new cases diagnosed each year. Cervical cancer arises from the "neck" of the uterus, also known as the cervix. The cervix is located at the lower end of the uterus, or womb, and is what dilates during labor to allow a baby to pass through the vaginal canal. The cervix is easy to see during a pelvic exam.

Risk factors for developing cervical cancer include infection with the human papilloma virus (HPV) and smoking. Also, if you've never had a Pap test or have Pap tests infrequently, you may miss detecting precancerous conditions of the cervix that could develop into cervical cancer. The average age of people with cervical cancer is 40 to 50 years.

Cervical cancer is diagnosed by examining a small piece of tissue (biopsy) of the cervix under a microscope. The biopsy is taken during a pelvic exam when a concerning growth is seen or when a person has had an abnormal Pap test. Many people with cervical cancer report symptoms such as vaginal bleeding after sexual intercourse or bleeding between menstrual periods. If you experience symptoms like these, it's important to tell your clinician right away.

CAN CERVICAL CANCER BE PREVENTED?

Yes, cervical cancer can be prevented through vaccination with the HPV vaccine and screening for precancerous conditions with regular Pap tests. It also helps to not smoke.

HPV vaccine

The cause of most cervical cancers is a virus called human papilloma virus (HPV). There are hundreds of different HPV types that can cause a variety of diseases, ranging from genital warts to cancers of the cervix, anus and mouth or throat. HPV is highly contagious. It's transmitted through skin-to-skin contact during vaginal, anal and oral sex. Most people will become infected with HPV within a year of initiating sexual activity. The majority of infections produce no symptoms and clear quickly, so people are not aware that they have had an infection. However, in a small percentage of

Cervical cancer

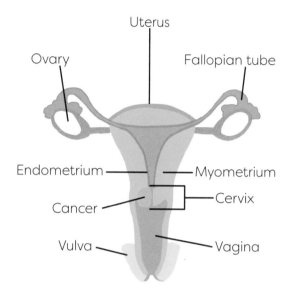

Uterus

Ovary

Fallopian tube

Endometrium — — Myometrium

Cancer — — Cervix

Vulva — — Vagina

people, HPV can linger and cause precancerous changes or cancer. Ongoing infection with two high-risk HPV types, HPV 16 and HPV 18, can be particularly worrisome, since these two types cause over 70% of all cervical cancers.

One of medicine's great success stories has been the discovery of HPV as the primary cause of cervical cancer. This discovery led to the development of the HPV vaccine. There currently are several vaccines on the market that target a range of common HPV types. The vaccines work by directing your immune system to make antibodies against HPV so that if an exposure to the virus does occur, your immune system will quickly recognize and prevent infection. Several large trials have shown that these vaccines are safe and effective in preventing both precancerous conditions of the cervix and cervical cancer.

The current recommendation from the Centers for Disease Control and Prevention (CDC) is for children and adults between the ages of 9 and 26 to receive the HPV vaccine, ideally between ages 11 and 12. In general, the HPV vaccine works better at preventing infections when given before sexual activity is initiated. But because older age groups may still benefit, the Food and Drug Administration (FDA) has also approved the HPV vaccine for adults aged 27 to 45. For children aged 9 to 15, the HPV vaccine is given as two shots spaced apart; for adolescents and adults aged 16 through 45, the vaccine is recommended as a series of three shots. The vaccine is safe. It may have mild side effects, such as arm soreness.

Pap test

One of the most common ways to prevent cervical cancer is through a screening test for pre-cancerous cells called a Pap test (previously called a Pap smear). A Pap test is easily done during a pelvic exam. Your clinician collects cells from your cervix to test for abnormalities and for HPV. If abnormal cells are found or HPV is detected, your clinician will likely refer you to an OB-GYN to obtain a biopsy of your cervix that can be examined in a lab for precancerous cells (dysplasia) or cancer. Testing for high-risk HPV types is usually done at the same time, as detection of these types can help identify an increased risk of developing either precancerous conditions or cancer in the near future.

Smoking cessation

It's well known that smoking cigarettes can have a lot of negative health effects. Smoking can also increase your risk of cervical cancer. One of the best ways you can reduce your risk of getting cervical cancer is by stopping smoking, or better yet, never taking it up!

HOW IS CERVICAL CANCER TREATED?

If a biopsy confirms cervical cancer, the next step is to visit with a specialist in gynecologic cancers (gynecologic oncologist) to discuss the best treatment plan for your circumstances. The gynecologic oncologist will take notes on your medical history and perform a physical exam, including pelvic and rectal exams, to look for any signs that the cancer has spread (metastasized). Imaging tests such as CT (computed tomography) or PET-CT (positron emission tomography) are done to look for cancer cells that may have spread to local lymph nodes and other body parts such as the lungs and liver.

The exams and test results will determine the extent (stage) of the cancer, which will help determine appropriate treatment options. Staging is a medical term that refers to where the cancer is found and how much it has spread. There are four stages. They range from stage 1, in which the cancer is only in the cervix, to stage 4, in which the cancer has spread to other parts of the body.

Surgery: Early-stage treatment
A tumor that is small and limited to the cervix with no evidence of spread (metastasis) on imaging tests is considered early stage and is a good candidate for surgical removal. The standard curative surgical treatment for early-stage cervical cancer is an extended hysterectomy, sometimes called a radical hysterectomy, which involves removal of the uterus, cervix, fallopian tubes and some extra tissue around the cervix. In addition, local lymph nodes may be removed to see if cancer cells have spread outside of the cervix.

The hysterectomy is done using an open surgical approach, usually with an incision low on the abdomen (bikini incision), and requires a stay in the hospital of several days. Minimally invasive hysterectomy (using a robotic or laparoscopic procedure) is not recommended, as several recent large clinical trials have shown a worse survival rate in women who underwent minimally invasive surgery for cervical cancer.

For women who are menopausal, removal of the ovaries is recommended at the same time to further reduce the risk of cancer recurrence.

For certain women who want to have children in the future and have very early cervical cancer with small tumors, fertility-sparing surgery may be an option. This is a type of surgery in which the cervix is partially or completely removed but the uterus is left in place. These are highly specialized cases that are best considered at cancer centers that specialize in these types of surgeries.

Most women with early-stage cervical cancer can be cured by surgery alone. Some may need radiation therapy after surgery depending on whether high-risk features were found during surgery, such as cancer in the lymph nodes. In general, survival rates for early-stage cervical cancer are high — over 85% at five years after diagnosis.

Radiation: Treatment for locally advanced cancer

When the tumor is large — 4 centimeters (cm) or greater — or the cancer has spread beyond the cervix, either into the vagina or into nearby tissues, it is considered locally advanced. The best treatment option in this case is pelvic radiation with low-dose chemotherapy. Pelvic radiation is given both externally, using radiation beams, and internally, using a device filled with radioactive materials, over the course of six to eight weeks. Low-dose chemotherapy with a drug called cisplatin is given weekly through a vein (intravenously or IV) during the radiation. Surgery is rarely recommended. Cure rates can be good, with survival rates of over 60% at five years.

Chemotherapy: Treatment for metastatic or advanced stage cancer

When cancer has spread to other parts of the body such as the lungs, it is called metastatic or stage 4 cancer. Recommended treatment for cervical cancer at this stage is intravenous chemotherapy with three drugs — paclitaxel, cisplatin and bevacizumab. Stage 4 disease is rarely curable in the long term — less than 16% of people survive five years after diagnosis — however, many people manage the disease and its symptoms for several years with treatment. Radiation may also be used to provide symptom relief for bleeding or pain.

Immunotherapy

Some women may be candidates for immunotherapy treatment, which involves receiving a medication designed to activate the immune system to fight the cancer. Some people do better with this type of therapy than other people do. Talk to your oncologist to find out if it's a possibility for you.

WHY DOES CERVICAL CANCER MATTER TO WOMEN?

Cervical cancer is a preventable cancer. The best way for women to protect themselves from cervical cancer is by getting the HPV vaccine. The next best way to prevent it is by getting pelvic exams annually and Pap tests every three to five years depending on your age to screen for precancerous conditions. Unfortunately, cervical cancer causes high rates of death and illness in women in many parts of the world who do not have access to screening or HPV vaccination. Of the 550,000 new cases of cervical cancer worldwide each year, the majority are in poor-resource countries with high rates of death — over 300,000 women a year. Advocating for women to have access to HPV vaccines and screening tests for cervical cancer is an important step in reducing this global disparity.

QUESTIONS TO ASK YOUR HEALTH CARE TEAM ABOUT CERVICAL CANCER

On prevention

- Am I a candidate for the HPV vaccine?
- When do I start getting Pap tests, and how often should I get them?
- What are the symptoms of cervical cancer that I should watch for?

- Besides the HPV vaccine and Pap tests, are there other ways I can reduce my risk of getting cervical cancer?
- I have a relative with cervical cancer — am I at increased risk?

If you have been diagnosed with cervical cancer
- What stage is my cancer?
- What are my options for treatment?
- Will I become menopausal with treatment?
- What are the side effects of treatment?
- Should I have immunotherapy?
- What will my sexual function be like after surgery? Radiation? Chemotherapy?
- What will my follow-up be after finishing treatment?
- What are the chances of the cancer returning?
- What are my chances of surviving the cancer?
- Are there resources to help me learn about nutrition and cancer?

PEARLS OF WISDOM

Cervical cancer is a preventable cancer! If women worldwide can be armed with knowledge, access to HPV vaccines and Pap test screening, the disease can be eradicated. If you are diagnosed with cervical cancer, seek help from a specialist in gynecologic cancers for the best treatment advice. With appropriate treatment, most women will be successful in beating cervical cancer.

"I believe in helping women facing cancer empower themselves with knowledge and novel therapies to overcome their illness."

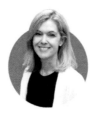

Heidi J. Gray, M.D. - she/her
Dr. Gray is Chief and Professor of the Division of Gynecologic Oncology in the Department of Obstetrics and Gynecology at the University of Washington in Seattle, Washington. She serves as the Director of Clinical Trials for Gynecologic Cancers at the Seattle Cancer Care Alliance as well as the NRG Principal Investigator for the UW/Fred Hutchinson Cancer Research Center. Her clinical expertise is ovarian cancer surgery and therapeutics as well as advanced robotic surgery for gynecologic cancers. She has extensive experience in clinical trials for cervical, endometrial and ovarian cancer.

19
Chronic fatigue syndrome (myalgic encephalomyelitis)

Marianna Gasperi, Ph.D., and Niloofar Afari, Ph.D.

WHAT IS CHRONIC FATIGUE SYNDROME (MYALGIC ENCEPHALOMYELITIS)?

Chronic fatigue syndrome (CFS), also referred to as myalgic encephalomyelitis (ME) or myalgic encephalomyelitis/chronic fatigue syndrome (ME/CFS), is a serious and debilitating illness. It is characterized by at least six months of extreme fatigue that does not get better with rest, may be worsened by physical or mental effort, and cannot be explained by another underlying condition.

ME/CFS affects 1% of the general population and is four times more common in women than men. The way in which ME/CFS affects individuals can vary widely. ME/CFS may come on suddenly in one person or develop gradually in another. Symptoms can be mild or severe, come and go slowly or suddenly, and last for a few weeks or years. A person with ME/CFS may have good days and bad days. ME/CFS symptoms can begin at any age but most commonly signs and symptoms start either between the ages of 10 and 19 or 30 and 39.

Not everyone with ME/CFS experiences the same symptoms or all symptoms simultaneously. And symptoms of ME/CFS can affect different body systems. Nonetheless, there are some key characteristics of ME/CFS that include:

- Profound exhaustion or fatigue that is not the result of ongoing excessive exertion and is not made better by rest.
  - › The fatigue is severe enough that you feel unable to engage in your previous level of activity.
  - › The fatigue often worsens after physical exercise or mental effort, a phenomenon known as post-exertion malaise.
  - › The fatigue is not relieved by rest and requires an extended recovery period.
- Trouble sleeping or feeling unrefreshed after sleeping.
- Frequently feeling faint or dizzy when sitting up or standing up (orthostatic intolerance).
- Trouble with concentration and memory, also known as brain fog.

While everyone feels deeply tired or fatigued on occasion, people with ME/CFS experience such symptoms for at least six

ME/CFS symptoms

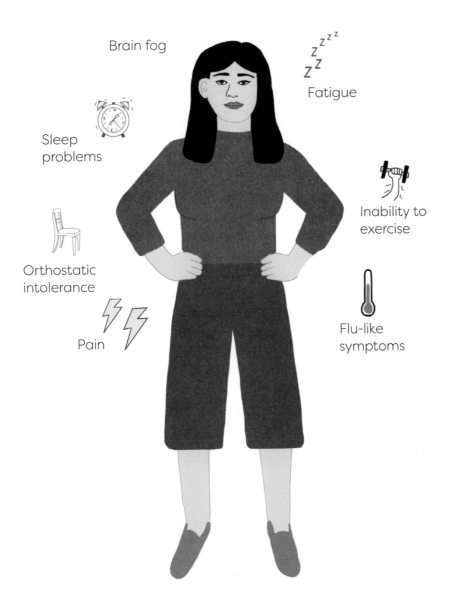

Brain fog

Fatigue

Sleep problems

Inability to exercise

Orthostatic intolerance

Pain

Flu-like symptoms

months and to a degree that prevents or significantly affects their ability to engage in activities related to work, school or social life. In addition, these symptoms represent a change in a person's ability to function compared with her abilities before symptoms began. Some have described ME/CFS as developing bad flu-like symptoms that just do not go away.

How is ME/CFS diagnosed?

The cause of ME/CFS is unknown, and there are no lab tests that can identify this condition. This makes a diagnosis of ME/CFS one of exclusion, meaning the diagnosis is made through a process of elimination, after tests for all other reasonably possible diagnoses reveal no other problems. Because of this, ME/CFS can be difficult to diagnose. Most clinicians rely on a set of criteria established by the National Academy of Medicine in 2015 to make a diagnosis of ME/CFS.

A diagnosis of ME/CFS also requires a collaborative relationship between clinician and patient. If you have symptoms of chronic fatigue, the first person you might seek help from might be your primary care clinician, who might refer you in turn to specialists in arthritis (rheumatology), heart disease (cardiology), sleep or diseases of the nervous system (neurology). Not all clinicians diagnose and treat ME/CFS. And because the symptoms of ME/CFS are often vague and transient, they may be overlooked. Carefully tracking a symptom timeline can be a helpful tool in guiding an ongoing conversation with your clinician, especially if you have trouble concentrating. The best thing you can do to reach a correct diagnosis is to:
- Find a clinician who listens and takes your concerns seriously
- Offer the clinician accurate information about your symptoms

Since the signs and symptoms of ME/CFS are like those of several other conditions, it's important to rule out other conditions using blood and urine tests, imaging tests or sleep studies — a process that can take time. Some commonly used tests to evaluate ME/CFS include:
- Orthostatic vital signs or measurements of heart rate and blood pressure in various positions (sitting and lying down). Testing that lasts longer than 10 minutes is the most accurate.
- A sleep study to check for disorders such as sleep apnea and restless leg syndrome.

- Blood and urine tests to rule out other reasons for fatigue, including anemia, underactive thyroid, diabetes, mononucleosis, lupus, low vitamin D and Lyme disease.
- Imaging scans to check for other conditions, such as multiple sclerosis.

About 70% of people with ME/CFS report that it took over a year and seeing four or more doctors to arrive at a diagnosis, and 29% said it took over five years to receive a diagnosis. It is believed that up to 90% of individuals with ME/CFS are not yet diagnosed.

ME/CFS is a complex illness and often includes other symptoms in addition to chronic fatigue. Many people with ME/CFS experience some or all of the following symptoms:
- Muscle pain
- Joint pain without swelling or redness
- Sore throat that is constant or that frequently comes and goes
- Headaches that are new or different from before
- Tender lymph nodes in the neck or upper arms

People with ME/CFS may experience other related medical conditions, including migraine headache (Chapter 44), tension headache, irritable bowel syndrome (Chapter 38), temporomandibular disorder (TMD), fibromyalgia (Chapter 29), painful sex or vulvodynia (Chapter 51), endometriosis (Chapter 28), and interstitial cystitis. These conditions are known as chronic overlapping pain conditions (COPCs). They tend to occur together and have many symptoms in common. A person who has one COPC is at a greater risk of being diagnosed with another. If you've been diagnosed with ME/CFS or are undergoing evaluation for ME/CFS be sure to report any additional symptoms that may be associated with one of these conditions — including pain, headache, digestive problems, sexual or reproductive concerns, or urinary symptoms — as this information may help your medical team understand and manage your symptoms better.

ME/CFS is not a mental health disorder. But people with ME/CFS may experience depression (Chapter 24) or anxiety (Chapter 12). They might feel stressed, overwhelmed or socially isolated. Depression or anxiety may be present before ME/CFS or may develop with ME/CFS. Whether they develop before or after an ME/CFS diagnosis, depression and anxiety can make ME/CFS worse and vice versa. There are many effective treatments for depression and anxiety, and it is essential to get the right help by starting a conversation with your clinician about it.

Symptoms of ME/CFS are real, and ME/CFS can cause significant impairment and disability. People with ME/CFS can be more functionally impaired than those with type 2 diabetes, multiple sclerosis or congestive heart failure. As many as 25% of individuals with this condition are housebound or confined to bed at some time during their illness.

CAN ME/CFS BE PREVENTED?

The causes of ME/CFS are still unclear, and ways to prevent it are yet unknown.

Research suggests that several factors might contribute to ME/CFS, including bacterial or viral infection, immune system dysfunction, hormonal imbalance, trauma and stress. However, no definitive cause or mechanism has been established.

Some people begin to experience symptoms after an infection such as the flu or with the Epstein-Barr virus that causes mononucleosis. But the reasons for a link between these viruses and ME/CFS are not clear. ME/CFS-like symptoms following coronavirus disease 2019 (COVID-19) have been reported, but more research is needed to understand this relationship. Others develop symptoms after extreme emotional or physical stress, including from another illness.

ME/CFS is not contagious and cannot be passed on to other people, though it can run in families. Research has suggested that genetic factors may play a role in why some people develop ME/CFS, but the mechanisms responsible for this vulnerability are not clear. It is most likely that ME/CFS is the result of multiple factors, rather than just one.

HOW IS ME/CFS TREATED?

There is no cure for ME/CFS, but a number of treatment strategies can help you manage and relieve symptoms. While it can be challenging to regain prior levels of functioning, most people do experience improvement in symptoms. Because symptoms are unique to each person and vary over time, supportive treatment is different from person to person. Communicating with your treatment team about how your symptoms change can help you find the right supportive therapy.

Treating fatigue and post-exertion malaise

ME/CFS can be worsened by exertion, so establishing appropriate personal limits for physical and mental activity is essential. Exhaustion cannot always be avoided, but pushing past your limit can lead to a flare-up and set you back. Physical activity is vital for health, but getting the right kind of exercise with ME/CFS can be challenging. Graded exercise therapy, a form of physical therapy that gradually increases physical activity over time, was once thought to be an effective strategy. However, research has shown that while some people with ME/CFS might find it helpful, others may be negatively impacted. Engaging in exercise within your physical limits is key. Yoga, even sitting yoga, has been shown to improve fatigue symptoms in some people and is generally well tolerated.

Activity management, also called pacing, is used to balance intervals of activity and rest. Minor adjustments, such as sitting down to perform a task or splitting up a large task into smaller tasks, can also help. Tracking symptoms, planning, prioritizing the most important activities, and learning to recognize early signs of exertion can help you work within your limits rather than fight them. Reducing flare-ups can give you a sense of being able to manage ME/CFS rather than having it manage you.

Improving sleep quality

One of the most common symptoms of ME/CFS is unrefreshing sleep. Addressing sleep problems can improve your ability to deal with other symptoms and reduce brain fog. Treatment may include changing sleep habits and taking appropriate medication. Alternative treatments, including meditation and yoga, may also help improve sleep.

Treating dizziness

Blood pressure medications may regulate blood pressure and heart rhythm to decrease orthostatic intolerance or dizziness associated with ME/CFS.

Relieving pain

ME/CFS pain is typically treated with nonprescription medications, such as ibuprofen (Advil) or naproxen sodium (Aleve). Talk to your clinician before starting or changing any nonprescription medication for ME/CFS. Opioid drugs are not recommended for ME/CFS. In some cases, other medications, including gabapentin, pregabalin, amitriptyline or duloxetine may be prescribed. Nondrug interventions such as cognitive behavior therapy (CBT) and acceptance and commitment therapy (ACT) are also effective methods for managing chronic pain.

Improving memory and concentration

Memory and concentration difficulties are common in people with ME/CFS. Tools such as calendars, alarms, notes and reminders on your smartphone can help you accomplish your goals and reduce frustration. Stimulant medications used for attention-deficit/hyperactivity disorder may be prescribed, but while they can aid concentration, they might also push you past your limit and worsen fatigue.

Improving mental health

People with ME/CFS may experience depression or anxiety, but that does not mean that mental health concerns cause ME/CFS or that ME/CFS is a psychological condition. Treating depression and anxiety symptoms is important, though, because it can help you cope with ME/CFS symptoms, including fatigue. Low doses of antidepressants may decrease pain and improve sleep in some people. Therapy and counseling, whether one-on-one or in a group setting, in person or virtually, can also improve symptoms of depression, anxiety, fatigue and pain, and should be considered in any treatment plan. Such sessions can include strategies such as CBT, ACT, mindfulness and meditation.

Alternative treatments

Many supplements, herbal remedies and alternative treatments claim to improve ME/CFS symptoms, including fatigue. However, none are approved for ME/CFS, and some might do more harm than good. Talk to your clinician before starting any alternative treatments or supplements.

WHY DOES ME/CFS MATTER TO WOMEN?

ME/CFS can affect people of any gender and of all ethnic, racial and socioeconomic backgrounds. Yet ME/CFS is two to four times more common in women than men. Research has shown that women's pain and fatigue symptoms may be ignored, resulting in delayed diagnosis and treatment. Women are more likely to be told that their symptoms are "normal." This is especially true for women of color and other minorities. While women may feel tired juggling multiple responsibilities, symptoms of ME/CFS go well beyond feeling run-down and need to be taken seriously, especially because ME/CFS is challenging to diagnose.

QUESTIONS TO ASK YOUR HEALTH CARE TEAM ABOUT ME/CFS

- Do you have experience treating people with ME/CFS? If not, can you recommend a specialist?
- Will you screen me for depression and anxiety?
- Should I see a sleep specialist or undergo a sleep study if I'm having trouble sleeping or I feel unrefreshed after sleeping?
- Should I have a neuropsychological evaluation if I've recently started having memory, thinking or concentration problems?

If you are unsure if you have ME/CFS
- What are other possible conditions that might explain my symptoms?
- Could my other symptoms have something to do with how I feel?

If you have been diagnosed with ME/CFS
- What can I do to manage my symptoms?
- What medications or supplements can I take?
- How can I best address other symptoms not related to ME/CFS?
- How can I safely increase my activity level?
- Would I benefit from physical therapy, rehabilitation or counseling?

PEARLS OF WISDOM

ME/CFS is not a psychological condition, but like people with other chronic conditions, such as diabetes, people with ME/CFS can greatly benefit from behavioral or psychological interventions. In addition to reducing anxiety and depression, psychological interventions may improve your ability to cope with ME/CFS symptoms, discover your limits and resources, and adjust to life with a condition that is unpredictable and disruptive.

Having a chronic health condition is challenging, and psychological interventions can give you evidence-based skills to get more out of life. It is also important to recognize the high degree of overlap between ME/CFS and other chronic overlapping pain conditions and to bring up any symptoms, even if they seem unrelated, to your clinician. Establishing a partnership with your clinician and clearly communicating your symptoms over time is key to reaching a correct diagnosis and effectively managing ME/CFS.

"Empathy for each woman's unique health needs and concerns is essential to promoting the best health care decisions and outcomes."

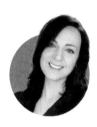

Marianna Gasperi, Ph.D. - she/her
Dr. Gasperi is an Assistant Professor of Psychiatry at University of California San Diego and a research psychologist at VA San Diego Healthcare System in San Diego, California. She specializes in the genetic epidemiology of chronic pain conditions, psychiatric disorders, and substance use.

"Accurate information is what empowers women to advocate effectively for their health care needs."

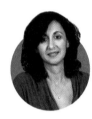

Niloofar Afari, Ph.D. - she/her
Dr. Afari is Professor of Psychiatry at the University of California San Diego and Associate Chief of Staff for Mental Health at VA San Diego Healthcare System in San Diego, California. She specializes in evaluation and behavioral interventions for chronic health conditions.

20
Chronic obstructive pulmonary disease

Dawn L. DeMeo, M.D., M.P.H.

WHAT IS CHRONIC OBSTRUCTIVE PULMONARY DISEASE (COPD)?

Chronic obstructive pulmonary disease (COPD) is a lung disease associated with limited flow of air through the lungs. COPD may also include emphysema and chronic bronchitis. COPD is a growing burden in women but has received minimal attention as a women's health concern. The number of women diagnosed with COPD continues to increase, and it is crucial to understand that COPD is not a disease of men only.

Outdated ideas persist that the "typical" patient with COPD and emphysema is a male smoker, and these ideas further perpetuate bias in diagnosing COPD in women. Women with COPD, compared with men with COPD, are generally younger, have smoked few cigarettes in their lives and may have more symptoms. Early diagnosis of COPD in women is a cornerstone of improving women's health.

HOW IS COPD DIAGNOSED?

If you have shortness of breath that has worsened over time and gets worse with exercise, don't assume this is because of aging or being out of shape. While women may make frequent excuses for shortness of breath, feeling short of breath when doing daily activities should not be ignored. Shortness of breath may indicate COPD. The same is true for persistent cough or wheeze or recurrent respiratory infections.

In considering your symptoms, ask yourself what circumstances cause you to feel short of breath. Tell your clinician if you are short of breath not only with exercise but also during everyday activities, such as hurrying along a sidewalk or walking up a hill or a flight of stairs. Share with your clinician details about these moments of breathlessness, such as needing to slow down while walking with a friend so that you can walk and talk simultaneously, or feeling short of breath when you're getting dressed or taking a shower. It is also important to tell your clinician about any risk factors you may have related to exposure and environment, including your

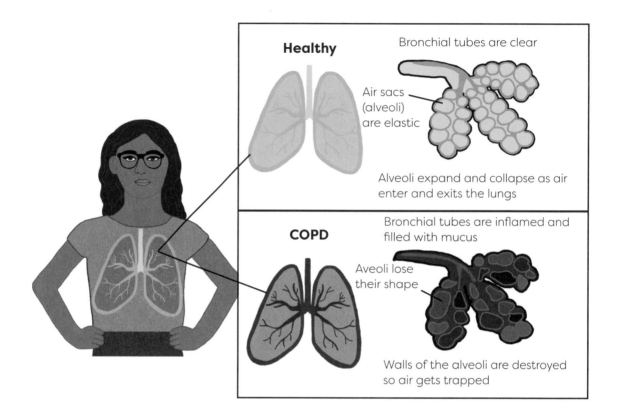

Healthy

Bronchial tubes are clear

Air sacs (alveoli) are elastic

Alveoli expand and collapse as air enter and exits the lungs

COPD

Bronchial tubes are inflamed and filled with mucus

Aveoli lose their shape

Walls of the alveoli are destroyed so air gets trapped

exposure to tobacco smoke or other indoor air pollutants. Other important factors to mention include being born prematurely or having family members with COPD, as these factors can provide context to your symptoms.

COPD is generally diagnosed using a simple noninvasive breathing test called spirometry. For this evaluation, you breathe out forcefully into a tube. The amount of air exhaled in one second provides a lot of information about limitations to your airflow. The spirometry test also measures something called vital capacity. Together, the spirometry measurements, sometimes called "breathing numbers," help your clinician identify the presence of COPD and

rate its severity. This simple test, often underutilized in primary care, can help diagnose COPD in a timely manner.

Similar to awareness of your blood pressure and cholesterol levels, knowing your breathing numbers by having a spirometry test will allow you to be a strong self-advocate for your lung health. Do not minimize your breathing problems.

CAN COPD BE PREVENTED?

Yes, in many cases COPD can be prevented by limiting exposure to tobacco and other inhaled products. Breathing in fresh air is fundamental to protecting lung health and preventing COPD. The risk of COPD is different for every person. A person's risk is linked to exposure to environmental risk factors, such as tobacco smoke and other pollutants, as well as genetics and family history. Although cigarette smoking is the leading cause of COPD in men and women in the developed world, occupational and indoor air pollutants are likely to be particularly relevant to COPD in women worldwide.

Quit smoking

Across the globe, lifetime nonsmokers with COPD are more likely to be women. Although the reason for this is not fully understood, evidence suggests that women are more susceptible to the lung-damaging effects of poor air quality, including second-hand smoke. Quitting smoking is important not just for the smoker's health but for those who live with the smoker. It is important to limit exposure to smoke-filled air overall. Researchers are working to understand the health effects of newer ways of inhaling nicotine and other substances, such as vaping and electronic cigarette use, but the general rule is to avoid inhaled substances.

Limit exposure to workplace pollutants.

Occupational exposures in women also pose a threat to lung health. Think about your workplace exposures to dust and fumes and take steps to limit inhalation of those substances. Be sure to talk to your clinician about your work environment, especially if it is in construction, mining, welding, manufacturing or painting. These are just a few occupations that are more common for women to have now than in prior decades.

Reduce household air pollution

Indoor air pollution is a global risk. Around the world, many women use biomass such as wood, sawdust, plant husks, seeds or cones for heating their homes or for cooking in poorly ventilated spaces. Household air pollution generated by using wood and other types of biomass as fuel may present an exposure risk that's not always readily apparent. It is important to consider these indoor threats to the air you breathe and minimize them. Although air purifiers may be helpful, it is better to avoid these exposures altogether, if possible, for example by opening windows to improve ventilation or moving cooking outdoors. Supporting clean household energy is an effective way to support women's lung health locally and around the world.

Alert your clinician to any family history of lung disease

Knowing your family history of lung disease is crucial. Let your clinician know if anyone in your family has or has had COPD or emphysema. COPD can run in families due to shared genetic material, and evidence suggests that women may in fact be genetically more susceptible to severe and early-onset COPD. One specific genetic form of COPD is called alpha-1-antitrypsin deficiency. Genetic testing can help identify this type of inherited COPD. Specific treatment for alpha-1-antitrypsin deficiency is available. Also ask your clinician about having spirometry testing or a chest CT scan to look for emphysema. And given that some genetic forms of COPD and emphysema are associated with liver disease or a skin disease called panniculitis, consider all aspects of your family health history as potentially informative.

Seek help for worsening symptoms

Additionally, seek out timely care when breathing problems get worse. Periodic worsening of COPD (COPD exacerbation) may be more common in women, and these exacerbations may lead to further breathing difficulty. Obtaining timely medical care for worsening of breathing is important.

Slow the progression of mild COPD

If you have mild COPD, you may wonder if it's possible to slow the progression of the disease. If you smoke, stopping smoking is crucial to slowing down the decline of lung function. Due to a decades-long lag time between starting smoking and the start of COPD symptoms, people aren't always aware of the lung damage taking place until many of the changes are irreversible. And it doesn't help that as women (and men) age, lung function naturally declines — a decline that's accelerated by menopause, research suggests. It is never too late to stop smoking, and the sooner you stop, the more you're able to slow down the progression of COPD from mild to severe.

HOW IS COPD TREATED?

COPD is a lung disease first and foremost, but there are relevant health management issues from head to toe. Treatment for COPD includes approaches with and without medications.

Smoking cessation and treatment for nicotine addiction

The most important part of treating COPD is not smoking. All women with a history of tobacco use need to stop smoking if they haven't already. In terms of lung symptoms, women may have greater benefit from smoking cessation than men. And some approaches may work better for women than they do for others. Women may be less responsive to nicotine replacement products such as nicotine patches or nicotine gum and may respond better to smoking cessation medications taken by mouth (orally) such as bupropion and varenicline. Talk with your clinician about different approaches to permanently quit smoking.

COPD medications

Medications for COPD include inhaled, oral and intravenous medications. Treatment with medications can relieve symptoms, treat exacerbations, improve overall health and increase physical endurance. When receiving treatment, prepare for your appointments by thinking about how the medications are impacting your symptoms and exacerbations and about any side effects the medications may be causing. Also consider how the costs of medications are affecting you.

Inhalers

COPD medication frequently is prescribed in the form of an inhaled mist. There are short-acting and long-acting inhaled medications, with one to three drugs delivered at a time depending on the formula. Many people are prescribed a rescue inhaler to use for sudden attacks of shortness of breath. Carry this inhaler with you. Your daily long-acting medicines help with long-term symptom management and will not help with breakthrough symptoms.

If you are prescribed an inhaler, ask your health care team to show you how to use the inhaler or recommend an instructional video. Review your inhaler technique with your clinician at each visit. Hand arthritis may impact the ability to effectively use inhalers. Alternative delivery can be arranged for some inhaled medications through a device called a nebulizer. Do not be embarrassed to tell your health care team if you are having difficulty using an inhaler.

Inhaled COPD medications may have side effects outside of the lungs such as increased heart rate, tremors or dry mouth. When you are prescribed a new inhaler, read the package insert to be aware of potential side effects. Report any new symptoms to your clinician.

Oral medications

Oral medications for COPD may include steroids or other drugs to manage lung inflammation. Other oral medications may help relax the airways or break down mucus in the lungs so the mucus is easier to clear. Sometimes antibiotics are recommended. Be sure you know what type of oral medication you are using and why.

Vaccination

Yearly flu shots and a pneumococcal vaccine are beneficial when you have COPD. In addition, ask your clinician about a pertussis vaccine if you were not previously vaccinated as a teenager. Getting vaccinated against COVID-19 will also support your lung health. Vaccination recommendations are updated frequently, so ask whether your vaccines are up to date at each visit with your clinician.

Pulmonary rehabilitation

An exercise prescription, called pulmonary rehabilitation, provides a supervised approach to increasing physical activity. Pulmonary rehabilitation programs can be done in person or virtually and combine structured exercise with education. These programs improve symptoms, functional abilities, mental well-being and quality of life. The programs may also lead to fewer hospital stays and can help with the management of COPD-related anxiety and depression. They may even introduce you to something new, such as learning to play the harmonica — a fun approach to doing something useful for the lungs that is not limited to musicians.

Oxygen therapy

Everyone needs the right amount of oxygen to live and function well; needing extra (supplemental) oxygen should not lead to feelings of shame. If a person with COPD has a low oxygen level at rest, extra oxygen can improve survival. Talk to your clinician about whether you need extra oxygen while awake or when asleep. Many different portable oxygen devices are available that will allow you to stay active. Talk to your health care team if you need help finding a device that fits well with your schedule and activities. A common misconception is that someone who uses supplemental oxygen cannot fly in a commercial airplane. Your clinician can work with you to secure the oxygen you might need for air travel. If you are short of breath during air travel, be sure to discuss this with your clinician.

Bronchoscopy and surgery

For symptoms of advanced COPD, usually with emphysema, a procedure called lung volume reduction surgery may be an option. The procedure removes some of the damaged tissue from the lungs to make room for healthier tissue. It can be done as open surgery or as a minimally invasive procedure using a scope and smaller incisions (endoscopically). In some situations, where lung function decline is severe and oxygen levels are very low, a lung transplant may be recommended. A lung transplant is not for everyone. But be sure to discuss all options with your clinician, so that you can be fully informed about the challenges of each of the surgical options and make decisions accordingly.

Alpha-1 augmentation

In women with alpha-1-antitrypsin deficiency, a genetic cause of COPD mentioned earlier in the chapter, intravenous replacement of the alpha-1 protein is available.

Nutrition

Balanced nutrition is an important component of COPD management, and visiting with a registered dietitian or nutritionist can be helpful. Lack of vitamin D is a very common deficiency, and taking supplemental vitamin D has been linked to fewer COPD exacerbations. Be sure to discuss your vitamin D levels with your clinician.

Sleep

Consistent and uninterrupted sleep patterns are crucial for women with COPD. Sometimes supplemental oxygen is needed during sleep to improve decreased oxygen levels. In addition, sleep apnea may become an issue for some people. It is important to discuss daytime fatigue and sleepiness with your care team. A sleep study may be needed to evaluate your sleep quality, quantity and oxygen levels.

Other medical conditions

Some medical conditions, not directly related to the lungs, are more common in women with COPD compared with men with COPD. Anxiety and depression occur more frequently in women with COPD, for example, but these conditions may not be actively screened for, recognized or treated. If you are feeling anxious or sad, be sure to bring it up with your clinician. Treating depression and anxiety can have a positive impact on your quality of life and may help you better manage your COPD symptoms.

WHY DOES COPD MATTER TO WOMEN?

Women with COPD may experience the disease differently than men with COPD do and may exhibit different signs and symptoms. Because COPD has historically been considered a disease of men, a diagnostic bias may exist that results in an incorrect diagnosis in some women. Sometimes women are diagnosed with asthma, for example, when they really have COPD. Asthma is another kind of lung disease that is associated with irregular lung function and shortness of breath (see Chapter 13). But in most cases, medication fully reverses the signs and symptoms of asthma. This is not the case for COPD, which requires a different treatment strategy. Although asthma and COPD can be present in the same person, women with COPD are more likely to receive an incorrect diagnosis and inadequate treatment.

As you've already read, lung function decline may accelerate around menopause. As a result, COPD symptoms may be mistaken for symptoms of menopause.

COPD also may have a greater impact on overall health and quality of life in women compared with men. Women are more likely to develop COPD earlier in life, in their late 40s or early 50s. They generally have more shortness of breath, increased depression and anxiety, and higher rates of osteoporosis compared with men with COPD. Overall, women have a lower history of smoking and are overrepresented among people with COPD who have never smoked. But clinicians may not routinely consider COPD in a woman without a smoking history. As the third leading cause of death for women, COPD should routinely be considered in women.

QUESTIONS TO ASK YOUR HEALTH CARE TEAM ABOUT COPD

If you smoke
- Can you help me stop?
  › What resources are available?
- What are my risk factors for COPD?
  › Should I have a genetic test?

If you have COPD
- How often should I have breathing tests (spirometry and lung capacity)?
- Should I have an X-ray of my lungs?
- Should I have a CT scan of my lungs to screen for lung cancer?
- Do I need medications and supplements such as inhalers or bronchodilators, steroids, anti-inflammatory medication, mucus controllers, antibiotics and

vitamins (such as vitamin D)?
- Do I need pulmonary rehabilitation?
  › What about supplemental oxygen?
- How do I best handle COPD exacerbations?
- What vaccinations should I have?
- Do I need to be evaluated for bone strength (osteoporosis), stomach acid reflux, anxiety, depression or lung cancer?
- Would surgery help me?

PEARLS OF WISDOM

Women of all ages need to understand that experiencing shortness of breath with daily activities or having a persistent daily cough are symptoms that should not be ignored or minimized. They may be a sign of lung disease such as COPD. Untreated COPD can greatly impact overall health and quality of life.

It is never too late to stop smoking or to modify occupational and environmental exposures when possible. Exercise and physical activity are crucial for staying strong and independent and go hand in hand with a healthy diet and quality sleep. Conditions such as depression, anxiety and osteoporosis are more common in women versus men with COPD, further impacting quality of life if left untreated.

When properly diagnosed, COPD is treatable, so it is important to be a self-advocate. Talk to your health care team about obtaining a spirometry test and a CT scan of the chest if a lung cancer screening is appropriate. Keeping active with COPD is as critical as routine preventive care that includes pneumonia, flu and COVID vaccination.

A lot of research is being focused on limiting risk, improving diagnosis and raising awareness about COPD in women. Educating women and girls — mothers, daughters, friends and all —about the importance of breathing clean air is integral to ensuring a healthy tomorrow for women everywhere.

Additional resources

COPD Foundation
www.copdfoundation.org

Alpha-1 Foundation
www.alpha1.org

Better Breathers Club/American Lung Association
www.lung.org

National Heart Lung and Blood Institutes
www.nhlbi.nih.gov

"Women's lung health must be an international priority."

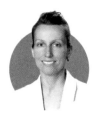

Dawn L. DeMeo, M.D., M.P.H. - she/her
Dr. DeMeo is a pulmonary and critical care physician and a respiratory epidemiologist, with a specialty in the genetics and epigenetics of obstructive lung diseases. She is an Associate Physician at Brigham and Women's Hospital, a researcher at the Channing Division of Network Medicine and Associate Professor of Medicine at Harvard Medical School.

21
Colorectal cancer

Lynn K. Symonds, M.D., and Stacey A. Cohen, M.D.

WHAT IS COLORECTAL CANCER?

Colorectal cancer is a tumor (malignancy) that grows from cells in the colon, also known as the large bowel or large intestine, or in the rectum, the section between the colon and anus. Though it can be uncomfortable to talk about, it is important to know about this common cancer!

Colon and rectal cancer are often lumped together (colorectal cancer), but the slight location difference sometimes matters for treatment. Regardless of the location, colorectal cancer often starts as an adenoma polyp, a small mass of cells growing on the inner lining of the colon. Over time, some colon polyps grow out of control and develop into colon cancer. Not all polyps are precancerous, however. Some, such as hyperplastic polyps, are noncancerous (benign).

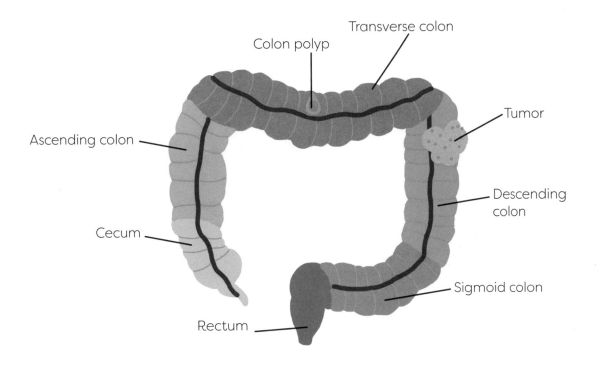

Symptoms of colorectal cancer are varied, but can include:

- Abdominal pain or discomfort or cramping
- Bloating
- Blood from rectum or dark bloody stools
- Changes in bowel movements (diarrhea or constipation)
- Fatigue
- Gas
- Loss of appetite
- Nausea or vomiting
- Pencil-thin, ribbon-like stools
- Unexplained weight loss (losing 10 pounds or more without knowing why)

In the early stages of colorectal cancer, many people experience no symptoms, which is why getting screened regularly is important. Colorectal cancer is more common with age, but it can occur in younger adults, too.

CAN COLORECTAL CANCER BE PREVENTED?

Colorectal cancer cannot always be prevented, but there are ways to lower your risk and screen for early signs of cancer. Early detection of colorectal cancer can be lifesaving!

Colorectal cancer screening

There are different ways to screen for colorectal cancer, but probably the most familiar is colonoscopy. Work together with your clinician to select the test that is right for you. Most important, if any of these tests are abnormal, it's critical that you follow up with a full colonoscopy to look for concerning polyps or cancer.

Colonoscopy This is the gold standard for colorectal cancer screening. A colonoscopy allows the doctor to see the lining of the bowel, remove polyps and take tissue samples of the tumor (biopsies) to test for cancer if needed. Before you have a colonoscopy, you'll need to complete a process called a bowel prep. The prep involves limiting your diet to clear liquids for one to two days, followed by "cleaning out" your colon with laxatives.

When you arrive for your colonoscopy, you'll receive a sedative medication to keep you comfortable during the procedure. Your doctor inserts a thin tube with a camera (colonoscope) through your anus so that the inside of the colon and rectum can be thoroughly examined. Most people say the bowel prep before the procedure is worse than the procedure.

Other screening tests (see tests that follow) may seem simpler than a colonoscopy but have limitations and must be done more often.

Flexible sigmoidoscopy This procedure is similar to a colonoscopy but requires less prep and examines only the rectum and end of colon.

Home-based tests There are several tests that you can do at home that screen for blood or tumor DNA in your stool. These often require wearing gloves while putting a small stool sample on a provided card or in a sample container that then gets mailed back for testing.

Computed tomography colonography (CTC) This is a specialized type of screening CT scan, though it is not commonly used.

Timing and frequency of screening The timing and frequency of screening depends on your risk of developing colorectal cancer and the type of test you choose.

- **Average risk** Most people have an average risk of developing colorectal cancer in their lifetimes. For these people, guidelines recommend starting screening at age 45. Colonoscopies are performed every 10 years if the results are normal. All other screening tests are done more frequently; the home-based tests may even be needed yearly. If a concerning polyp is ever found, more frequent screening is typically recommended.
- **High risk** Some people have a higher risk of developing colorectal cancer because of an underlying medical condition, such as a genetic condition (most commonly Lynch Syndrome or familial adenomatous polyposis), a history of colorectal cancer in a close blood relative, or a personal history of cancer or adenoma polyps. If you have a higher-than-average risk, it's important to be screened for colorectal cancer with a colonoscopy. You may also need to begin screening at an earlier age and have screening performed more often.

Lifestyle changes

Exercising regularly, maintaining a healthy weight and following a diet rich in fruits, vegetables, whole grains and fiber may help lower your risk of developing cancer. Avoiding red and processed meat is also important because these are linked to an increased risk of colorectal cancer. Maintaining adequate vitamin D levels, avoiding or minimizing alcohol use and not using tobacco are additional ways to reduce your risk of colorectal cancer.

HOW IS COLORECTAL CANCER TREATED?

When a person is diagnosed with cancer, doctors start by collecting information about the cancer to guide the treatment plan. This may include getting answers to these questions:

- **What type of cancer is it?** A biopsy is needed to confirm the cancer diagnosis. For a localized tumor, this is typically done with a colonoscopy. If the cancer has already spread, another site may be biopsied, depending on accessibility. A doctor who specializes in looking at tissue samples (pathologist) looks at the cells under a microscope to determine the cancer type — often an adenocarcinoma — and where it came from. Additional features of the tumor may be described in a full pathology report, some of which can guide the kinds of treatment recommended.
- **Where is the cancer?** The cancer stage helps summarize where the cancer is located at the time of diagnosis. The higher the stage, the more advanced the cancer. Staging for colorectal cancer ranges from 1 to 4.
  - › A stage 1 or 2 cancer is small and confined to the colorectum (localized cancer).
  - › A stage 3 cancer has spread to nearby lymph nodes.
  - › A stage 4 cancer means the cancer has

spread to other parts of the body (typically through the bloodstream).

› A full body CT scan is often used to determine the cancer's stage. An MRI of the pelvis is needed for rectal cancers. Positron emission tomography (PET) scans are rarely needed.

• **Is genetic testing useful?** Why someone develops colorectal cancer often remains unknown. However, some people have a higher risk because they are born with a genetic alteration that they inherit from a parent. There are also genetic changes that occur only within cancer cells. These changes develop over time and don't run in families. Depending on your personal and family medical history, your doctor may suggest testing for one or both types of genetic alterations to determine your risk of other cancers, to see if your blood relatives are at risk and to guide treatment.

Types of treatment

Colorectal cancer treatment is individualized based on the stage of your cancer, other medical conditions you may have and your goals. Early-stage colon or rectal cancers may be treated with polyp removal or surgery alone. If a cancer is more advanced, it may be treated with some combination of surgery, radiation and chemotherapy. After treatment is complete, your doctor will follow up regularly with exams, labs, scans and periodic colonoscopies to check that the cancer hasn't come back or spread.

If cancer has metastasized, it is usually considered incurable. In these cases, the goal of treatment is to help someone live as long and as well as possible. Chemotherapy is the backbone of treatment to control metastatic cancer. Surgery or radiation are typically only used to help relieve symptoms, rather than to try to get rid of the cancer. If quality of life is reasonable and there are available drug options, treatment usually is ongoing to maintain control of the cancer.

Surgery to remove the original (primary) tumor When a cancer is very small or found only in a polyp, removing the polyp may be all the treatment that's needed. However, most people with localized cancer need surgery to remove the cancer and surrounding tissues, including nearby lymph nodes. The type of surgery depends on the size and location of the tumor. If the tumor is at the end of the rectum, the intestine cannot be reconnected to the rectum after tumor removal. In this case, the surgeon will attach the intestine to an opening (ostomy) created in the skin of the abdomen. A bag is then placed over the ostomy to collect stool. This may be temporary or permanent. People live normal and active lives with an ostomy, but it can take some time to adjust to it. Some nurses specialize in helping people learn to care for their ostomies. In addition, many support groups are available where people can talk with others who are in similar situations.

Radiation therapy Radiation involves targeting high-energy beams at a tumor to kill its cells. Radiation is used mostly for rectal cancer, since its location in the pelvis makes it challenging to remove. Giving radiation before surgery can shrink the cancer and make removal easier. Radiation treatment typically involves 1 week or 5.5 weeks of daily radiation treatment sessions targeted to the tumor. These may be combined with chemotherapy, which makes the tumor more sensitive to radiation. Common side effects include fatigue, skin rash, diarrhea and nausea. Infertility after radiation therapy is common for premenopausal women. To avoid early menopause and preserve fertility, surgically moving the ovaries away from the radiation field may be recommended.

Chemotherapy For localized cancers, chemotherapy may be recommended, either before surgery to help shrink the tumor or after surgery to decrease the chances of the cancer returning. For cancers that have spread to other parts of the body (metastasized), chemotherapy is the main treatment. Most medicines for colorectal cancer are given through an IV line (intravenously). Chemotherapy is usually given in dose cycles every two to three weeks. Side effects vary, depending on the person, the drugs used and the duration of treatment. Common side effects include fatigue, nausea, diarrhea, low blood counts, and numbness or tingling of the hands, feet or mouth (neuropathy). Chemotherapy can also have temporary or lasting effects on fertility. Egg stimulation and harvesting for storage is recommended prior to treatment for women who want to have a baby later.

Targeted and immunotherapy treatments Chemotherapy drugs work by affecting how fast-growing cells divide and grow. Depending on the results of genetic testing and the stage of the tumor, additional treatments, such as targeted therapies (drugs that target a specific genetic change in the tumor) or immunotherapy (drugs that "rev up" the immune system to try to get it to attack the cancer) may be recommended. These are most common for metastatic colorectal cancer.

Alternative therapies Unfortunately, there is limited data to support alternative options for the primary treatment of colorectal cancer. However, certain procedures or supplements may be reasonable complements to established treatments. For example, acupuncture may help decrease neuropathy from chemotherapy. If you are considering taking supplements or participating in complementary medicine techniques, it is important to discuss them with your doctor or pharmacist to make sure that there are no safety concerns involved.

WHY DOES COLORECTAL CANCER MATTER TO WOMEN?

Colorectal cancer is very common. Approximately 1 in 25 women will develop colorectal cancer during their lifetimes. In the U.S., colorectal cancer is the third most common type of cancer among women. Fortunately, there are many screening options. It is important for women to get age-appropriate screening and be aware of potential signs of colorectal cancer, including blood in the stool, any significant change in bowel habits, unexplained weight loss and new abdominal discomfort.

QUESTIONS TO ASK YOUR HEALTH CARE TEAM ABOUT COLORECTAL CANCER

For anyone without a diagnosis of colorectal cancer

- Would you consider me to be at average or high risk of colorectal cancer?
- What is the best type of screening test for me?
- I was told I had a polyp. Was it the precancerous type?

For someone with a diagnosis of colorectal cancer

- Will you connect me with someone who has been through a similar treatment?
  - › Are there any support groups you recommend for patients and caregivers?
- Will treatment impact my ability to get pregnant or deliver a baby?
- How will treatment impact my sexual health?
- Are there any clinical trials that I should consider?
- Will I be able to work, exercise, travel and engage in other activities during treatment?
- Is there someone who can help me talk to friends, family members or children about my diagnosis?
- Do you offer financial assistance for treatment?

PEARLS OF WISDOM

The best "treatment" for colorectal cancer is prevention and early diagnosis. It's important for women to get age-appropriate cancer screening and adopt a healthy lifestyle to help prevent cancer. Many colorectal cancers are originally misdiagnosed as hemorrhoids or irritable bowel syndrome. If you have ongoing symptoms that might suggest colorectal cancer, ask your clinician about colorectal cancer screening (even if you are younger than the usual screening age).

If you have been diagnosed with colorectal cancer, it's common for the initial diagnosis to feel overwhelming and scary. Your health care team will review the details of your diagnosis with you and discuss your treatment options, including the expected length of treatment and possible side effects. Write down questions you have and bring the list with you, especially when you meet your doctor for the first time. This will help your health care team learn about you and your cancer and help you determine the right treatment strategy together.

Cancer care may be improved when clinicians are specially trained in this type of cancer. For example, it can help to have surgery with a colorectal cancer surgery specialist or to be treated at a specialty cancer clinic. It's OK to ask about your team's experience with colorectal cancer. If you're not feeling confident about your treatment plan, it's also OK to ask for a second opinion. Your team wants you to feel good about your care!

"Women deserve to be empowered decision makers on their health care journey."

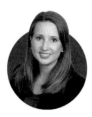

Lynn K. Symonds, M.D. - she/her
Dr. Symonds is senior hematology/oncology fellow at the University of Washington in Seattle, Washington. She is specializing in women's cancers.

"Women deserve excellent medical care and a safe space to discuss their concerns."

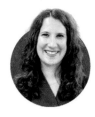

Stacey A. Cohen, M.D. - she/her
Dr. Cohen is an Associate Professor at the University of Washington and Fred Hutchinson Cancer Research Center. She is a gastrointestinal (GI) medical oncologist, specializing in the care of colorectal cancer patients and using tumor genetics to individualize care.

22
Constipation

Xiao Jing (Iris) Wang, M.D., and Jean C. Fox, M.D.

WHAT IS CONSTIPATION?

Constipation means different things to different people.

Constipation is formally defined as fewer than three bowel movements a week, with stools that are hard or lumpy, or difficult to pass. This can result in a need to push or strain when trying to defecate, which can be painful. Some people also feel a sense of incomplete emptying of the bowels or a feeling that they have something blocking the bowel movement. Some people may even need to use a finger to manually remove stool.

Almost everyone has experienced constipation at some point in their lives, and these formal definitions are relative. If you have a bowel movement regularly every day, skipping one day may make you feel constipated. On the other hand, if you usually have a bowel movement every two to three days, then fewer than three bowel movements a week may not bother you. It is also common to experience short-term constipation during times of travel or illness, which usually goes away after returning to your regular schedule and lifestyle.

Constipation as a medical condition refers to long-term (chronic) constipation, which can lead to other symptoms throughout your gastrointestinal tract. Constipation is considered chronic if it has lasted at least 12 weeks in the last 12 months. Importantly, constipation can not only lead to discomfort in the lower abdomen before and during stool passage, but can often cause symptoms in the upper belly including nausea, bloating and decreased appetite. (When considering your bowel habits, keep in mind that if you experience significant weight loss without trying, or if you see blood mixed in with stool, or if you are over 50 years old with a new change in your bowel habits, it's important to seek care with a clinician.)

Reasons for constipation

While constipation can happen for many reasons, all of them lead to too little water in the colon, producing firm or hard stools that move more slowly through the colon. Some reasons for constipation include:

Diet too low in fiber Diets that are low in fiber from sources such as grains, fruits and vegetables, or low in water, can lead to constipation. Fiber in the diet holds on to water to keep stools soft and helps increase the bulk of the stool, which helps it move through the colon.

Not drinking enough water When you do not drink enough water, your body will reclaim water to maintain your blood pressure from any sources available, including the colon, which can lead to harder stool.

Medications Certain medications can slow down movement in the colon, which leaves more time for water to be absorbed back into the body and delays the stool reaching the rectum.

Medical conditions Conditions such as irritable bowel syndrome cause constipation in many ways, including by creating changes in the gut bacteria (microbiome) and possibly producing low levels of inflammation that are not detectable by testing. This inflammation leads to more water in the colon being absorbed back into the body and is accompanied by pain that is relieved by a bowel movement.

Pelvic floor dysfunction This is a common cause of chronic constipation that is under-recognized. Pelvic floor dysfunction can prevent easy passage of stool out of the rectum even if the stools are not hard.

Stress Stress can alter nerve signals throughout the body and lead to changes in bowel habits, including constipation for some people and diarrhea for others. Chronic levels of stress can lead to the development of irritable bowel syndrome or other gut disorders, as well.

Aging Older people have higher rates of constipation for a number of reasons,

including use of more medications with side effects, other systemic or nervous system diseases that can slow down the bowels, development of pelvic floor dysfunction, and lower activity levels. Prevention of constipation in later years is particularly important because straining to produce a bowel movement can stress the nervous system and lead to symptoms of lightheadedness, dizziness or even fainting.

Sedentary lifestyle Physical activity helps stimulate the bowels to move. Sedentary lifestyles remove this important trigger for bowel function and can also lead to constipation in other ways if accompanied by poor food choices, such as low-fiber snack foods.

Pregnancy Pregnancy is known to cause constipation through changes in hormones throughout the pregnancy, slowing down the entire GI system, and through loosening connective tissues that can lead to pelvic floor issues. As the pregnancy progresses, the growing uterus can put physical pressure on the colon, preventing stool from moving easily in the colon.

CAN CONSTIPATION BE PREVENTED?

Some of the causes of constipation can be prevented or improved by diet and lifestyle changes. Good self-care is critical. Eating regular meals helps to stimulate colon motion. Eating a good amount of dietary fiber and drinking enough water throughout the day can prevent constipation. It is also very important to stay active because regular physical activity and exercise help maintain bowel regularity.

Often, you cannot stop taking medications needed for other health conditions. But being aware of the potential side effects of your medications is important. If constipation occurs as a side effect of a medication you are taking, discuss it with your clinician, who may be able to recommend an alternative. In some cases, the side effect of constipation may need to be accepted and treated.

It is important to know that constipation can lead to more constipation. As your colon fills with stool, it sends signals to slow down the delivery of more stool, decreasing movement and causing more constipation. Therefore, it is important to treat constipation early on to prevent the development of a vicious cycle.

In situations where constipation might be anticipated — such as after an elective surgery, during hospitalization, or while pregnant or traveling — extra hydration and stool softeners such as docusate sodium may be helpful to maintain soft stools and help promote regularity.

HOW IS CONSTIPATION TREATED?

Constipation starts with dietary changes. Other steps also may be helpful.

Fiber and water
Constipation treatment starts with adequate fiber and water intake, which is both preventive and used as early treatment. Dietary intake should include at least 25 grams (g) of fiber a day with accompanying water intake, according to the American Heart Association. Other experts recommend 20 to 30 grams of fiber a day for women and up to 38 grams a day for men. Recent studies have shown that two kiwi fruit (with skin on) a day or four prunes daily are effective in managing mild constipation.

Laxatives
When dietary measures are not enough, the next step is to add a nonprescription laxative. These can be divided into two categories:

Osmotic laxatives Osmotic laxatives pull water into the colon. Some examples are polyethylene glycol (MiraLAX) and milk of magnesia. Osmotic laxatives tend to be gentler and should be taken on a regular basis.

Prokinetic laxatives Prokinetic laxatives, such as bisacodyl and sennakot, make the colon move. These can be added as needed if osmotic laxatives are not producing enough results. Prokinetic laxatives do not have to be continued once bowel movements are regular.

Treatment of pelvic floor dysfunction
Pelvic floor dysfunction, which is discussed further in the next section, can be treated effectively with pelvic floor retraining under the guidance of a physical therapist. Use of a step stool around the toilet to help raise the knees above the level of belly button, simulating a squatting position, can help improve pelvic floor muscle dynamics. These are commercially available to purchase, but regular footstools, or even bricks, can be used to achieve the same goal!

Alternative therapies
Alternative therapies such as yoga and

Using pelvic position to relieve constipation

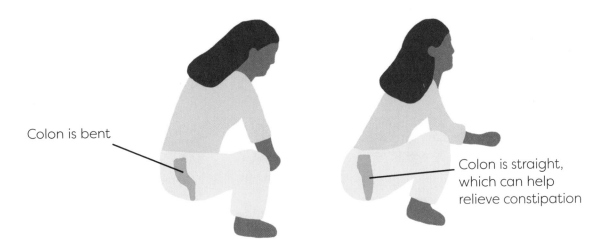

Colon is bent

Colon is straight, which can help relieve constipation

acupuncture have also been shown to help constipation by stimulating bowel movements. These interventions have minimal side effects and are quite safe to pursue. On the other hand, while there are herbal supplements that can be beneficial, use them with caution as many of these preparations are not FDA approved and the composition and other ingredients added are not regulated.

WHY DOES CONSTIPATION MATTER TO WOMEN?

Women are particularly at risk for constipation because of changes in hormones and the impacts of pregnancy and childbirth. In general, estrogen and progesterone can decrease the strength of colon contractions, slowing movement. Hormonal changes that occur during ovulation and pregnancy can lead to constipation. Relaxin, a hormone produced at about 10 weeks of gestation, softens the pubic symphysis to prepare room for the growing uterus — and decreases

smooth muscle activity in the bowel, slowing down movement. This hormone can increase slackness in the pelvic floor, which in addition to the weight of an enlarging uterus, can lead to pelvic floor dysfunction and constipation from obstruction.

Thyroid function also has a strong influence on the speed of bowel movements, with lower levels of thyroid hormone leading to constipation. Thyroid issues are common in women, particularly after childbirth; sudden changes in stool frequency with feelings of sluggishness and weight gain could suggest a thyroid issue.

Women who have had children, especially those who have had multiple vaginal deliveries, are more likely to have pelvic floor issues leading to constipation. This is particularly the case when active labor is prolonged and a long time is spent pushing, when the mother has high-degree vaginal tears, or when forceps or vacuums are needed to help deliver the baby.

Symptoms of pelvic floor dysfunction, particularly in women, can include needing to urinate frequently, difficulty emptying the bladder or frequent urinary tract infections. Women with pelvic floor dysfunction can also experience pain with intercourse because of irritation in the pelvic floor muscles. If you have these symptoms along with constipation, consider discussing testing of your pelvic floor with your clinician.

Importantly, anyone who has experienced sexual trauma or assault can develop pelvic floor dysfunction with constipation. If this is part of your history, making sure your clinician knows about this is very important, as it can change the testing you need. Pelvic floor therapists should also be told about any history of trauma, as it may influence the type of therapy used.

Depending on the cause of constipation, outcomes may be different for women. While both men and women can develop hemorrhoids, fissures or diverticular disease because of their constipation, women are more likely to develop pelvic organ prolapse (see Chapter 53). This is particularly true if the woman has experienced prior birthing trauma. Even without birth trauma, women can develop pelvic organ prolapse because of chronic prolonged straining from constipation. Pelvic organ prolapse is due to weakening and subsequent outpouchings (herniation) of pelvic organs such as the bladder, vaginal canal or rectum. These outpouchings can develop because of straining, but then can worsen constipation by further obstructing the rectum, creating a harmful cycle of greater straining and obstruction.

QUESTIONS TO ASK YOUR HEALTH CARE TEAM ABOUT CONSTIPATION

- Are any of my medications potentially contributing to constipation?
- Should I ask a dietitian to assess my diet and help me find ways to increase fiber intake?
- Are there signs of pelvic floor dysfunction, and would I benefit from therapy?
- Should I have my thyroid checked?
- What is a reasonable laxative regimen for me, and when do we consider prescription medications?

If you have a family history of colon cancer
- Should I be screened for this with a colonoscopy; or, am I up to date on my screening?

Your clinician may need to ask you some difficult questions, such as whether you experienced any physical or sexual trauma. There is no need to share the specific details about the event; however, it is important to be honest about what you experienced, as it might impact your treatment plan in the setting of pelvic floor dysfunction.

PEARLS OF WISDOM

There are many causes of constipation including diet, medications and pelvic floor dysfunction. Be proactive about discussing medication side effects with your clinician, as well as your prior medical and social history. Prevention is key! Physical activity stimulates your colon, so keep moving. Eat well, get plenty of fiber and stay hydrated.

Additional resources

- American Gastroenterological Association
  www.gastro.org

- International Foundation for Gastrointestinal Disorders:
  www.iffgd.org

"Women are not like men — health care providers should understand and treat the unique health care needs of women."

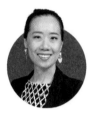

Xiao Jing (Iris) Wang, M.D. - she/her
Dr. Wang is an Assistant Professor at Mayo Clinic in Rochester, Minnesota, and a general gastroenterologist with a passion for teaching. She specializes in disorders of the gut brain axis (DGBA) and chronic abdominal pain.

"Self-care is not selfish. You are worth caring for."

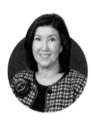

Jean C. Fox, M.D. - she/her/they
Dr. Fox is an Assistant Professor at Mayo Clinic in Rochester, Minnesota. She specializes in gastrointestinal motility disorders. Dr. Fox is the associate vice chair for diversity and equity and inclusion for her division. She is passionate about patient education and empowerment.

23
Dementia

Zelde Espinel, M.D., M.A., M.P.H., and Elizabeth A. Crocco, M.D.

WHAT IS DEMENTIA?

Dementia is not a part of normal aging. It is a disease of the brain that causes problems with cognition — the mental processes that allow you to think, talk, problem-solve, make judgments and remember. There are many different causes of dementia, and they occur fairly commonly in older adults. Although dementia can occur suddenly, as a consequence of a traumatic head injury, for example, most dementias progressively worsen over time.

Alzheimer's disease, a neurological disease, is the most common cause of dementia. In Alzheimer's disease, there is a buildup of a protein called beta-amyloid in the spaces between the nerves of the brain. There is also an abnormal form of a protein called tau within the nerve cells. Initial symptoms of Alzheimer's are typically forgetfulness and memory lapses. Because Alzheimer's accounts for at least two-thirds of dementia cases, people often use the term Alzheimer's synonymously with dementia.

The remaining third of dementias, those not due to Alzheimer's disease, include:
- Vascular dementia, which is caused by strokes and diseases of the blood vessels in the brain (cerebrovascular diseases)
- Lewy body dementia, which builds up a protein in nerve cells called alpha-synuclein and is very similar to Parkinson's disease
- Frontotemporal dementia, which is related to cell death in very specific parts of the brain. Frontotemporal dementia leads to behavioral changes and problems with language as the condition progresses. It is a less common type of dementia.

Dementia is diagnosed by a doctor based on an assessment of the affected person's thinking processes and interviews with family members who have observed the person firsthand. A medical and neurological examination is also required to properly diagnose the type of dementia. Blood tests and imaging of the brain, such as MRI or positron emission tomography (PET) scan, are also used to make the diagnosis.

In addition to problems with cognition, dementia causes a range of neurological, psychiatric and functional symptoms:
- Neurological symptoms include problems with memory, movement or sensation that can lead to difficulty walking or urinary incontinence.

Dementia symptoms

Trouble completing familiar tasks

Difficulty remembering or prouncing words

Mixing up time and location

Unfounded emotions

Poor judgment

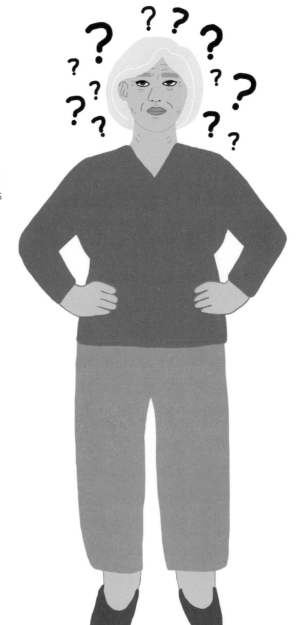

Withdrawing from social activities

Dimished problem-solving skills

Losing or misplacing items

Trouble with images and spaces

Memory loss

- Psychiatric symptoms include problems with mood, such as anxiety and depression; behavior, such as agitation or disinhibition; and psychosis, such as paranoia or hallucinations.
- Functional symptoms include the inability to perform activities of daily living, such as caring for one's household chores or personal hygiene.

CAN DEMENTIA BE PREVENTED?

Recent research developments show that the earliest changes in the brain may occur 20 to 25 years before the outward appearance of Alzheimer's signs or symptoms. Some of the most influential risk factors for Alzheimer's disease cannot be controlled, such as aging and genetics. Aging is the biggest risk factor for developing Alzheimer's disease and its related dementias.

However, 35% to 40% of the risk of Alzheimer's disease in most people is linked to select behaviors and lifestyle changes that can be controlled. For example, many of the risk factors for diseases of the heart and blood vessels (cardiovascular disease) also apply to diseases of the brain, including Alzheimer's disease. Prevention of Alzheimer's disease and other dementias involves rigorously diagnosing and managing cardiovascular risk factors, such as high blood pressure, diabetes and unhealthy cholesterol levels. What is good for the heart is good for the brain.

Other lifestyle behaviors that optimize health and longevity include:
- Maintaining a healthy diet that is high in fiber and low in fats and sugar
- Engaging in moderate to vigorous physical activity on a regular basis
- Moving and standing up frequently throughout the day
- Staying mentally active and socially engaged
- Moderating alcohol consumption
- Quitting smoking

To lower your risk of dementia, it is also important to have preventive checkups that include monitoring blood pressure and blood fats (lipids). Making careful changes in your lifestyle, in addition to seeking appropriate medical care, can help lower your risk of dementia.

HOW IS DEMENTIA TREATED OR MANAGED?

While there is no cure for most dementias, identifying and treating other possible causes of a person's symptoms, such as depression or vitamin deficiencies, can help slow the progression of dementia. This is why it's important to undergo a medical evaluation as soon as symptoms arise.

Management of dementia focuses on keeping the person's symptoms from worsening and keeping the person as independent as possible for as long as possible.

Medications
There are three different types of medications that are approved for the treatment of the cognitive symptoms of Alzheimer's disease.

Cholinesterase inhibitors These medications, such as donepezil, rivastigmine and galantamine, can slow the progression of cognitive decline for a limited amount of time in people with mild, moderate and severe Alzheimer's disease. Cholinesterase inhibitors also help alleviate cognitive symptoms in people with Lewy body dementia.

Memantine This drug is used for people who are in the more moderate to severe stages of Alzheimer's disease. Memantine works by decreasing overstimulation of nerve cells, which can lead to damage.

Aducanumab When used in the earliest phases of Alzheimer's disease, this recently approved drug may help slow the disease process by removing beta-amyloid plaques.

Management of vascular changes

The management of vascular dementia is focused on slowing vascular changes in the brain through the steady management of high blood pressure, diabetes and cholesterol levels, as well as by taking steps to prevent stroke.

Management of behavioral symptoms

Often it's the behavioral symptoms that are the most disruptive and upsetting to both the person with dementia and the caregiver. Behavioral symptoms include agitation, anxiety, depression, irritability, delusions, hallucinations, and sleep and appetite changes. Such behavioral symptoms are associated with a faster progression of disease and increase the likelihood that the person will need to be placed in a long-term care facility.

Despite the advertisements and marketing claims of numerous vitamins, supplements and other pharmaceuticals, there are currently no approved medications that specifically target behavioral symptoms. Nevertheless, psychiatric medications, particularly antidepressants, may be very helpful in easing depression, anxiety or agitation. When symptoms of agitation and psychosis — such as seeing, hearing or believing things that are not real — are severe, other psychiatric medications, such as sedatives or antipsychotics, may be necessary. These last drugs should only be used with extreme caution, however, as they can lead to increased risks of falls, strokes and death in people with dementia.

Behavioral management with proper daily structure and the use of adult day care centers can be very beneficial. As the disease progresses, it is important to keep the person with dementia as active — and interactive — as possible. Home care or placement in a long-term care facility may be necessary when loved ones can no longer provide care. When Alzheimer's is diagnosed at an early stage, the person with the diagnosis can have an active say in discussions regarding future medical, financial and functional issues, including questions about when to stop driving.

WHY DOES DEMENTIA MATTER TO WOMEN?

Dementia is more common in women than in men — women with dementia outnumber men two to one. Although women are more likely to live longer than men, this alone does not fully explain why the number of cases seen in women is greater. Brain scans show that brain cells die at a faster rate in women than in men as they age. However, as in other illnesses, neurological diseases such as dementia have not been as well-studied in female animals as they have been in male animals. Animal studies are often the initial step in understanding brain conditions and finding effective treatments to manage these conditions.

Current research shows that the production of estrogen appears to be protective against Alzheimer's. It is believed that after menopause, the marked drop in estrogen production in women's bodies may be a significant risk factor for developing dementia later in life. Thus, women who experience early menstruation and later menopause may be at lower risk because they've been exposed to estrogen longer. Hormonal replacement therapy (HRT) used to be more commonly prescribed for women and was seen as a potential way to protect against dementia. However, the data is mixed, with some studies suggesting HRT decreases the risk of Alzheimer's disease and others saying that it increases the risk. Overall, any potential benefit provided by long-term use of HRT after menopause in reducing Alzheimer's disease does not outweigh the added risks of other conditions, such as cancer, stroke and cardiovascular disease. Thus, this strategy is prescribed less commonly now.

Dementia care providers

Most care providers for people living with dementia are women. They are typically family members, such as wives or daughters, who are often caring for their own children and working outside the home in addition to caring for a loved one with dementia. Caregivers frequently support people living with dementia without any financial compensation or aid. Compared with male caregivers, female caregivers tend to spend more time in the role and are more likely to experience stress and depression.

As symptoms of dementia progress over time, the demands of caregiving increase and, eventually, care may be required around the clock. To make informed, workable decisions regarding how to support their loved ones, it's important for caregivers to know about the declining future course of dementia, including financial and legal issues that arise as the cognitive impairment worsens. Caregivers themselves often need support to prevent the burden of caregiving from negatively impacting their own physical and mental health.

QUESTIONS TO ASK YOUR HEALTH CARE TEAM ABOUT DEMENTIA

For all family members

- What is the cause of the dementia?
- What lifestyle changes can help decrease the risk of dementia?
- Is the diagnosis Alzheimer's disease or dementia? What is the difference?
- What stage is the dementia?
- What resources are available to help with caregiving?
- How quickly do symptoms tend to progress?
- How long can my loved one remain living at home?

For the person with early-stage dementia

- Is there any medication that will help me?
- What symptoms can I expect as the disease progresses over time?
- What are the chances that my relatives will get dementia?
- Are the advertised supplements and programs that are promoted as a cure for dementia useful?

PEARLS OF WISDOM

Dementia is typically a progressive and debilitating illness that disproportionately affects older adults, particularly women. Most cases of dementia are caused by neurological disorders such as Alzheimer's disease, which is by far the most common cause of dementia.

When symptoms occur, such as forgetfulness and memory loss, it is important to undergo an evaluation in a timely manner. Although there is no cure for these illnesses, management with medications and behavioral interventions can improve distressing symptoms.

People who provide care for loved ones with dementia are most likely to be women, who often have little support. These caregivers are at risk of developing harmful stress levels and depression that could affect their day-to-day functioning and ability to care for their loved ones. For caregivers, reaching out and obtaining needed education and support is essential in assisting those with dementia.

"Female patients have unique mental health needs based on their biology, life cycle, and psychosocial stressors, and this requires a different approach to psychiatric history, diagnosis, and treatment."

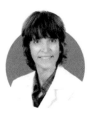

Zelde Espinel, M.D., M.A., M.P.H. - she/her
Dr. Espinel is Assistant Professor in the Department of Psychiatry and Behavioral Sciences at the University of Miami, Miller School of Medicine. She is a psychiatrist based at Sylvester Comprehensive Cancer Center. She specialized in geriatric and consultation liaison psychiatry.

"Women are essential to improved health outcomes. They not only come to us as patients, but they also make up the majority of care providers assisting and advocating for those who are elderly and chronically ill."

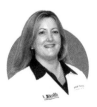

Elizabeth A. Crocco, M.D. - she/her
Dr. Crocco is the Medical Director of the Center for Cognitive Neuroscience & Aging, and Professor and Chief of the Division of Geriatric Psychiatry in the Department of Psychiatry and Behavioral Sciences at the University of Miami Miller School of Medicine.

24

Depression

Jennalee S. Wooldridge, Ph.D., and Kanwal L. Haq, M.S.

WHAT IS DEPRESSION?

Depression, also known as clinical depression or major depressive disorder, is a mood disorder that affects how you feel, think and act. It also impacts your ability to function and perform daily activities, such as sleeping, eating or working.

Depression is common. It impacts 1 in 15 adults in any given year, and 1 in 6 people will experience depression at some time in their lives. Depression can begin at any time, but it tends to first appear during the late teens to mid-20s.

Depression can show up in different ways, in mental and emotional ways as well as not-so-obvious physical ways. In addition to feelings of sadness, for example, depression can increase feelings of physical pain, including headaches, back pain and abdominal pain.

Someone with depression will experience some of following symptoms for at least a two-week period:
- Feelings of sadness, emptiness or hopelessness most of the day
- Loss of interest or pleasure in activities once enjoyed
- Changes in appetite

- Weight loss or weight gain unrelated to dieting
- Changes in sleep, such as trouble sleeping or sleeping too much
- Increase in purposeless physical activity, such as handwringing or pacing
- Slowed movements and speech, noticed by others
- Loss of energy or increased fatigue
- Feelings of worthlessness, guilt or self-loathing
- Difficulty thinking, concentrating or making decisions
- Thoughts of death or suicide

Because of the complex biological system that is responsible for a person's moods, perceptions and experience of life, depression can look very different from one person to another. There are many chemicals inside the brain that can interact with each other and with other substances in millions of different ways that impact a person's mood. Thus, while two people may have very similar outward symptoms of depression, they could have very different chemical changes going on inside their brains. This is why it can take some time to figure out which treatment is best for each person.

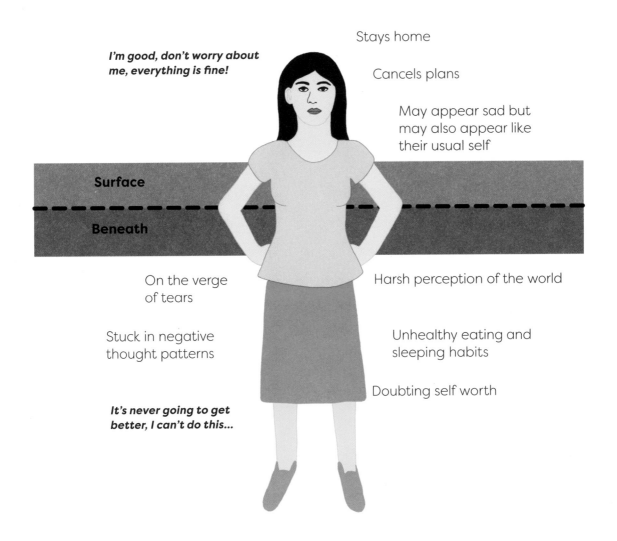

Stays home

Cancels plans

May appear sad but may also appear like their usual self

I'm good, don't worry about me, everything is fine!

Surface

Beneath

On the verge of tears

Harsh perception of the world

Stuck in negative thought patterns

Unhealthy eating and sleeping habits

Doubting self worth

It's never going to get better, I can't do this...

The chemicals inside the brain act as little messengers, called neurotransmitters, that carry messages to different parts of the brain and body. When these messengers can't get to where they need to go and their path is disrupted, depression can result. When enough neurotransmitters (the triangles and circles in the image on page 148) are being released, most people are able to go about their daily lives without too much difficulty. If only a few neurotransmitters are present, the neurotransmitters have to work much harder and can't always make the right connections, resulting in feelings of "being depressed." Low levels of neurotransmitters can also impact other parts of the body and cause a range of problems, including chronic pain, stomach issues, inflammation, loss of sexual desire and increased risk of heart disease.

Normal **Depression**

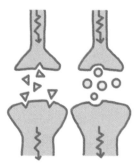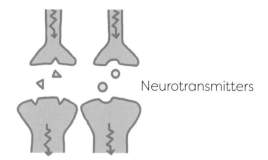

Neurotransmitters

Fewer neurotransmitters in the brain can contribute to depression.

CAN DEPRESSION BE PREVENTED?

Depression can't always be prevented, but there are ways to reduce your risk of depression. Current research suggests that there are many factors that make people more likely to experience depression. The most common risk factors are genetics, chronic health conditions, major life changes and a history of trauma or stressful experiences. Other factors also play a role, including your personality, your social support networks and your environment (such as how much sunlight you get).

While many risk factors are outside of your control, there are some factors you can work on to help prevent depression.

Proper sleep
Poor sleep can make depression worse, and depression can disrupt sleep. Keeping a regular sleep schedule and maintaining healthy sleep habits can help you break that cycle.

Physical activity and exercise
Even small amounts of regular physical activity and exercise can promote healthy changes in the brain that help improve your mood and your body's responses to stress.

Healthy diet
People who eat a lot of fruits and vegetables are less likely to be depressed. On the other hand, people whose diets contain a lot of processed meats, sugar and fried food are more likely to be depressed.

Thoughtful consumption of alcohol
Many people use a glass of wine or a cocktail to unwind and sometimes to cope with symptoms of depression. However, drinking alcohol can lead to depression and make symptoms of depression worse because alcohol belongs to a group of drugs known as depressants. Most health experts recommend that women limit alcohol to one serving a day, if any. If you are at risk of depression or are having symptoms of depression, you may want to avoid alcohol altogether.

Mindfulness meditation
This is a mind-body practice that focuses on being more aware of experiences in the

present moment and less distracted by your thoughts and what is happening around you.

Social support

There are a lot of benefits to having friends and family who can help you when you're facing a difficult situation. It's good to reach out when you need help or someone to talk with.

Proactive prevention

You don't have to wait for depression to become severe to get help. If you are experiencing even mild symptoms of depression or are at risk of depression — because you've just had a baby, for example, or you have a personal or family history of depression — consider asking your clinician about depression prevention. For example, attending a cognitive behavioral-based depression support group can help you learn skills for coping with depression and staying engaged in life.

Complementary and alternative practices

Researchers continue to investigate alternative and complementary practices (such as acupuncture and herbal remedies) for depression. Often these practices can be combined with other depression prevention and treatment approaches to enhance your well-being. Be aware, however, that alternative and complementary practices can have negative interactions with certain medications you may be taking. For example, some vitamins and supplements can interact with prescription medications. Before trying any new approach or practice, always first discuss it with your clinician.

HOW IS DEPRESSION TREATED?

Successful treatment of depression depends on an accurate diagnosis. Before recommending treatment, your clinician will conduct an evaluation that identifies the specific symptoms you are experiencing, your medical and family history, and relevant cultural and environmental factors. A comprehensive evaluation typically includes a screening questionnaire, a physical examination and a blood test to rule out other underlying conditions. You may be referred to an appropriate mental health professional — such as a psychologist, psychiatrist, psychiatric nurse practitioner, clinical social worker or licensed counselor — for a more detailed evaluation that can help identify the best treatment options for you.

Treatment options include the following.

Exercise

Among non-medical treatments for depression, exercise has one of the broadest bases of scientific support. Many experts recommend adding exercise, even in small doses, to treatment plans for depression.

Psychotherapy

Administered by a licensed professional, psychotherapy, — also known as talk therapy — helps you learn skills for managing depression and engaging in meaningful activities. Significant improvement through talk therapy can be made in 10 to 15 sessions. There are several types of talk therapy but one of the most common is cognitive behavioral therapy (CBT), which helps you become more actively involved in life as well as recognize and modify negative thought patterns. Other types of talk therapy that can help with depression are mindfulness-based cognitive behavioral therapy (MBCT), acceptance and commitment therapy (ACT) and interpersonal psychotherapy (IPT). It is important to work with a psychotherapist you feel comfortable with, and it is completely OK to try more than one therapist until you find the right fit. Talk therapy is typically used alone for mild depression and can be used alongside medications for moderate to severe depression.

Medications

Since brain chemistry can contribute to depression, that factor might also need to be addressed during treatment. The medications for depression, called antidepressants, can help release the right amount of neurotransmitters in your brain to restore healthy brain chemistry. Antidepressants are not addictive. They are also not sedatives, tranquilizers or "uppers." In fact, antidepressants do not have any type of stimulating effect on people who are not experiencing depression. Their whole purpose is to restore balance to the brain. Antidepressants may provide some improvement to mood within two weeks, but usually their full benefits are not seen for about two months.

Because there are many different types of neurotransmitters and five major types of antidepressants (selective serotonin reuptake inhibitors, serotonin and norepinephrine reuptake inhibitors, atypical antidepressants, tricyclic antidepressants, and monoamine oxidase inhibitors), it may take some trial and error to find the right medication and dosage that works for you.

Medication and talk therapy together can be a highly effective way to treat depression, especially when symptoms are severe or certain symptoms, such as suicidal thoughts, hopelessness or a marked inability to feel pleasure, are present.

Electroconvulsive therapy (ECT)

Some people with severe depression may not respond to talk therapy and medications. They may benefit from ECT. ECT is a safe treatment that delivers a small amount of electricity through the brain. This electrical current causes chemical changes in the brain that can help reduce symptoms of depression. Most people need 6 to 12 treatments but frequently start experiencing the benefits after a few sessions. ECT is less scary than it is often portrayed in movies. The procedure only takes about 5 to 10 minutes and does not require staying in a hospital.

WHY DOES DEPRESSION MATTER TO WOMEN?

Research shows that women are more likely than men to experience depression, with some studies showing that 1 in 3 women will experience a major depressive episode in their lifetimes. Women are more prone to seasonal depression, and they are more prone to depression during reproductive years. It is also more common for women than men to experience physical symptoms of depression, such as changes in appetite, sleep and fatigue.

The exact reasons for these differences are unclear, but the interactions between biological sex differences, life circumstances and culture are known contributors. Unequal power and status, work overload and higher rates of physical and sexual abuse may make depression more common in women. The good news is that even though depression is more common in women, women and men seem to benefit equally from treatments for depression, such as psychotherapy and medication.

QUESTIONS TO ASK YOUR HEALTH CARE TEAM ABOUT DEPRESSION

- Do you think I need medications for my depression and why?
  › What type of antidepressant do you recommend and why?
  › What should I expect when I start this type of medication?
  › How long does the medication take to improve depression symptoms?
  › What side effects should I expect from the medication I've been prescribed?
  › Will this medication affect my daily functioning, such as my sex life, sleep, appetite or weight?
  › What can I do to ease the side effects of this medication?
- What depression treatments are available that don't include antidepressant medications?
  › Should I see a therapist as part of my depression treatment?
  › What type of psychotherapy do you recommend?
  › Do you have referrals for psychotherapists that take my insurance?
- Do any of my depression symptoms need special treatment?

- › Should another type of health specialist be involved in my care?
  › Do I need to get blood tests or any other tests done?
  › Could other health conditions be contributing to my symptoms of depression?
  › Could my depression be causing me physical pain?
- What else should I do to relieve my depression and keep it from coming back?
  › What kinds of behavioral changes will help with my symptoms of depression?
- Should I (or a member of my family) alert you if there are any changes in my behavior?
  › What should I do if I am in a crisis or an emergency, or if I feel suicidal?

If you are ever in danger of hurting yourself, you — and your family — need to know what steps to take. Some resources include:

- › National Suicide Prevention Lifeline **1-800-273-8255**
- › Veteran and Military Crisis Line **1-800-273-8255**
- › Crisis Text Line **www.crisistextline.org**

PEARLS OF WISDOM

Depression is very treatable, and there are lots of treatment options available. But treating depression can involve some trial and error, and it's common to try multiple psychotherapists and medications before finding the right fit for you.

In addition to receiving treatment for depression, you may benefit from treatments for other conditions that commonly occur alongside depression. For women, anxiety often accompanies depression. Having difficulty sleeping is also common in women with depression. These conditions can and should be treated as well.

While depression can make even small things feel difficult, many people feel better after taking action — whether that's getting outside for a walk, calling a friend or scheduling a first therapy appointment — even if they don't feel like taking action at first. It is possible to stop struggling with depression and to live a full and meaningful life.

"Mental health is health."

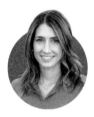

Jennalee S. Wooldridge, Ph.D. - she/her
Dr. Wooldridge is a Clinical Psychologist at VA San Diego Healthcare System in San Diego, California, and Clinical Assistant Professor at University of California San Diego. She specializes in behavioral medicine, particularly the behavioral and emotional factors associated with chronic health conditions.

"Whether an illness affects your heart, your leg or your brain, it's still an illness, and there should be no distinction."
– Michelle Obama

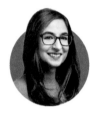

Kanwal L. Haq, M.S. - she/her
Kanwal is a medical anthropologist passionate about creating more connected, more informed, and more equitable systems of care. She specializes in community-based participatory research and builds accessible tools, resources, and programs for women around the globe. Kanwal currently leads the NYC women's health programs at the Arnhold Institute for Global Health at Mount Sinai's Icahn School of Medicine.

25
Diabetes

Samar Hafida, M.D., and Sarah Knapp, M.D.

WHAT IS DIABETES?

Diabetes is a disease that develops when your body is unable to process food for energy in an appropriate manner. It is a complex medical condition that results in high blood sugar. This happens because the carbohydrates that you eat — foods that contain sugar, fiber and starches — are not properly converted to fuel.

To understand diabetes, it is important to know how carbohydrate metabolism works. Insulin, a hormone made by the pancreas, is the most important player in carbohydrate metabolism. As you digest food, the carbohydrates and sugars you eat are broken down into a sugar known as glucose. Glucose is absorbed from the gut and used for energy in cells everywhere in your body. However, sugar can't get into cells without the help of insulin. Think of insulin as a key that opens the door for sugar to get inside cells. If your body can't make insulin, or isn't able to use it properly, then sugar will be stuck in the bloodstream. The result is high blood sugar — also known as high blood glucose or hyperglycemia — which is the hallmark of diabetes.

There are several types of diabetes.

Type 1 diabetes

About 5% to 10% of people living with diabetes have type 1 diabetes, a condition in which the pancreas stops making insulin altogether. This happens because the immune system attacks and destroys cells in the pancreas that produce insulin. People with type 1 diabetes often develop this disease when they are children or adolescents. However, anyone at any age can develop type 1 diabetes.

Type 2 diabetes

About 90% to 95% of people living with diabetes have type 2 diabetes. This type of diabetes mostly happens because your body isn't able to use the insulin it makes. This is often referred to as insulin resistance and is linked to weight gain, especially in the belly area. Other risk factors that may increase your chances of developing type 2 diabetes are:

- A family history of diabetes
- Belonging to certain ethnic and racial groups including African Americans, Latinos, Native Americans, Asian Americans and Pacific Islanders
- Having high blood pressure
- Having high cholesterol

- Leading an inactive lifestyle
- Being older than 45
- Having developed diabetes during pregnancy (gestational diabetes)
- Having polycystic ovary syndrome

Gestational diabetes

Some women who have never had diabetes before may develop this type of diabetes during pregnancy. This is because hormone changes that happen during pregnancy can cause the body to become insulin resistant. Although this is a temporary type of diabetes that usually goes away after delivery, women who get gestational diabetes have a high risk of getting type 2 diabetes later in life.

CAN DIABETES BE PREVENTED?

Prevention of diabetes depends on what type of diabetes a person has. So far, there is no evidence that type 1 diabetes can be prevented. However, type 2 diabetes can be prevented or slowed down, and with the right steps, diabetes-related complications can almost always be avoided. Type 2

Glucose production and absorption

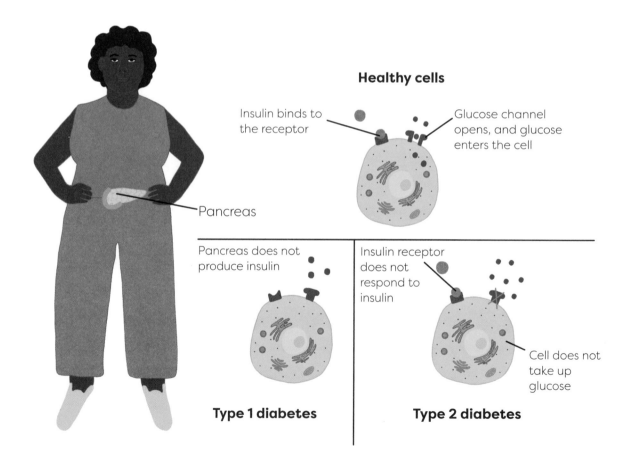

Healthy cells

Insulin binds to the receptor

Glucose channel opens, and glucose enters the cell

Pancreas

Pancreas does not produce insulin

Insulin receptor does not respond to insulin

Cell does not take up glucose

Type 1 diabetes

Type 2 diabetes

diabetes is a slowly progressive disease that takes many years to fully develop. The stage before diabetes is called prediabetes, in which insulin resistance first shows up as mild irregularities in blood sugar levels, but these sugars don't rise enough to make the cutoff points that doctors use to diagnose type 2 diabetes. During both the prediabetes stage and the early stages of type 2 diabetes, it is possible to reverse the course of disease. With the following measures, you can stop diabetes.

Nutrition

By making simple changes to the way you eat — for example, avoiding foods and drinks with added sugar, ultraprocessed foods, and foods that are high in starches — you can lower your risk for developing type 2 diabetes. There are many "diets" or eating patterns that claim to be the best for people with diabetes. In reality — whether it's a Mediterranean, a low-carb or even a plant-based diet — all of these have similar benefits in lowering the risk of diabetes and improving blood sugars. Whatever changes you decide to make to your eating patterns, they must be practical, sustainable, based on your preference and culture, and most of all, enjoyable.

Physical activity

Moderate physical activity, such as brisk walking, swimming, dancing or even yardwork, has been shown to prevent or delay the onset of type 2 diabetes. You can lower your risk of getting type 2 diabetes and lower blood sugar levels by making sure to avoid periods of prolonged sitting and by exercising for at least 150 minutes a week — about 30 minutes a day.

Healthy body weight

Maintaining a healthy body weight is one of the most powerful actions you can take to prevent diabetes. A healthy body weight can reduce your risk of diabetes by 58%. Lifestyle changes, which include adopting healthy eating patterns, increasing physical activity, getting enough sleep and addressing mental health stressors, are the foundation of weight loss. Medical and surgical weight loss options are also important and very effective ways to help you lose weight, and thus, prevent diabetes.

HOW IS DIABETES TREATED?

Treatment of diabetes starts with diagnosis and understanding what your blood sugar numbers should be. Your doctor may order a lab test called hemoglobin A1C, or A1C for short. This test tells your doctor your average blood sugar over the past three months. An A1C of 6.5% or higher means you have diabetes.

Because the underlying cause of type 1 is different from that of type 2 diabetes, it is treated differently. Type 1 diabetes is treated only with insulin, given either through many injections per day under the skin, or in some cases, an insulin pump.

The foundation of type 2 diabetes treatment is lifestyle changes that help with weight loss. In addition, your doctor may prescribe medications that work in different ways. If you are treated with medication, your doctor will tell you what your target A1C should be. Some medicines help your body become more sensitive to its own insulin, some help you make more insulin, some eliminate sugar from your body, and some lessen the absorption of sugar from the gut. The type of medicine your doctor prescribes depends on how high your blood sugars are and whether you have or are at high risk of kidney or heart disease.

Sometimes, people living with type 2 diabetes have very high blood sugars or have had diabetes for many years and need insulin. This does not mean type 2 diabetes turns into type 1 diabetes — it just means your diabetes may be difficult to manage with noninsulin medications.

Primary care doctors are skilled at taking care of people living with type 2 diabetes, but some people with diabetes may need to see a diabetes specialist called an endocrinologist. People living with diabetes should also meet with a diabetes educator, also referred to as a certified diabetes care and education specialist, when first diagnosed and periodically throughout their care.

Your blood sugar goals will depend on many things including your age, whether you are pregnant, what type of diabetes you have, what medications you take and your general lifestyle. Managing diabetes includes treatments designed to lower blood sugar and manage risk factors such as high blood pressure, high cholesterol, and overweight and obesity.

If diabetes is not treated in a timely or effective way and your blood sugar stays high, over time this may damage your nerves (neuropathy), eyes (retinopathy), kidneys (nephropathy), heart, large blood vessels and brain. Damage to these vital organs may result in foot pain, ulcers, deformities, vision loss, kidney failure needing dialysis, heart attacks and strokes.

Additional problems resulting from diabetes are preventable with self-care and regular follow up with your medical team. Monitoring and recording your blood sugar are important ways to know if your lifestyle changes and treatment are working.

Lowering blood sugar with lifestyle changes and medication is not the only goal of diabetes management. It is important for people living with both type 1 and type 2 diabetes to also treat additional risk factors that may worsen the complications mentioned earlier. This can be achieved by:
- Managing blood pressure and high cholesterol
- Keeping body weight in a healthy range
- Addressing mental health issues
- Avoiding tobacco

In addition, you should plan to have:
- Yearly eye doctor visits
- Regular blood tests
- Regular urine tests
- Regular cholesterol level checks
- Visits with a foot doctor (podiatrist) to monitor your feet for neuropathy and get counsel on foot care.

WHY DOES DIABETES MATTER TO WOMEN?

Diabetes matters for women because 16 million women in the U.S. are living with diabetes as of 2018. Women with diabetes often have more to manage because they typically carry the responsibilities of caring for their families, communities and careers all while managing the complex demands of diabetes. Some of the factors relevant to women living with diabetes include these:

- Compared with men, women with diabetes are at a higher risk of having a heart attack or a stroke. This may result in serious medical complications and even premature death.
- Women living with diabetes experience mood disorders, such as depression, twice as often as men do, which can have a serious impact on their ability to care for themselves.
- Eating disorders are twice as common in women with diabetes compared with women without diabetes, and studies suggest this complication is often overlooked by their health care team.
- Women living with diabetes are also at higher risk of having urinary tract infections and genital yeast infections than women without diabetes are.
- During a woman's pregnancy, having diabetes can put both the mother and her baby at risk for severe complications. After delivery, about half of women with gestational diabetes will develop type 2 diabetes in the next ten years. If you've had gestational diabetes, work with your doctor to monitor your blood sugar closely — at least every year — for signs of diabetes after you give birth.
- Women are vulnerable to feeling shame because of the stigma associated with having diabetes or with being over-weight. Feeling embarrassed about diabetes or obesity may become a barrier that prevents women from trusting their health care team or being comfortable discussing important topics with them.

QUESTIONS TO ASK YOUR HEALTH CARE TEAM ABOUT DIABETES

- Can I reverse diabetes?
  - › If so, how?
- How can you support me in making changes to my diet and daily activities, with the goal of losing a modest amount of weight?
  - › Should I see a dietitian?
- Can I meet with a diabetes educator who can provide more details about my condition?
- Do I need to start a medication to help manage my blood sugar?
  - › Which is the one best for me?
  - › What are the benefits and what are the risks of these medications?
- What are my goals for A1C, blood sugars, blood pressure and cholesterol levels?
- When is it safe to become pregnant?
  - › Do I need birth control?
- I had gestational diabetes; how are we monitoring for diabetes now?
  - › How are we going to prevent the onset of type 2 diabetes?
- Do I need to see an endocrinologist? Or other specialists such as an eye, kidney or heart specialist?

PEARLS OF WISDOM

Diabetes affects the lives of many women worldwide. Although women may experience higher rates of complications than men do, it is a very manageable condition. By learning about this disease and asking the right questions, you can be an active part of your health care team. If you have diabetes, it is important to not feel shame, to speak up for yourself and to ask for help when you need it. Remember, diabetes does not define you — you are in control!

"Supporting the health and well-being of women is essential to the health and well-being of our society and future generations. It's time women take the lead on their self-care and be taken seriously by health care providers."

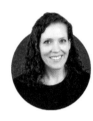

Sarah Knapp, M.D. - she/her

Dr. Knapp is an endocrinologist at the Joslin Diabetes Center and Beth Israel Deaconess Medical Center, and an Instructor in Medicine at Harvard Medical School in Boston, Massachusetts.

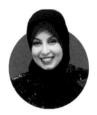

Samar Hafida, M.D. - she/her

Dr. Hafida is an endocrinologist and Instructor in Medicine at Harvard School of Medicine. She specializes in diabetes and medical weight management.

26
Diverticulitis

Riann B. Robbins, M.D., and Jessica N. Cohan, M.D., M.A.S., FACS

WHAT IS DIVERTICULITIS?

Diverticulitis is the inflammation or infection of small, balloon-like pouches that can form in the large intestine (colon). These pouches, called diverticula, develop when the inner lining of the colon pushes out through the outer wall. Diverticula may form when high pressure within the colon strains the colon wall. Diverticula can occur anywhere in the colon, but in the United States the most common location is on the left side (sigmoid colon and descending colon).

The presence of diverticula in the colon is called diverticulosis, a very common condition. The chances of developing diverticulosis increases with age, occurring in approximately half of people over age 60, and two-thirds of people over the age of 80. Most people with diverticulosis do not have any symptoms.

Diverticulosis can lead to diverticulitis if one or more diverticula become infected or inflamed. Clinicians often divide diverticulitis into two categories: uncomplicated and complicated.

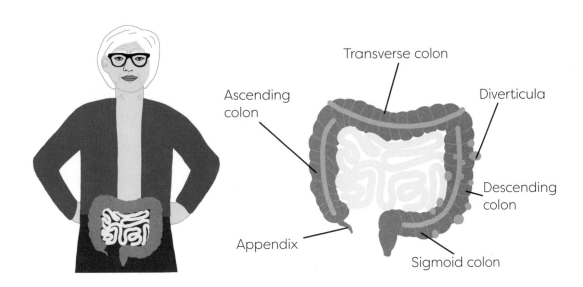

- **Uncomplicated diverticulitis** is an infection and inflammation located within the colon.
- **Complicated diverticulitis** occurs when the infection or inflammation causes a more severe problem, such as:
    › A serious infection in the abdomen (abscess)
    › A blockage of the intestine (bowel obstruction)
    › A hole in the colon (perforation)
    › An abnormal passageway (fistula) between sections of bowel or the bowel and other organs, such as the bladder, vagina, uterus, and other parts of the intestine or the skin.

Symptoms of diverticulitis depend on the severity and complications of the disease. Mild diverticulitis usually causes abdominal pain in the lower left part of the belly, although the pain can occur in other areas. Other common symptoms include low-grade fever, decreased appetite, nausea or change in bowel movement patterns (for example, from constipation to diarrhea).

Moderate or severe cases of diverticulitis will develop more significant symptoms, such as unmanageable pain, high fevers or inability to stay hydrated. Moderate cases of diverticulitis may also lead to one or more problems related to complicated diverticulitis.

In order to make a diagnosis, a clinician will perform an examination and may use blood tests, a CT scan or both. A few other diseases can cause symptoms similar to those of diverticulitis, including colorectal cancer, Crohn's disease and poor blood flow in the colon (ischemic colitis). These other diseases are relatively rare in people who have been diagnosed with diverticulitis, but your clinician may recommend a colonoscopy to rule out additional causes of your symptoms, especially if you're due for a colonoscopy.

CAN DIVERTICULITIS BE PREVENTED?

In the past, experts believed certain types of foods caused diverticula. More recent research has shown that a combination of factors likely increases the risk of developing diverticulitis. These include your family history, immune system, gut bacteria (microbiome), environmental exposures, diet, and exercise.

Diet and exercise

Healthy foods such as nuts, grains, corn and popcorn were once believed to cause diverticulitis by blocking the diverticula. However, research has shown that these foods are safe and may even help protect your colon. In fact, a fiber-rich diet is thought to be one of the best ways to prevent both diverticulosis and diverticulitis. Research suggests that a diet that includes at least 32 grams of fiber per day reduces the risk of developing diverticulosis and diverticulitis. For example, several studies have found lower rates of diverticulitis among African and Asian populations with high-fiber diets compared with Western populations eating a low-fiber diet.

Research also shows that avoiding or limiting red meats and processed meats in your diet can reduce the risk of diverticulitis. Other important prevention strategies include exercising regularly and maintaining a healthy weight.

Smoking

Avoiding or reducing tobacco smoking may also reduce the risk of diverticulitis. In one study, women who smoked were 24% more likely to be hospitalized with complications from diverticulitis compared to women who didn't smoke. Risk is even higher among people who smoke more frequently and for longer periods in their lives. In contrast, alcohol and coffee consumption do not appear to increase the risk of developing diverticulitis.

Medications

Blood pressure and cholesterol medications, such as calcium channel blockers and statins, may reduce the risk of diverticulitis.

On the other hand, medications such as aspirin and nonsteroidal anti-inflammatory drugs may increase the risk of developing diverticulitis.

HOW IS DIVERTICULITIS TREATED?

If you're diagnosed with diverticulitis, your treatment will depend on how severe your symptoms are.

Mild diverticulitis

Most cases of diverticulitis are mild. In mild cases, the pain is manageable and treatment usually consists of dietary changes. Your clinician may recommend consuming a diet based on liquids or soft, easily digestible foods until the pain improves. Although antibiotics were once the main treatment for

To prevent diverticulitis

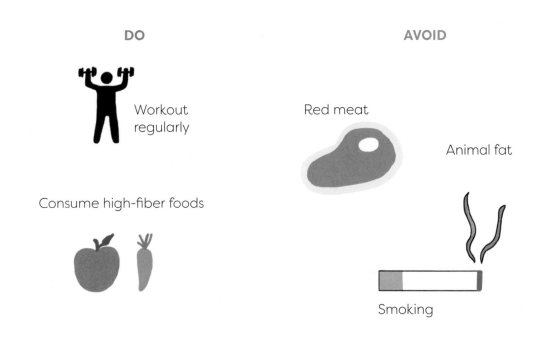

DO

Workout regularly

Consume high-fiber foods

AVOID

Red meat

Animal fat

Smoking

mild diverticulitis, recent studies have challenged the idea that antibiotics help people with mild symptoms feel better faster. However, further research about antibiotics is needed. Your clinician will discuss whether antibiotics are recommended for your condition if you develop mild diverticulitis.

Moderate to severe diverticulitis

If you experience a moderate or severe case of diverticulitis, your clinician will likely prescribe a course of antibiotics. If your symptoms don't improve after a few days, you may undergo repeat blood tests or a CT scan to determine if the disease has worsened.

Moderate or severe disease is more likely to occur in people who are older, have other medical problems, such as diabetes or cancer, or have a weakened immune system due to certain health conditions or medications. If you fall into any of these categories, your clinician may perform blood tests and CT scans to detect whether you have developed complicated diverticulitis, in which an abscess in the abdomen, blockage in the intestine, perforation of the colon or fistula is present. These complications may not be severe enough to require an emergency surgery, but may require hospitalization. During a hospitalization, a period of bowel rest may be necessary (often nothing to eat or drink by mouth). Clinicians may also prescribe IV fluids, antibiotics and pain medication.

If a severe infection leads to an abscess, your clinician may recommend a drainage procedure. In this procedure, sometimes called percutaneous drainage, a radiologist puts a tube through the skin to help drain fluid from the abscess into a collection bulb on the outside of the body. This drainage tube can stay for days or weeks depending on the severity of the infection.

After recovering from mild or moderate diverticulitis, your clinician may consider an elective surgery to remove the diseased segment of bowel. Unlike emergency surgery for severe disease, elective surgery doesn't need to be performed urgently or within a specific time period.

Elective surgery Elective surgery is considered when symptoms don't go away after being treated with medication or other less invasive procedures (such as a drain), or in people with multiple episodes of diverticulitis that require treatment. Recent medical trials show that elective surgery can improve quality of life in certain cases of diverticulitis, especially for patients with persistent or recurrent symptoms. Another reason to consider elective surgery is if the diverticulitis forms complications, such as a fistula or a bowel narrowing (stricture), which can occur later in your recovery.

Elective surgery for diverticulitis is an inpatient procedure. It is typically minimally invasive, meaning it involves small incisions. During the procedure, a surgeon removes the affected segment of the colon and reconnects the ends. In rare cases, the surgeon may attach your colon or small intestine to an opening created in your abdomen (ostomy). This allows waste to leave your body through the opening and collect into an attached bag. The opening may be permanent or temporary.

After surgery, there is still a small risk of developing diverticulitis (about 5%), but this rarely requires another surgery. Surgery does not typically cause major long-term bowel habit changes, but some people find that they have an additional bowel movement per day.

Very severe diverticulitis

The most severe complications occur when the inflammation from diverticulitis is significant. This can cause a large hole in the colon (free perforation) that leaks stool and infected material into the abdomen outside the colon. A large perforation can make people very sick and usually requires an emergency surgery. Another situation that can require emergency surgery is a bowel obstruction.

Emergency surgery Emergency surgery for diverticulitis involves removing the diseased segment of bowel. This may be done through a minimally invasive procedure or through a large incision (open surgery). In some cases, emergency surgery for diverticulitis may involve an ostomy, such as an ileostomy (small bowel ostomy) or colostomy (large bowel ostomy). Sometimes the ostomy is temporary and another surgery is performed to reverse the procedure after all the inflammation in the colon has calmed down. Rarely, the procedure cannot be reversed and becomes permanent. Even in these situations, patients are able to live relatively normal lives. Severe episodes of diverticulitis requiring emergency surgery are relatively rare, occurring in only about 1 in 20 of people with diverticulitis.

WHY DOES THE CONDITION MATTER TO WOMEN?

Generally speaking, diverticulitis is not considered to be significantly different in women compared to men. However, some studies show that diverticulitis may be more common in women as age increases. Women may also be more likely to be hospitalized.

QUESTIONS TO ASK YOUR HEALTH CARE TEAM ABOUT DIVERTICULITIS

- What are the symptoms of diverticulitis?
- What can I do to prevent diverticulitis?
- When do I need to call my doctor or go to the hospital if I think I have diverticulitis?
- Will I need surgery to treat my diverticulitis?
- Are any other tests, such as a colonoscopy, needed for my diverticulitis?

PEARLS OF WISDOM

Diverticulosis is a very common condition in the Western world that sometimes causes problems, such as diverticulitis. It can range from mild disease that is managed at home (common) to severe disease that requires hospitalization or surgery (rare). You can reduce your risk of developing diverticulitis by eating a diet high in fiber and low in red meat, avoiding smoking and exercising regularly.

"Women belong in all places where decisions are being made."

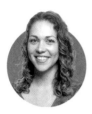

Riann B. Robbins, M.D. - she/her
Dr. Robbins is a general surgery resident at the University of Utah Health. She will complete her training in general surgery and proceed to fellowship training in surgical critical care.

"The best medical care is patient-centered care."

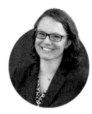

Jessica N. Cohan, M.D., M.A.S., FACS - she/her
Dr. Cohan is an Assistant Professor of Surgery at the University of Utah in Salt Lake City. Her clinical practice includes the treatment of cancers of the small bowel, colon, and rectum, as well as inflammatory bowel disease, diverticulitis, fistulas, and many other diseases of the digestive tract and anal area. She is trained in minimally invasive techniques as well as complex and revisional surgery. She specializes in colon and rectal surgery.

27
Endometrial cancer

Mona Saleh, M.D., and Leslie R. Boyd, M.D.

WHAT IS ENDOMETRIAL CANCER?

Endometrial cancer, the most common type of uterine (womb) cancer, is also the most common cancer related to the female reproductive system (gynecologic cancer) in the United States. Endometrial cancer occurs when the cells lining the inside of the uterus transform from healthy endometrial cells into cancerous cells.

Precancerous cells in the uterine lining have the potential to transform into cancerous cells. A common sign of this transformation is a change in a woman's bleeding pattern. For this reason, if you have any type of abnormal uterine bleeding, tell your doctor or gynecologist (a doctor who specializes in the female reproductive system) as soon as possible.

An abnormal uterine bleeding pattern includes postmenopausal bleeding, having more than one period per month, skipping periods, bleeding after sexual intercourse and unusually heavy vaginal bleeding. Women know their menstrual cycles. If you feel like there is a change in your bleeding pattern, make sure to see your gynecologist promptly.

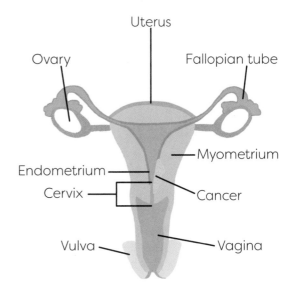

Endometrial cancer occurs more often with age. Most women are diagnosed in their 60s or later. Bleeding after menopause (postmenopausal bleeding) is the most common early sign of endometrial cancer. However, 25% of endometrial cancers are diagnosed in younger women who have not yet experienced menopause. Whatever your age, it's important to bring any change in vaginal bleeding patterns to the attention of a gynecologist.

Other symptoms of endometrial cancer, and of gynecologic cancers in general, include unintentional or unexplained weight loss, nausea, vomiting, feeling full quickly or having decreased appetite, abdominal pain, and a change in urination or bowel habits. In more advanced stages of endometrial cancer, women may feel a mass in their abdomen.

It is critical to have a relationship with a gynecologist throughout your life, even if you have never been sexually active, and even if you think you have no risk factors for endometrial cancer. Having an established relationship with a gynecologist will enable you to be seen more rapidly if you develop symptoms of endometrial cancer. If you do not have a gynecologist, bring these symptoms to the attention of your primary care clinician and request a referral to a gynecologist.

Endometrial cancer is often diagnosed by an in-office procedure called an endometrial biopsy. This involves taking cells from the uterine lining and sending them to a lab for assessment with a microscope. If you are diagnosed with endometrial cancer, your gynecologist will likely refer you to a surgeon who specializes in treating gynecologic cancers (gynecologic oncologist). When endometrial cancer is caught before it has spread outside the uterus (early-stage endometrial cancer), the overall survival rate is 80% to 90%. The more advanced the cancer is at diagnosis, the lower the rate of survival. Endometrial cancer that has spread outside of the pelvis (metastatic endometrial cancer) has a survival rate of approximately 20%.

Uterine sarcomas, a less common but more aggressive form of uterine cancer, will not be discussed in detail in this chapter.

Uterine sarcomas are rare and tend to occur in women with a history of pelvic radiation, long-term use of tamoxifen (a medication often used after breast cancer therapy) or certain hereditary syndromes. However, uterine sarcomas cause symptoms that are similar to endometrial cancer, so it's important to tell your gynecologist if you experience any of the symptoms described in this chapter.

HOW CAN ENDOMETRIAL CANCER BE PREVENTED?

Many cases of endometrial cancer can be prevented by addressing other related conditions. The most common type of endometrial cancer, for example, is related to obesity. Women with obesity experience constantly high levels of estrogen instead of the usual ebb and flow of estrogen levels throughout the menstrual cycle. These high levels of estrogen cause a buildup of endometrial tissue in the uterus, which may begin to harbor cancerous or precancerous cells. Losing weight can help bring estrogen levels back to regular patterns, thereby reducing the buildup of endometrial tissue and helping prevent the development of endometrial cancer. Even if you have been diagnosed with endometrial cancer, losing weight can help prevent a return of the cancer after treatment. Studies show that bariatric surgery can significantly decrease the risk of endometrial cancer and, in some cases, even reverse the course of the disease.

Diabetes, high blood pressure (hypertension), certain types of estrogen-only hormone replacement therapy and treatment with tamoxifen are also risk factors for the development of endometrial cancer. For many women, weight loss improves diabetes and hypertension, which will decrease endometrial cancer risk. Switching to hormone replacement therapy that contains the hormone progestin and being on the lowest effective dose possible also will decrease the risk of endometrial cancer.

A genetic disease called Lynch syndrome increases the risk of developing several cancers, including endometrial cancer. If you've been diagnosed with Lynch syndrome, work with your gynecologist to obtain endometrial biopsies every one or two years, starting at age 30 to 35, or even earlier in some cases. These biopsies can detect early precancerous changes in the uterus, and early treatment will prevent transformation into endometrial cancer.

If you have parents, siblings, children or other blood relatives who have been diagnosed with endometrial, colon or ovarian cancer, tell your gynecologist about this family history. If there is an abundance of these or other types of cancers in your family, your gynecologist may recommend that you or your relative undergo genetic testing.

HOW IS ENDOMETRIAL CANCER TREATED?

For early-stage endometrial cancer, treatment is primarily surgical, with removal of the uterus and the cervix (total hysterectomy), both Fallopian tubes and both ovaries. Your surgeon may also remove lymph nodes to see if the cancer has spread beyond the reproductive organs. Depending on the size of the uterus, the skill of the surgeon, and the capabilities of her medical center, this surgery may be done in a minimally invasive fashion with several small incisions on the abdomen, or it may be done with a larger incision requiring a longer hospital stay. A small-incision surgery is recommended for most patients. In early-stage endometrial cancer, total hysterectomy leads to a cure. For later stage or more aggressive forms of endometrial cancer, treatment may also include radiation therapy and chemotherapy.

If you want to preserve your ability to have children, a personalized treatment plan created by your health care team can help you meet your fertility goals while ensuring that your cancer is treated. If your cancer meets certain early stage criteria, you may be treated with progestin, either in oral form or through an intrauterine device (IUD). Your health care team will monitor you closely, with endometrial biopsies every three months to ensure that the cancer does not progress. Progestin therapy is also a treatment option for some people with precancerous changes in the uterus.

After treatment, even if you've been cured of endometrial cancer, you will need to see your gynecologic oncologist or gynecologist at least once a year to detect signs of cancer recurrence as early as possible.

If your doctor determines that your form of endometrial cancer may be genetic, you will likely be referred to a genetic counselor to discuss genetic testing for you as well as for other family members.

WHY DOES ENDOMETRIAL CANCER MATTER TO WOMEN?

Anyone with a uterus is at risk of developing endometrial cancer, especially in later life. Women with a uterus carry this risk even if they have had no children, have never been sexually active, are transgender or have no family history of endometrial cancer.

Endometrial cancer matters to women because it is curable when caught early. Some women may believe that after child-bearing or after menopause, there is no longer a need to see a gynecologist every year. This is not true. Having an established relationship with a gynecologist may lead to earlier identification of endometrial cancer symptoms, and earlier evaluation and referral. In fact, it's essential for all women — regardless of their status in terms of childbearing, sexual activity or menopause — to schedule an annual gynecologic visit. This is true even for women who have had their uterus removed.

Discussions of menstrual bleeding and menopause may be taboo among some groups of women. This often leads to a harmful lack of knowledge on these topics. For example, there's a common misperception that menopause has more to do with hot flashes and other symptoms than the full stop of monthly menstrual bleeding.

Some studies show that Black women may normalize abnormal bleeding patterns and may even, unfortunately, not have their symptoms taken seriously by their clinicians, which may account for later detection and a more advanced cancer at diagnosis. The fact of the matter is that topics such as menstruation and menopause are universal, and women should not be embarrassed to discuss them, least of all with their clinicians. All women should also feel empowered to seek a second opinion from another clinician if they feel that their symptoms are not being addressed or given enough attention. In the U.S., Black women are more likely to have aggressive forms of endometrial cancer and have worse outcomes with all forms of endometrial cancer, regardless of stage. For this reason, it is particularly important for Black women to seek care as soon as possible if they have symptoms of endometrial cancer.

QUESTIONS TO ASK YOUR HEALTH CARE TEAM ABOUT ENDOMETRIAL CANCER

- What are my risk factors for developing endometrial cancer?
  - › If my risk is related to being over-weight or obesity, can you refer me to a dietitian or nutritionist and a personal trainer?
  - › What are ways that I can lose weight?

For women who have been recently diagnosed with endometrial cancer
- Is my form of endometrial cancer genetic?
  - › If so, are my daughters or other female relatives at risk?
- What type of treatment do you recommend?
  - › If I need surgery, can I have a minimally invasive option?
- What if I feel depressed by the diagnosis?
  - › Can you refer me to a mental health clinician?

- › Can you refer me to support groups for women diagnosed with and undergoing treatment for endometrial cancer?
- Can you help me make a plan about how to inform my family and friends about my cancer?
- After initial treatment, what will my follow-up and surveillance be like?
  - › What are the signs or symptoms that the endometrial cancer may have returned following treatment?

For women who are diagnosed with endometrial cancer before menopause
- Will I develop any menopausal symptoms if my ovaries are removed?
  - › Are there any therapies to help decrease these symptoms?
- What are my options if I still wish to have children?

PEARLS OF WISDOM

Bleeding after menopause, even just spotting, is never normal. Be sure to see your primary care doctor or gynecologist right away if you experience this symptom.

Maintaining a healthy weight will help you prevent many types of endometrial cancer. Enlist the help of your primary care clinician to help you lose weight if you are overweight or obese. The most common form of endometrial cancer, when detected early, is curable with surgery. The sooner you seek care, the more likely you are to have an excellent outcome. Get a second opinion if you do not feel comfortable with the plan set forth by your doctor, or if you simply want a second set of eyes on your case.

Bring a trusted family member or friend to your gynecologic oncology appointments. Having someone else there with you will help you remember information and ask important questions. It's easy to feel overwhelmed during these visits; having support is critical. Even though your endometrial cancer will be treated by a gynecologic oncologist, enlist the help of your primary care clinician for ways to treat and improve conditions such as diabetes, hypertension and obesity.

"Women need to boldly, shamelessly, and selfishly advocate for themselves."

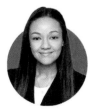

Mona Saleh, M.D. - she/her
Dr. Saleh is a gynecologic oncology fellow at the Icahn School of Medicine at Mount Sinai in New York City. She will graduate in 2024 and looks forward to providing equitable gynecologic cancer care to all women, especially to those who have been systematically disenfranchised.

"Compassion is the foundation of all healing."

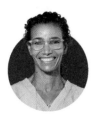

Leslie R. Boyd, M.D. - she/her
Dr. Boyd is the director of the division of Gynecologic Oncology at the NYU Grossman School of Medicine, where she is an Associate Professor of Obstetrics and Gynecology. She specializes in advanced surgery and chemotherapy for gynecologic cancers.

28
Endometriosis

Christine E. Hur, M.D., and Lisa Green, M.D., M.P.H.

WHAT IS ENDOMETRIOSIS?

Endometriosis is a chronic condition defined by the presence of endometrial tissue — the tissue that makes up the inner lining of the uterus — in an area outside of the uterus. Abnormal areas of tissue (lesions) or aggregations of cells (nodules) can lead to intense pain, particularly during menstruation, and may contribute to infertility.

Endometriosis lesions are most commonly found in the pelvis, involving the lining of the pelvis (peritoneum), the ovaries and fallopian tubes or the posterior cul-de-sac, the area behind the uterus but in front of the rectum. Less often, some women have endometriosis that involves their bowel, bladder or even diaphragm.

With each menstrual period, endometriosis lesions become stimulated by estrogen, the same hormone that stimulates the lining of the uterus. This can cause bleeding and inflammation where the endometriosis lesions are located.

Endometriosis lesions on the ovaries can cause endometriomas — dark, fluid-filled cavities, also called chocolate cysts — that destroy normal ovarian tissue and can result

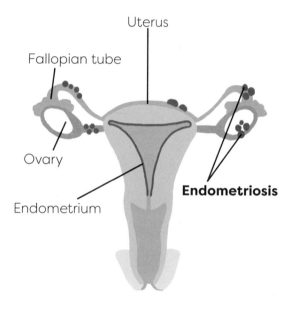

in lower quality and quantity of eggs within the ovary. Lesions on the fallopian tubes can change the fallopian tubes' normal location or block the opening of the tubes, which negatively affects their function.

Endometriosis can also contribute to adhesions, which are thick bands of fibrous tissue that can make tissues and organs stick to each other. These adhesions can lead to pain during intercourse and pain and difficulty with daily bodily functions, such as urination, depending on where the adhesions formed.

The American Society of Reproductive Medicine (ASRM) describes four stages of endometriosis, determined by the size and depth of endometriosis lesions present, as well as the severity of adhesions associated with the endometriosis.

- **Stage 1:** Minimal disease — isolated superficial lesions on the inner lining of the abdomen or pelvis without significant surrounding scarring
- **Stage 2:** Mild disease — multiple superficial lesions with no significant associated adhesions
- **Stage 3:** Moderate disease — multiple lesions that are both deep and superficial, including smaller endometriomas (cysts of endometriosis within the ovary) with associated adhesions involving the fallopian tubes, ovaries or both
- **Stage 4:** Severe disease — multiple lesions, both deep and superficial, including larger endometriomas, and more significant scar tissue involving the fallopian tubes, ovaries and posterior cul-de-sac

It is important to acknowledge that the severity of endometriosis does not always relate to the severity of symptoms. Some women with endometriosis may have no symptoms at all. Others experience a wide range of symptoms, and for some women, symptoms can be severe and life-altering.

The most common signs and symptoms of endometriosis are:
- Pain in the lower back, abdomen or pelvis during the menstrual cycle
- Pain with intercourse
- Infertility

Less common signs and symptoms may include:
- Pain or bleeding with urination Pain with bowel movements
- Nausea with menstruation
- Heavy menstrual periods
- Bleeding between periods

CAN ENDOMETRIOSIS BE PREVENTED?

Many factors involved in endometriosis are not preventable. Nonetheless, certain steps may keep it from getting worse.

Risk factors
Risk factors that may increase your risk of developing endometriosis include:
- Having a first-degree relative (mother, sister or daughter) with endometriosis
- Starting your period at an early age
- Low body mass index (BMI)
- Short menstrual cycles (lasting less than 27 days)
- Heavy menstrual periods that last longer than 7 days
- Never giving birth or giving birth for the first time after age 30
- Going through menopause at an older age
- Having an abnormal shape of the uterus or cervix
  › Risks are increased further if there is a structural cause, such as scarring (stenosis) of the cervix, preventing menstrual outflow.

Theories on how endometriosis happens
Emerging theories as to how endometrial tissue forms outside of the uterus include the following.

Retrograde menstruation This theory has the most support and is thought to account for most endometriosis cases. Retrograde menstruation is very common in women and occurs when endometrial cells are pushed through the fallopian tubes during a period instead of exiting through the cervix. In women with increased risk of endometriosis, these cells then implant in different locations within the pelvis, such as the ovary, fallopian tube, bowel or bladder, causing inflammation, scarring and pelvic pain.

Coelomic metaplasia There have been reports of endometriosis found in young girls prior to their first menstrual cycle. This hypothesis suggests that cells located within the pelvis kept their ability to become different types of tissue and changed into endometrial tissue in the wrong location.

Spread outside of the uterus by way of the lymph nodes or blood This theory is supported by the discovery of endometrial cells within the lymph nodes of women with moderate to severe endometriosis, as well as endometrial cells found in locations far from the pelvis, such as the brain and lungs.

Steps to lessening progression
While there are no known strategies to prevent endometriosis, there are ways to lessen the progression of endometriosis.

Stopping periods (suppress menses) There are multiple options to stop the menstrual cycle, including hormonal birth control methods, which include birth control pills, patches, vaginal rings and intrauterine devices (IUDs).

Exercising Exercising at least four to five hours a week helps keep body fat at a healthy level and decreases the amount of estrogen circulating through the body.

Avoiding alcohol Alcohol raises estrogen levels. Limit consumption to no more than one drink a day.

Avoiding caffeine Drinking more than one caffeinated drink a day, especially sodas and green tea, can raise estrogen levels.

HOW IS ENDOMETRIOSIS TREATED?

Endometriosis is first diagnosed through a careful medical history and physical examination. If your doctor finds a hardening beneath the uterus (cul-de-sac), an inability to move the uterus or a displaced cervix, this suggests endometriosis.

Identifying endometriosis
Methods to identify endometriosis include the following.

Endometrial biopsy A tissue sample of the lining of the uterus can be tested to see if there are findings suggestive of endometriosis, such as increased BCL6 expression. BCL6 is a protein that is found in inflamed tissue. When found within the uterus, BCL6 is highly associated with endometriosis.

Imaging studies Ultrasound is a widely available and relatively inexpensive tool used to look at the pelvis. A doctor or ultrasound technician (sonographer) who has experience with endometriosis can reliably diagnose endometriosis that involves the ovary. MRI can sometimes show evidence of endometriosis. However, MRIs are more expensive than ultrasound, and small lesions are easily missed. MRI can be more helpful in trying to identify other cysts, such as dermoid or hemorrhagic cysts.

Blood tests Many doctors and researchers have searched for a blood test to diagnose endometriosis. However, many of these tests rely on markers commonly found in other disorders. This makes it difficult to diagnose endometriosis solely on a blood test. Suggested blood tests have included CA-125 and CA 19-9.

Surgery Surgery is the gold standard for diagnosing as well as treating endometriosis. Despite this, surgery should be considered carefully for both diagnosis and treatment because it carries risks of bleeding, infection and injury to internal organs.

Treatment options

Treatments for endometriosis include these.

Surgery The goals of endometriosis surgery are to restore normal anatomy, remove or destroy all endometriosis tissue and clear adhesions and scar tissue. Again, surgery should be considered thoughtfully, as it carries risks of bleeding, infection and injury to internal organs. Surgery can often be performed laparoscopically, even in the setting of severe disease. Laparoscopic surgery is performed using a tiny camera and several small instruments, which are inserted through three to five small incisions. The benefits of this approach include decreased blood loss, lower risk of infection and shorter recovery time.

Nonsteroidal anti-inflammatory medications (NSAIDs) These are typically the first-line treatment for endometriosis, together with birth control pills that contain both estrogen and progesterone (combination oral contraceptive pills). Popular NSAIDs include ibuprofen, aspirin and naproxen.

Combination oral contraceptive pills (COCPS) COCPS are commonly used to treat endometriosis. They are often the treatment of choice for women with symptomatic endometriosis who also desire contraception to prevent pregnancy. Studies show that two-thirds of women with endometriosis have relief of symptoms with COCPs, especially when taken continuously (skipping the sugar pills).

Progestins Progestins are a synthetic form of the hormone progesterone. They treat endometriosis by preventing endometrial growth and may also cause periods to stop by preventing ovulation. Several progestins are available to effectively treat endometriosis. Progestins can be administered as an oral tablet, an intramuscular shot, an intrauterine device or an implant placed just below the skin in the upper arm.

GnRH agonists and antagonists GnRH agonists and antagonists work by causing a "pseudomenopause," a temporary state of menopause. In menopause, the ovaries do not produce the hormones needed to stimulate endometrial tissue. A state of pseudomenopause can bring relief from symptoms of endometriosis. Menopausal side effects such as hot flashes, night sweats, fatigue, headaches and changes in mood and libido may occur with the use of GnRH agonists. Bone loss is a major concern with the long-term use of GnRH agonists. If you are doing a long course of GnRH agonists or antagonists, your clinician may recommend "add-back" hormonal therapy to prevent the loss of bone density.

Aromatase inhibitors Aromatase is an enzyme that blocks the conversion of testosterone, the male hormone, to estrogen, the female hormone. Women with endometriosis have an abnormal expression of aromatase within their endometrial cells, and aromatase inhibitors can improve the symptoms of endometriosis.

Other strategies that can help you improve symptoms of endometriosis include:
- Regular exercise
- Warm baths
- Rest and use of a hot water bottle or heating pad on the abdomen
- Acupuncture
- Chiropractic therapy
- Increase in dietary fiber and antioxidants; a high-fiber diet can lower estrogen levels, and antioxidants can reduce inflammation

WHY DOES ENDOMETRIOSIS MATTER TO WOMEN?

Endometriosis is a very common chronic disease that impacts an estimated 200 million women worldwide and 6.5 million women in the U.S. Approximately 10% of reproductive-aged women have endometriosis. The true percentage is unknown because a definitive diagnosis of endometriosis requires surgery. Evidence of endometriosis can be found in 12% to 32% of women who have surgery for pelvic pain.

Between 30% and 50% of women with endometriosis experience issues with fertility. Endometriosis is the cause of chronic pelvic pain in up to half of adolescents with pelvic pain and painful periods.

The estimated global economic burden of endometriosis is $22 billion. Women with endometriosis are also more likely to be diagnosed with other conditions, such as:
- Depression
- Disorders of inflammation
  - Irritable bowel syndrome
  - Irritable bowel disease
  - Interstitial cystitis
  - Myofascial pain
- Autoimmune diseases
  - Multiple sclerosis
  - Lupus
  - Thyroid disease
  - Chronic fatigue syndrome
  - Fibromyalgia
- Increased risk of certain cancers
  - Ovarian
  - Breast
- Vulvodynia
- Asthma

QUESTIONS TO ASK YOUR HEALTH CARE TEAM ABOUT ENDOMETRIOSIS

- How will endometriosis impact my quality of life?
- How will endometriosis change as I age?

For those planning to conceive
- How will endometriosis affect my fertility?
- What steps can be taken to preserve my future fertility?

For those with painful periods, painful intercourse or chronic pelvic pain

- What treatments can help with pain?
  › What are the short- and long-term implications of each of these treatments?
- Are there other causes of pain?
  › If so, are there also treatments to target those causes?

PEARLS OF WISDOM

The way that women experience endometriosis varies widely. Keep a diary of your symptoms and how they relate to your menstrual periods. Endometriosis may only be diagnosed surgically, although often a doctor may suspect endometriosis purely based on a woman's symptoms. If you feel unheard, seek a second opinion and continue to advocate for yourself!

"As physicians and health care providers, our job is to empower women to make informed decisions regarding their health."

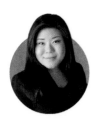

Christine E. Hur, M.D. - she/her
Dr. Hur is a current Reproductive, Endocrinology and Infertility (REI) fellow at the Cleveland Clinic in Cleveland, Ohio. She has a special interest in health literacy, endometriosis, fibroids, and polycystic ovary syndrome and the effects they have on reproduction and a woman's overall well-being.

"Your health is your most valuable possession, so entrust your care to someone who makes you feel heard and always advocate for yourself."

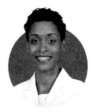

Lisa Green, M.D., M.P.H. - she/her
Dr. Green is the Assistant Program Director of the OBGYN residency program at Prisma Health in Greenville, SC. She specializes in Reproductive Endocrinology and Infertility.

29
Fibromyalgia

Carmen Gota, M.D.

WHAT IS FIBROMYALGIA?

Fibromyalgia is a chronic, stress-related condition defined by the presence of widespread body pain, fatigue, non-refreshing sleep, difficulty with memory and concentration, and increased tenderness to touch. The pain is felt in muscles, in joints or in both, and it almost always involves the lower back, upper back or both. Most people diagnosed with fibromyalgia have experienced persistent pain and other symptoms for years.

People with fibromyalgia hurt more at night and in the morning, as well as after periods of prolonged inactivity and after exercise. Some ways people with fibromyalgia describe the pain include "severe," "being hit by a truck," "stabbing," "burning," "tingling," or "feeling like someone took an ice pick to my joints." Along with pain, someone with fibromyalgia may experience:
* Morning stiffness, often lasting more than an hour
* Headaches

Tender Points

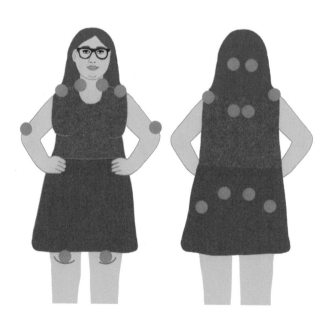

Fibromyalgia symptoms

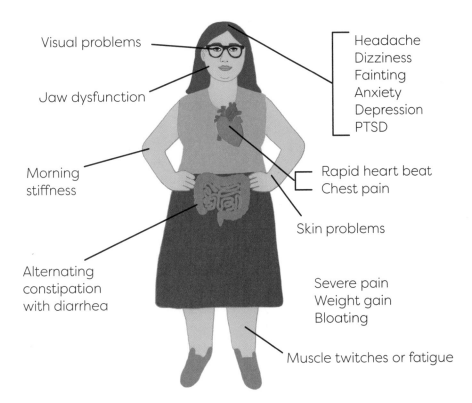

Visual problems

Jaw dysfunction

Morning stiffness

Alternating constipation with diarrhea

Headache
Dizziness
Fainting
Anxiety
Depression
PTSD

Rapid heart beat
Chest pain

Skin problems

Severe pain
Weight gain
Bloating

Muscle twitches or fatigue

- Symptoms of irritable bowel syndrome, such as alternating diarrhea with constipation, abdominal pain, bloating and heartburn
- Symptoms of autonomic dysregulation, such as dizziness, fainting and rapid heartbeat
- Depression, anxiety and or other mood disorders or post-traumatic stress disorder

Many people incorrectly believe that fibromyalgia is a catchall diagnosis that doctors make when they can't find anything else to explain a person's symptoms. In reality, fibromyalgia is a diagnosis of inclusion, not one of exclusion, meaning the diagnosis requires a person to have specific symptoms.

If you've experienced widespread pain and other common fibromyalgia symptoms for at least three months and a physical examination doesn't uncover other causes, you can be confident in a fibromyalgia diagnosis. There's no need for extensive tests — such as numerous blood tests, radiographs, CT scans or MRIs — to rule out other causes.

CAN FIBROMYALGIA BE PREVENTED?

Certain factors may increase your risk of developing fibromyalgia, including:
- Genetic factors, such as a family history of fibromyalgia

- The ability to move joints beyond the usual range of motion (hypermobility)
- Prolonged stress
- Traumatic events
- Mood disorders such as depression and anxiety
- Disorders that impair your ability to sleep
- Lack of exercise
- Maladaptive responses to pain

The good news is that a number of strategies can help reduce your chances of developing full-blown fibromyalgia, even if the condition runs in your family. These strategies include:
- Exercising regularly
- Getting enough sleep
- Managing stress

HOW IS FIBROMYALGIA TREATED?

A general principle in fibromyalgia is that "one size does not fit all." The best treatment for you may be different from the treatment needed by another person with fibromyalgia. To ensure that treatment is tailored to your needs, work with your clinician to understand the factors that impact your symptoms.

Compared with treatments for conditions such as lupus or rheumatoid arthritis, which involve taking prescription medications, the treatment for fibromyalgia is more complex. Treating the pain with the usual pain medications will not work. Opioid drugs are not recommended and can actually make the pain worse. Instead, treatment involves addressing you as a whole person in a partnership between you and your clinician. The role of your clinician is to diagnose fibromyalgia, provide information about it and about available resources, and determine if there are any symptoms that need specific treatment, such as depression and poor sleep. Your role is much more "hands on."

Be sure to read informational material your clinician gives you about fibromyalgia to better understand the condition. You may also want to seek out other reliable information about fibromyalgia and its treatment. For example, a useful website from the University of Michigan offers guidelines on how to be active, set goals and pace yourself, relax, reframe negative thoughts and communicate with others. Visit online at: **https://fibroguide.med.umich.edu.**

Educating yourself about your condition will help you better explain it to your family and friends. Pain is a subjective experience. Your loved ones may have difficulty understanding what you're feeling. When communicating with others, speak with confidence about what you are going through. It helps to think ahead of time what you want to say and to be specific about the kind of help you're asking for.

Current guidelines for the treatment of fibromyalgia highlight the role of different strategies to reduce symptoms, including:

Exercise
Exercising regularly is the staple of fibromyalgia care. Aim to do a combination of aerobic, strengthening and mind-body exercises (for example, yoga, Pilates, tai chi).

Be aware that pain and fatigue after exercise are common in people with fibromyalgia and are a major barrier for many who want to work out but find themselves achier and stiffer after trying. Ask your primary care clinician to help you develop a plan to overcome the physical limitations you may initially experience. Start slow, at a level that does not make you feel worse the next day, and gradually build from there. Try low-impact exercise to begin with, preferably in a warm pool. Starting with water-based aerobic therapy can be very helpful because the warm water can help the muscles relax. Consider using a smart watch, step tracker or a journal to help you document your daily progress.

Mental health support

Experts recommend a type of psychotherapy called cognitive behavioral therapy (CBT) for people who have fibromyalgia. Finding a clinician who has experience with CBT and with treating chronic pain can be extremely helpful.

Many people with fibromyalgia experience depression, anxiety or other emotional disorders, such as attention deficit disorder, bipolar disorder or personality disorders. If you experience significant mood disorders that impair your day-to-day life, talk to your primary care clinician about seeing a psychiatrist. A psychiatrist can help you choose an antidepressant medication as part of your initial treatment, which may help improve your mood and reduce pain.

Stress management

In people with fibromyalgia, the brain is wired in a stress mode that results in over-activation of the "fight or flight" response. This automatic stress response can increase fibromyalgia symptoms. Learning to reduce stress in your life can help you feel better. Try relaxation techniques such as meditation or deep breathing. Reduce stressors where possible. For example, avoid overly negative or stressful people or change a difficult work environment. Other stressors can't be eliminated, such as trauma you experienced in the past. Although you can't change the past, psychological interventions such as psychotherapy can help you come to terms with the trauma or help lessen its impact on your life.

Sleep management

Most people with fibromyalgia do not sleep well at night, and it is well known that sleep deprivation leads to fatigue, difficulty concentrating, worsening depression and increased pain. The first step to improving your quality of sleep is to implement good sleep hygiene. Sleep supplements such as melatonin or valerian root may also promote better sleep. If these are ineffective, drugs such as low-dose tricyclic antidepressants or trazodone have been shown to help.

Medication

The U.S. Food and Drug Administration has approved two antidepressant drugs, duloxetine and milnacipran, for the treatment of fibromyalgia. These medications work by raising the levels of two chemicals in the brain, serotonin and norepinephrine, which have a role in preventing people from feeling pain. Studies show that these drugs don't work for everybody. They may be more likely to be effective if you also have depression, anxiety or both. If these drugs aren't effective or cause side effects, your clinician may recommend other antidepressants.

Gabapentinoids are a class of medications also proven to decrease pain. Two drugs in this category, gabapentin and pregabalin, are widely used to treat chronic pain. They may also benefit sleep, so your clinician may recommend taking these drugs at bedtime.

Management of flares

Sudden flares in fibromyalgia symptoms are triggered by lack of sleep, lack of exercise, worsening stress and worsening depression and anxiety. Useful strategies include continuing to be active, learning to pace yourself and learning to relax. Another important strategy is reframing negative thoughts. A flare may make you think that your fibromyalgia will only get worse, which can make the pain itself feel worse. Learning to think in realistic terms and challenge negative thinking can help diminish pain intensity.

WHY DOES FIBROMYALGIA MATTER TO WOMEN?

Women are at greater risk of developing fibromyalgia than men. Studies show that women may be two to nine times more likely than men to experience the condition. We do not know why women are more likely than men to develop fibromyalgia, but hormonal, cultural, and genetic factors may all play a role. Women also experience more symptoms in fibromyalgia compared to men. Women with fibromyalgia have more tender points, experience more fatigue and more pain, and are more likely to have irritable bowel

syndrome. Further research is needed to determine if a person's gender impacts the ability to get better with fibromyalgia.

QUESTIONS TO ASK YOUR HEALTH CARE TEAM ABOUT FIBROMYALGIA

- What is fibromyalgia, and how can I get better?
- How should I manage a fibromyalgia flare?
- What is the most appropriate treatment for me?
- How can I exercise when I experience increased pain after exercise?
- How do I explain to my family and friends that my condition is real and not "in my head"?

PEARLS OF WISDOM

Think of fibromyalgia as a manifestation of chronic stress that expresses itself in physical symptoms. The first steps toward getting better are understanding what fibromyalgia is and accepting the diagnosis. Exercising on a regular basis, learning how to pace yourself, using relaxation techniques and reframing negative thoughts are some of the most important steps in managing fibromyalgia.

Carmen Gota, M.D. - she/her
Dr. Gota is a rheumatologist at Cleveland Clinic in Cleveland, Ohio. She specializes in fibromyalgia.

30
Gastroesophageal reflux disease

Lora Melman, M.D., FACS, FASMBS

WHAT IS GERD?

Gastroesophageal reflux disease (GERD) is a common condition that occurs when the liquid (and usually acidic) content of the stomach refluxes backward up into the esophagus, the tube connecting the mouth to the stomach. Usually when you swallow, a circular band of muscle around the bottom of your esophagus called the lower esophageal sphincter acts as a valve that opens, allowing food and liquid to flow into your stomach. The sphincter then closes again.

In order to do its job effectively, the sphincter must do two things properly:

1. It must close, and close tightly, after it has let food pass to the stomach. If the sphincter opens or relaxes when it shouldn't, stomach acid can flow back up into the esophagus. This constant backwash of acid irritates the lining of your esophagus, often causing it to become inflamed.
2. The sphincter must also remain in its proper location at the hiatus (opening) of the diaphragm. The diaphragm is the

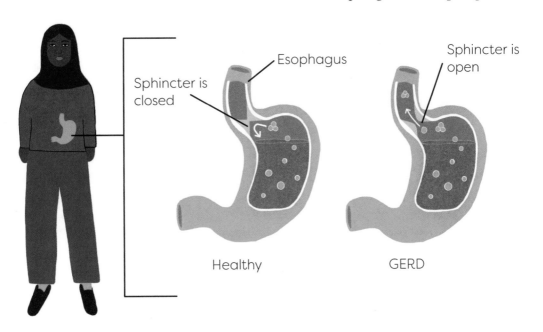

Sphincter is closed

Esophagus

Sphincter is open

Healthy

GERD

muscle that separates the chest cavity (containing the lungs) from the abdominal cavity (containing the stomach).

If the hiatal opening of the diaphragm becomes unusually enlarged, the sphincter can move out of its proper location, creating a hiatal hernia. The hernia can disrupt the function of the anti-reflux barrier, which consists of the sphincter and hiatal opening of the diaphragm. When the anti-reflux barrier no longer functions properly, stomach acid can reflux backward up past the sphincter.

The esophagus, anti-reflux barrier and stomach are like a musical trio: If all are playing their parts correctly, everything works together in harmony. But if one of them is off-tempo or playing the wrong tune, problems start to arise. In particular, the anti-reflux barrier must function in conjunction with the tightening and relaxation of the muscles in both the esophagus and stomach.

The main symptoms of GERD are typically heartburn (burning in the middle of the chest sometimes associated with a sour taste in the mouth) and regurgitation of food. People with GERD can also experience chest pain, hoarseness of voice and asthma-like symptoms from the gastric acid refluxing up to the vocal cords or into the lungs. If you experience chest pain symptoms, be sure to see your clinician right away to make sure the pain isn't being caused by heart disease or a heart attack.

GERD symptoms can also result from other conditions, including:
- **Esophageal disorders** Conditions in which the muscles of the esophagus spasm.

- **Achalasia** A condition that occurs when the lower esophageal sphincter does not open properly due to a loss of nerve cells. As a result, the sphincter doesn't open as it should when food moves down the esophagus toward the stomach, causing food to reflux back up from the esophagus.
- **Visceral hypersensitivity** A general increase of pain in the esophagus.
- **Dysfunctional anti-reflux barrier** A condition caused by a hiatal hernia and a sphincter that isn't properly functioning.
- **Gastric disorders** Conditions resulting from a slow emptying of the stomach.

Complications
GERD affects millions of people worldwide and can lead to significantly decreased quality of life, particularly through heartburn, interrupted sleep and intolerance of certain foods. If left untreated, GERD can potentially lead to:
- **Stricture** This is scar tissue that builds up and narrows the esophagus, which can cause problems with swallowing.
- **Ulcers** These painful, open sores can form in the esophagus due to the reflux of stomach acid. Ulcers can bleed, causing pain and also making swallowing difficult.
- **Esophagitis** This inflammation and irritation of the esophagus can lead to a condition called Barrett's esophagitis, in which the cells that line the esophagus become abnormal. Barrett's esophagitis can lead to esophageal cancer.

Diagnosis
Your clinician may diagnose GERD using one or more of the following methods:

Upper endoscopy An upper endoscopy is performed under sedation. Your doctor inserts a flexible camera into your mouth, guiding it down the esophagus into your stomach. This allows your doctor to detect evidence of GERD, including esophagitis and, in some cases, a hiatal hernia.

pH testing During this test, a doctor temporarily places an acid sensor near your lower esophageal sphincter. The sensor remains in place for 24 to 48 hours and records when, and for how long, stomach acid regurgitates in your stomach. During this period, you're asked to push a button every time you experience GERD symptoms. The information from this test can help your doctor determine if you have GERD, the severity of your condition and the best treatment options.

Manometry test is performed to detect how well the muscles of your esophagus constrict and relax. A doctor inserts a thin, flexible tube (catheter) with pressure sensors through your nose, down your esophagus and into your stomach. The sensors can detect if your esophageal muscles aren't functioning properly and if they're spasming or, in rare cases, if the lower esophageal sphincter isn't opening properly.

CAN GERD BE PREVENTED?

Yes, sometimes. The risk of developing GERD increases due to:
- Advancing age after the age of 50
- Obesity (a BMI greater than 30)
- Pregnancy
- Smoking

- Anxiety and depression
- Decreased physical activity

Not all causes of GERD are yet known. In some cases, people with few risk factors can still develop the condition. However, you can reduce your risk of GERD by exercising regularly, maintaining a healthy body weight and permanently stopping use of all products containing nicotine, including vaping.

Your eating habits can also help prevent GERD symptoms. Eating close to bedtime, eating large amounts of food and consuming acidic foods may trigger symptoms. For example, a big meal with tomato sauce and red wine right before bed is a classic trigger for heartburn that persists into the early morning hours, prevents a good night's rest and may even cause symptoms that last throughout the next day. Avoiding such triggers, and staying upright for at least 60 minutes after eating, can help you avoid or reduce GERD symptoms. Sleeping with your head elevated 30 degrees with a wedge pillow or sleeping in a recliner also helps reduce the amount of stomach content that can reflux up into the esophagus.

HOW IS GERD TREATED?

Most cases of GERD are caused by an anti-reflux barrier that isn't working properly and fails to prevent gastric acid from flowing up from the stomach. GERD is rarely caused by the acid itself or overproduction of stomach acid. For that reason, the goal of treating the condition is to keep acid out of the esophagus and in its proper compartment, the stomach. Treatment options include the following.

Medications

GERD is traditionally first treated with acid-reducing medications, which decrease the amount of acid made by the stomach. These medications include:

- Antacids, such as TUMS and Rolaids
- H2 receptor blockers (H2RBs), such as Pepcid or Zantac 360°
- Proton pump inhibitors (PPIs), such as Prilosec OTC and Nexium 24 HR

There are a multitude of antacids, H2RBs and PPIs available, and you can purchase many of them without a prescription. Antacids are considered the mildest medications, followed by H2RBs. Both types of medication are taken on an as-needed basis. PPIs are considered the strongest GERD medication and are designed to be used regularly instead of as needed.

It's important to notice how well the medications treat your symptoms. If heartburn symptoms are occasional, mild, and resolve with medication alone, generally you can use antacids or H2RBs as needed, and no further treatment or testing is required. If your symptoms are more severe, your doctor may recommend taking a twice-daily PPI for a period. If your symptoms do not improve enough to stop taking the medication, or if the medication stops working, your doctor may recommend other treatment options.

Surgery

In many people with GERD, the condition is caused by a structural problem, such as a hiatal hernia. If that's the case for you, your doctor may recommend surgery to correct the problem and restore the anti-reflux barrier so it can function properly.

Surgery to treat GERD is typically minimally invasive, meaning it involves small incisions. These procedures include:

- **Fundoplication** During this surgery, the upper part of the stomach is wrapped partially or fully around the sphincter to reinforce the sphincter and create less reflux.
- **LINX procedure** This procedure involves placing a magnetic beaded ring around the lower esophagus to help keep the acid from refluxing up into the rest of the esophagus. To determine if you would benefit from this procedure, your doctor may use a manometry test.

Most people do very well after these procedures and experience significant relief from their symptoms. However, some people develop ongoing dysphagia (difficulty swallowing) after surgery. Most cases of ongoing dysphagia after surgery are due to an incorrect diagnosis of GERD. For example, sometimes gallstone disease can be misdiagnosed as GERD. In such instances, surgery for GERD can lead to worsening symptoms rather than improvement. Work with your clinician to rule out other causes for your symptoms early to ensure that you receive the proper treatment.

WHY DOES GERD MATTER TO WOMEN?

GERD is more common among women. Structural changes to the anti-reflux barrier can begin during pregnancy and can lead to a higher risk of GERD as women advance past the age of 50. There is evidence that estrogen may play a role in the development of GERD, possibly due to changes that

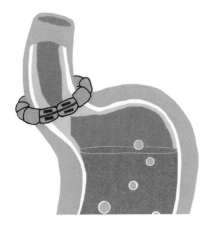

Closed Linx device

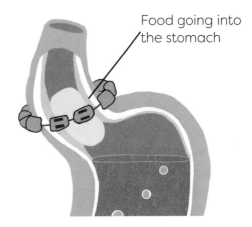

Food going into the stomach

Open Linx device

happen in the tissues of the anti-reflux barrier in response to that hormone.

In addition to being at increased risk of developing GERD, women taking PPIs for an extended period increase their risk of developing other conditions. One reason is that continuously taking PPIs can neutralize the acids in the stomach that protect the body from harmful bacteria and viruses. For example, people who continuously take PPIs are more than twice as likely to con- tract C. difficile, a bacteria that can cause a life-threatening infection in the colon.

Ongoing studies also suggest an association between long-term PPI medication use and increased risk of osteoporosis and bone fracture, as well as the development of chronic kidney disease, which further worsens osteoporosis. Thus, proper man- agement of GERD is necessary for women.

QUESTIONS TO ASK YOUR HEALTH CARE TEAM ABOUT GERD

For everyone
- What are my risk factors for GERD?

If you need help with weight loss
- Can you help me achieve a healthy weight?
- Can you refer me to someone who can help me lose weight and keep it off (nutritionist, weight loss program, bariatric surgeon)?

If you use nicotine
- Can you help me with nicotine cessation?
- Can you refer me to someone who can help me permanently quit (nicotine cessation specialist, quit center)?

If you have GERD
- Do I need an upper endoscopy?
  › If not now, when?

PEARLS OF WISDOM

If mild medications aren't enough to control your symptoms, seek out a surgeon who has specialty training in anti-reflux procedures to help you determine your best treatment options. When done properly, anti-reflux surgery is extremely safe and effective at helping people achieve long-term relief from GERD symptoms. Ask your primary care clinician or another trusted source to recommend an experienced surgeon. Your chances of a successful outcome are greatest if you work with a reputable surgeon who regularly performs anti-reflux procedures.

"Women need female surgeons to advocate for their health and the health of their families."

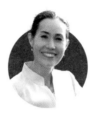

Lora Melman, M.D., FACS, FASMBS - she/her
Dr. Melman is the director of The Hernia Center of New Jersey at Advanced Surgical & Bariatrics in Central New Jersey. She specializes in minimally invasive surgery for GERD and reflux disease, as well as advanced hernia repair and weight loss surgery.

31

Hand and thumb pain

Clare E. Wise, M.D., and Amy L. Ladd, M.D.

WHAT IS THUMB PAIN?

Thumb pain is a common problem for many women throughout the course of their lives. The majority of thumb pain in middle-aged and older women is due to osteoarthritis of the carpometacarpal (CMC) basal joint of the thumb.

Your joints are protected by cartilage, a natural cushion between the joints. Osteoarthritis, or more simply, arthritis, develops when cartilage wears down. When bones start to rub together without cartilage in between, swelling and pain develop. In your thumb, wear and tear to the cartilage over time and the resulting arthritis causes additional deforming changes to your thumb.

These changes can cause the metacarpophalangeal (MCP) joint to move beyond its natural range of motion (hyperextend) and can sometimes cause the numbness and tingling of the thumb, index, and middle fingers that characterizes carpal tunnel syndrome (see Chapter 17). Additionally, thumb arthritis, also called CMC arthritis, can lead to decreased strength in your hands, particularly your pinch grip, making it difficult to do everyday activities such as hold a pencil or button your shirt.

Arthritis of the thumb can progress to include several bones in your wrist, known as STT arthritis (between the scaphoid, trapezium, and trapezoid bones). Arthritis at the end of the finger joints can also develop and commonly leads to thumb pain, usually in the distal interphalangeal (DIP) joint. Over time these joints can become less flexible due to the arthritis, which can lead to decreased range of motion. Painful, bony nodules on the backs of the finger joints, called Heberden's nodes, can also develop and are a common sign of arthritis.

CAN THUMB PAIN BE PREVENTED?

Maintaining a healthy weight can decrease stress on all joints of the body, including the hand and thumb, which can help decrease thumb pain. Excess stress contributes to the breakdown of cartilage and arthritic changes in the joints. Using your hands for strenuous and repetitive activities may also contribute to arthritis, but common tasks such as smartphone texting probably don't cause arthritis.

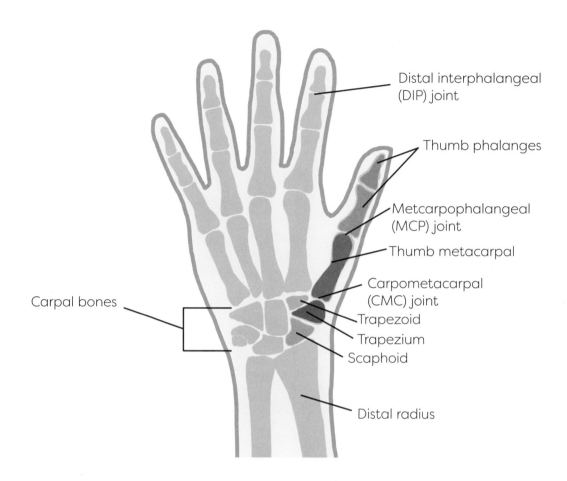

Distal interphalangeal (DIP) joint

Thumb phalanges

Metcarpophalangeal (MCP) joint

Thumb metacarpal

Carpometacarpal (CMC) joint

Trapezoid

Trapezium

Scaphoid

Distal radius

Carpal bones

HOW IS THUMB PAIN TREATED?

There are a number of ways to treat thumb pain due to arthritis.

Activity modification and thumb braces

Though it might seem like a no-brainer, try to avoid repetitive motions or activities that aggravate your thumb pain. Thumb braces, sometimes called splints, are also available to treat thumb arthritis pain. They help by stabilizing the arthritic joint and putting your thumb in a functional position. Thumb braces are usually one of two types: long (includes the thumb and crosses the wrist) or short (includes the thumb only). Both types may be either soft or rigid. Rigid braces provide more support, whereas soft ones permit some motion. There are advantages to both depending on the amount of pain and hand usage. A brace is usually a good treatment option to start with and is available online or through your physical therapist.

Hand or physical therapy

An occupational or physical therapist can help you learn how to strengthen the muscles around your thumb to decrease pain. A therapist can also provide options for avoiding or altering hand motions that aggravate your pain (such as opening jars or engaging in repetitive motions at your workstation) and provide custom braces for specific activities.

Medication

If your pain is preventing you from doing everyday activities, you can try nonprescription medications such as acetaminophen, or nonsteroidal anti-inflammatory drugs (NSAIDs) such as naproxen or ibuprofen. Prescription pain medication is usually not needed. Heat or ice can also help alleviate pain in your thumb joint. When using ice, apply it to your thumb over a thin cloth to prevent frostbite. Typically, you'll use the ice for about 15 minutes at a time.

Injections

Your doctor may recommend an injection into the thumb joint, which can help relieve pain. Usually these injections contain a steroid, sometimes with numbing medication added, such as lidocaine. Your doctor will inject the solution into the joint space, the source of the pain, in order to decrease the inflammation of the joint. This can be done at an office visit, and there are usually no restrictions after the injection, though your thumb may feel sore for the rest of the day.

Injection success can be variable. Some people feel relief from the injection for many months or years, whereas others experience only temporary and partial relief. If you experience significant relief from a first injection and your symptoms return, your doctor may consider a second steroid injection. However, recent studies suggest that people who undergo thumb surgery may experience more complications if they received prior steroid injections into the thumb joint. For that reason, some surgeons caution against receiving multiple injections.

Surgery for severe thumb (CMC) arthritis

If you experience severe symptoms of thumb arthritis, surgery may be recommended. Surgery for thumb arthritis typically involves removing one of the wrist (carpal) bones, specifically the trapezium. The trapezium is the part of the CMC joint where the pain is generated due to the severe bone-on-bone arthritis. This procedure is known as a trapeziectomy. Variations of trapeziectomy surgery include reconstructing the tendons of the wrist and thumb to provide further support to the bones of the thumb, allowing them to freely move and function. People usually have reduced pain after surgery but may not regain the full strength that they had before their arthritis symptoms began.

Nontraditional therapies

People may try nontraditional therapies, which include acupuncture, chiropractic treatment and application of medicines other than NSAIDs and acetaminophen. No scientific studies demonstrate success of these treatments for severe thumb arthritis.

WHY DOES THUMB PAIN MATTER TO WOMEN?

Osteoarthritis of all joints is common as we age. Women, particularly postmenopausal women, have a higher incidence than men of thumb arthritis. X-ray evidence of thumb arthritis is found in up to 40% of women over the age of 75 compared with 25% of men in the same age range. Joint looseness, which is more common in women, may contribute to arthritis development and progression. This looseness may be due to several factors, including hormonal differences between men and women, but there's not a lot of good scientific evidence to support that theory yet. Women may also develop thumb arthritis at higher rates because of the way they move their thumb joints compared to the way men do. Fortunately, surgical treatment such as trapeziectomy has been shown to effectively reduce thumb pain for both men and women.

QUESTIONS TO ASK YOUR HEALTH CARE TEAM ABOUT THUMB PAIN

For mild thumb CMC arthritis
- What type of activity modification do you recommend to decrease the pain?
- Are there braces available that would help my pain?
  › If so, when should I wear them?
- Would hand or physical therapy benefit me?
- What types of pain control medications do you recommend?
  › Is it safe for me to take NSAIDs?

For moderate to severe CMC arthritis
- Would a steroid injection help my pain?
  › (If you have diabetes) Would a steroid injection be appropriate given my diabetes?
- What kind of relief can I expect from a steroid injection?
  › What are the next steps if the injection is not effective?

- What surgical options are available for this condition?
  › At what point do you typically recommend surgery for people with my condition?

If the decision is to proceed with surgery for severe CMC arthritis
- How long will the surgery take?
- What type of restrictions will I have after surgery?
- What is the recovery time like after surgery?
- Which symptoms that I currently have will you expect to go away after surgery?

For finger joint (DIP joint) arthritis
- Are there braces available that would help my pain?
- What kind of surgical options are available?

PEARLS OF WISDOM

Hand and thumb pain can be debilitating and make it difficult to perform everyday activities. Make sure you tell your health care team about activities that you do with your hands that are important to you (computer work, baking, gardening, sports or other activities) so they can better understand your goals and form a treatment plan specific to your needs.

Unfortunately, arthritis is a progressive disease. While there's no magic wand available to "turn back the clock" on joint disease, many arthritis treatments can decrease your hand pain.

If you have swelling and pain in multiple joints, ask your clinician if you should be evaluated for systemic (whole body) conditions, such as rheumatoid arthritis, gout or pseudogout (CPPD). Your health care team can help connect you with the right specialty clinicians to treat all aspects of your joint pain.

"Build good habits for everlasting health, and inspire other women to do the same!"

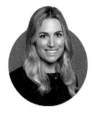

Clare E. Wise, M.D. - she/her
Dr. Wise is an orthopedic surgery resident at Stanford University in Palo Alto, California.

"A woman's bone health is critical to a functioning, vibrant lifestyle."

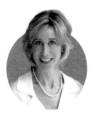

Amy L. Ladd, M.D. - she/her
Dr. Ladd is the Elsbach-Richards Professor of Surgery, Vice-chair, Department of Orthopaedic Surgery at Stanford University in Palo Alto, California. Dr. Ladd specializes in surgery and research of the pediatric and adult hand and upper limb.

32
Heart disease

Leslie Yingzhijie Tseng, M.S., and Erica S. Spatz, M.D., M.H.S.

WHAT IS HEART DISEASE?
WHAT IS A HEART ATTACK?

Heart disease is the leading cause of death in the United States for both women and men. The most common type of heart disease is coronary artery disease, which affects the blood vessels that supply blood to the heart (coronary arteries). Cholesterol and inflammation lead to fatty deposits called plaque that build up in the arteries in a process called atherosclerosis. As plaque builds up over time, the arteries can narrow, reducing the flow of oxygen-rich blood to the heart muscle. Restricted blood flow can cause chest pain and shortness of breath due to diminished oxygen supply to the heart muscle (angina).

In some cases, a plaque can rupture and form a blood clot that abruptly blocks blood flow to the heart. Without sufficient oxygen, the heart becomes damaged. This is called a heart attack, or myocardial infarction.

CAN HEART DISEASE BE PREVENTED?

Heart disease is common, but it can also be prevented. The first step is to understand your personal risk. Starting around menopause and continuing as women age, the risk of heart disease increases. If you have a parent or sibling who was diagnosed with heart disease before age 60, your own risk increases.

You can't change your age or genetics. But knowing they are risk factors can help you to be more attentive to symptoms and more proactive about your cardiovascular health.

Here are ways you can lower your risk of heart disease:

Know your heart disease risk factors
It's important to have a conversation about your lifestyle and medical history with your clinician. You can also use an online calculator, such as the ASCVD Risk Estimator recommended by the American Heart Association and American College of Cardiology, to estimate your risk of heart disease and stroke over the next 10 years. (Visit **http://tools.acc.org**)

Some additional risk factors not included in the calculator are specific to or more common in women. These include:

- A history of preeclampsia during pregnancy or preterm birth
- Early menopause
- An autoimmune disease, such as rheumatoid arthritis

If you have a somewhat elevated risk or intermediate risk of developing heart disease in the next 10 years, consider talking to your clinician about getting a calcium score. A calcium score is calculated from a CT scan of the chest that shows the degree of plaque buildup in the heart arteries. It can be a helpful piece of information when you and your clinician are making decisions about different strategies for preventing heart disease.

Manage blood pressure

High blood pressure (Chapter 34) occurs when the force of blood flowing through blood vessels is consistently too high. High blood pressure is called the "silent killer" because it often causes no symptoms but can lead to heart attacks, strokes, kidney disease and premature death if left uncontrolled. Thus, it's important to maintain a healthy blood pressure — typically under 130/80 millimeters of mercury (mmHg) — to reduce damage to blood vessels and other organs and to prevent heart disease.

Control cholesterol

Cholesterol is a waxy substance made by the liver that travels in the blood. The body needs cholesterol to make new cells, vitamins and hormones. There are a few types of cholesterol:

- LDL (low-density lipoprotein) is the "bad" cholesterol because it accelerates plaque buildup in the arteries and leads to heart disease. Fortunately, diet and medication can help lower LDL. If you have heart disease, are at high risk of heart disease or already have a diagnosis of heart disease, a lower LDL level is recommended.
- HDL (high-density lipoprotein) is the "good" type of cholesterol because it helps absorb LDL from blood and carry it back to the liver. Your genetics largely determines your HDL levels. Changes to lifestyle and medication tend to have a small effect.
- Lipoprotein(a), sometimes called Lp little a or Lp(a), is a third type of cholesterol. Lipoprotein(a) is not checked routinely, but higher levels may contribute to heart disease. High lipoprotein(a) runs in families. Medications that target this type of cholesterol are in development.

A cholesterol test can help determine your risk of heart disease and whether a change in diet or medication is warranted.

To get a more complete picture of the total cholesterol particles that can lead to heart disease, your clinician may also test for Apoliprotein B (apoB). Apoliprotein B is a structural protein in the blood that attaches to the lipoprotein particles that cause plaque buildup in the arteries.

Reduce blood sugar

Women with diabetes (Chapter 25) are twice as likely to have heart disease as women without diabetes are; moreover, disease occurs at a younger age than it does in women without diabetes. High blood sugar levels drive inflammation and slow blood flow, which speeds the process of plaque buildup. Maintaining a healthy diet, exercising and taking diabetes medication can help avoid or reduce these complications from diabetes. Recently, several medications developed to treat diabetes have been shown to also reduce heart disease.

Get regular physical activity
Physical activity can lower blood pressure, cholesterol and blood sugar. It can also help you maintain a healthy weight, manage stress and make staying tobacco-free easier. The American Heart Association recommends at least 150 minutes of moderate-intensity aerobic activity each week for adults and 60 minutes of daily physical activity for children and adolescents.

Choose healthy foods and drinks
Overall, diets that are more plant-based and include whole grains, fruits, vegetables, limited or no meat and low-fat or no dairy can lower the risk of developing several conditions, including heart disease. Also keep in mind these dietary tips:
- Avoiding foods high in saturated and trans fat can lower cholesterol.
- Reducing salt and alcohol intake can lower blood pressure.
- Limiting sugar intake, including sugary beverages, can keep blood sugar levels in a healthy range.

Avoid smoking or vaping
Toxic chemicals in tobacco can injure the heart. They increase inflammation and damage blood vessels, triggering plaque buildup. They also thicken the blood and raise blood pressure, making the heart work harder than normal. If you don't smoke, don't start, and avoid secondhand smoke. If you do smoke, quitting lowers your risk of heart disease no matter how much or how long you have smoked in the past.

Focus on mental well-being
Positive psychological states, such as feeling happy, optimistic and mindful, are associated with a decreased risk of heart disease. In contrast, negative psychological states, such as depression, anxiety, anger and loneliness, are associated with increased risk. What's more, reducing negative states of mind or promoting positive psychological well-being can help to prevent heart disease.

To support your well-being, engage in self-care. For example, practice good sleep hygiene, mindfulness techniques such as meditation, and mood-boosting activities, such as bonding with family and friends (even four-legged ones!). Doing so can help decrease the risk of developing or worsening heart disease.

HOW IS HEART DISEASE TREATED?

There are several strategies to treat heart disease.

Lifestyle changes
The same lifestyle behaviors that help prevent heart disease are important for treating heart disease. Diets that are more plant-based can prevent or slow the progression of plaque buildup and promote artery relaxation. With respect to physical activity, being active and getting exercise count. Maintaining a healthy weight, avoiding tobacco and excessive alcohol, and sleep quality are also important. Finally, adopting a healthy psychological mindset is critical.

Medications

Medicines are very important in preventing and treating heart disease. These can include:

- **Cholesterol-lowering medications** These medicines, such as statins and PCSK9 inhibitors, decrease not only cholesterol but also inflammation, and they lower the risk of future cardiovascular events.
- **Anti-ischemic medications** These drugs (beta-blockers, calcium channel blockers and nitrates) treat chest pain and lower blood pressure.
- **Antiplatelet medications** These medications (aspirin and P2Y12 inhibitors) prevent blood cells from sticking together and forming clots.
- **Glucose-lowering medications** These drugs, such as GLP-1 receptor agonists and SGLT2 inhibitors, lower blood sugar (glucose) and help prevent heart attack and other adverse cardiovascular events. They are increasingly being used in people without diabetes. GLP-1 receptor agonists are also used in people with obesity and other risk factors for heart disease.

Your clinician may recommend starting with a low dose of one or more of these medications, gradually increasing the dose until you achieve your goals for cholesterol levels, blood pressure and glucose management.

Revascularization (stenting or surgery)

Your doctor may recommend a procedure to restore blood flow to the part of the heart that is not getting enough blood. This procedure is called revascularization, and it can be accomplished in two ways:

Stenting During this minimally invasive procedure, a cardiologist inserts a tiny mesh tube, called a stent, in a blocked artery to hold it open. The cardiologist begins by performing a cardiac catheterization. This involves inserting a very thin, flexible catheter into the wrist (radial) or groin (femoral) artery to reach the heart arteries. Contrast dye is then injected to reveal any blocked heart arteries. If a blockage is determined to be severe, a tiny balloon on the catheter inflates and opens up the blockage site. When the catheter is removed, a stent is left behind to hold the artery open.

Coronary artery bypass surgery Also known as CABG (pronounced "cabbage"), coronary artery bypass surgery is an open-heart surgery. During the procedure, a surgeon attaches healthy arteries and veins from other parts of the body, called grafts, to the heart to provide alternate channels for blood flow. Specifically, the surgeon reroutes arteries from the chest cavity to the heart and harvests veins from the legs to reimplant into the heart. Coronary artery bypass surgery is typically the preferred surgery if there are extensive blockages throughout the heart arteries.

Cardiac rehabilitation People who have had a heart attack are encouraged to participate in structured cardiac rehabilitation (exercise) programs in a monitored setting. These programs can improve endurance, strength and balance, build confidence and decrease complications from heart disease. It is also increasingly recognized that cardiac rehab is important for people with cardiac conditions other than a heart attack and for the prevention of heart disease.

WHY DOES HEART DISEASE MATTER TO WOMEN?

Heart disease is the leading cause of death in women in the U.S., contributing to one in three deaths each year. Yet women are less likely to be diagnosed with heart disease or receive appropriate and timely treatment and are more likely to have a worse outcome.

Among women, the risk of heart disease can differ depending on race, ethnicity and age. In comparison with white women, Black women have more cardiovascular risk factors, develop heart disease at an earlier age and have higher mortality rates. For Hispanic and Asian women, the ethnic groups for whom we have data, heart disease is less prevalent compared with white or Black women. Still, cardiovascular disease remains the leading cause of death among Hispanic women. South Asians, American Indians and Alaska Natives also experience higher rates of cardiovascular risk factors and earlier cardiovascular mortality. East Asian women tend to experience lower rates of cardiovascular risk factors, disease and mortality. Finally, younger women who exhibit heart disease are at higher risk of poor outcomes; for example, women 55 years or younger who have a heart attack are twice as likely to die than similarly aged men with a heart attack.

Women have different biological risk factors for heart disease than men. A decline in estrogen during menopause increases women's risk. Pregnancy complications, such as preeclampsia and gestational diabetes, also increase risk. Women are more likely to develop autoimmune disease, in which the immune system attacks healthy cells — another risk factor for heart disease. Additionally, risk factors that impact everyone, including smoking, diabetes, inactivity, and depression and anxiety, tend to be more common in women.

The underlying causes of heart disease in women may also be different from those for men. Though plaque buildup in arteries is still the most common cause of heart disease and heart attacks, women are more likely than men to experience disease of the small blood vessels (microvascular dysfunction) and sudden tightening of a heart artery (coronary vasospasm). Broken heart syndrome, a temporary heart condition brought on by stress and extreme hormonal output, is another recognized condition that occurs more often in post-menopausal women. These problems often go undetected, and many women may be told that their symptoms are unrelated to heart disease. This results in missed opportunities to improve symptoms and prevent or treat serious heart conditions.

Another issue is that symptoms of heart disease can differ for men and women. While the most common heart attack symptom in women is chest pain (angina) or chest discomfort, women are also likely to experience other symptoms, particularly shortness of breath, nausea or vomiting, back or jaw pain, unusual fatigue, cold sweat and dizziness. These other symptoms can be vague and less noticeable than chest pain, which makes it harder for women to recognize warning signs. As a result, women may delay seeking medical care and experience worse health outcomes. You can help head off these problems by learning the

Symptoms common in women

Pain in jaw, neck, shoulder(s), or arm(s)

Palpitations
Shortness of breath

Indigestion
Nausea

Symptoms common in men and women

Dizziness
Lightheadedness

Chest pain, pressure, tightness, or discomfort

Sweating
Weakness/ fatigue

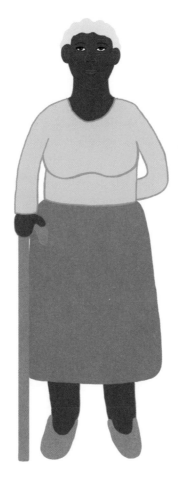

common warning signs of heart disease in women, listening to your body and seeking care if something does not feel right.

QUESTIONS TO ASK YOUR HEALTH CARE TEAM ABOUT HEART DISEASE

- Can you help me learn more about my personal risk of heart disease?
  › Does my family history increase my risk of heart disease?
  › What is my blood pressure and cholesterol level?
  › Do I have diabetes or am I likely to develop diabetes?
  › Would a calcium score be helpful in understanding more about my risk of heart disease?
- What can I do to lower my risk?
  › Do you recommend I take a medication to lower my risk of heart disease?
- What resources can you recommend to help me improve my diet, exercise more, quit smoking or manage stress?

If you have heart disease
- What are my treatment options?
- What lifestyle changes can I make to improve my health?
- How do the medicines you prescribed help me with my heart disease?
  › Do they have any side effects?
- Will a revascularization procedure or surgery help me live longer or reduce my chances of having a heart attack?
- What symptoms should prompt me to seek emergency medical attention?

If you recently had a heart attack
- How likely am I to have another heart attack?
  › What can I do to reduce that risk?
- What activities can I do safely?
  › Can I go back to work, exercise on my own, drink alcohol and have sex?
- Would I benefit from attending a cardiac rehabilitation program?
- What should I do if I feel sad or worried?
  › Is there a support group I can join?
  › Can you refer me to a therapist?

PEARLS OF WISDOM

Heart disease impacts women's health, quality of life and longevity — as it does in men. Yet, advances in the management of heart disease have not benefited women equally. We now know that women have different biological and life experiences and require a more personalized approach. More women-focused research is needed to advance equity in women's health.

Fortunately, you can take charge of your cardiovascular health. More than 80% of heart disease can be prevented with knowledge and action. Talk to your clinician about your risk, no matter which stage of life you're in. Encourage the other women in your life to do so as well. Together, we can improve women's heart health.

"In medical school, I learn facts from books and classes, but I learn medicine from the conversations that I have with patients."

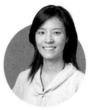

Leslie Yingzhijie Tseng, M.S. - she/her
Leslie is a third-year medical student at Yale School of Medicine in New Haven, Connecticut. She is passionate about women's health research, reproductive justice, and health care in low-resource settings.

"Conversations about women's risk of heart disease can be empowering, giving women the information and tools to make good decisions about their health and health care."

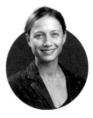

Erica S. Spatz, M.D., M.H.S. - she/her
Dr. Spatz is a cardiologist and researcher at Yale School of Medicine, and Director of the Preventive Cardiovascular Health Program at Yale Heart and Vascular Center. Her research focuses on patient engagement, women's cardiovascular health and health equity.

33
Hepatitis C

Mary Davies, M.D., and Lauren A. Beste, M.D., M.S., FACP

WHAT IS HEPATITIS C?

Hepatitis C is a viral infection of the liver. It is a leading cause of liver transplantation, liver cancer and liver-related death in the United States. The number of new hepatitis C virus (HCV) infections is rising, especially among women. The Centers for Disease Control and Prevention estimates that more than 7 million women in the United States have HCV infection.

HCV can only be spread by blood contact with someone who has the virus. People are usually not aware when the infection first happens, although a small percentage develop symptoms such as muscle aches, yellow skin and dark urine. Severe damage also causes confusion, a higher risk of bleeding and bruising, and swelling in the abdomen and legs. After many years, HCV infection can lead to liver scarring. HCV causes a long-term infection for most people, lasting until a person takes medication to cure it. However, for 15%-45% of people with HCV, the body can cure HCV on its own. This means that for a minority of people, the body clears the virus within a few months, even without treatment. Studies have shown that women are more likely than men to clear the virus on their own.

Because long-term (chronic) HCV infection usually causes no symptoms, people can live with the infection for years without being aware of it. Over time, the virus may damage the liver and lead to permanent liver scarring (cirrhosis), which increases the risk of liver failure and liver cancer.

HCV infection can be diagnosed with a simple blood test. All adults should get screened at least once before age 65. It's important to know that before 1992, the virus was unintentionally spread through blood transfusions and organ donations. Since 1992, transmission has been prevented by screening all donated blood products, tissues and organs for HCV. But if you received a blood transfusion, a Rho(D) immune globulin (RhoGAM) injection that is sometimes given during pregnancy, or an organ transplant before 1992, it is critical to get tested for HCV.

CAN HEPATITIS C BE PREVENTED?

HCV can be transmitted through any kind of blood-to-blood contact. The most important way to prevent HCV exposure is to stop transmission in the first place, since there is no vaccine to protect against HCV infection.

You cannot transmit HCV to others through routine physical contact, saliva or the air. Hugging, kissing and sharing food, drinks and utensils are all safe. However, people who have HCV should not share their personal hygiene items such as toothbrushes and razors with others, and blood spills should always be cleaned up with bleach. Here are other steps you can take to prevent HCV transmission and protect your liver from damage.

Use clean needles

Today, transmission most commonly occurs when people share needles or other supplies to inject drugs. People can protect themselves by always using clean needles and syringes if they inject drugs, and by disposing of used needles safely. Transmission can also happen by sharing straws to inhale drugs into the nose or when other types of sharp objects are shared, such as unsterilized needles for tattoos or body piercings.

Use condoms

A very small amount of virus is present in semen, so transmission during sexual activity is possible but extremely rare. A large study looked specifically at heterosexual couples in which only one person was infected with HCV, and found the risk of transmission was 7 cases per year for every 10,000 persons. Since the risk of sexual transmission is so low, long-term monogamous couples do not necessarily need to change their sexual practices. However, condoms are always recommended among non-monogamous couples as a general measure to prevent HIV and other sexually transmitted infections. Little is known about HCV transmission between female sexual partners, but the risk is believed to be extremely low.

Get pre-pregnancy testing

HCV can be transmitted from mother to child during pregnancy. On average, transmission happens in about 4% to 5% of pregnancies when the mother has HCV, although the rate is higher in mothers who have both HCV and HIV infections. Medications to cure HCV infection are not recommended during pregnancy. Therefore, the most important way to prevent mother-to-child transmission is to diagnose and treat the virus before conception. If HCV infection is discovered during pregnancy, the baby will be tested after delivery to determine if the infection was transmitted. If transmission occurred, a pediatrician can help decide on the right time for a child to be treated. The virus does not spread through breastmilk, so mothers infected with HCV can breastfeed safely.

Limit alcohol use

Alcohol use, even a small amount, can cause liver damage from HCV to happen faster. Reducing the amount of alcohol you drink, and ideally stopping completely, is crucial to prevent liver damage from getting worse.

Eat a healthy diet

In general, following a healthy diet helps protect the liver. Drinking a cup of coffee every day may also be beneficial by potentially reducing the risk of liver cancer. Always let your clinician know about any vitamins or supplements you are considering, since some may be harmful to the liver or interact with medication.

HOW IS HEPATITIS C TREATED?

Before 2015, HCV infection was very difficult to cure. Treatment required 6 to 12 months of injectable medication, but these regimens had serious side effects and often did not work. Fortunately, excellent medications have been available to treat HCV infection since 2015.

Today, the pills used to treat HCV infection cure 95% to 99% of people with the condition, if taken as directed. The HCV pills work even if people have had the virus for many years. These pills are extremely safe and cause few side effects. Successful treatment eliminates the risk of transmission to others and greatly reduces the chance of complications from HCV. There are many types of HCV pills available, no matter which version (genotype) of HCV you have.

To select the best option for you, your clinician may ask questions about your medical history and recommend blood tests. These tests will check for other blood-borne viruses, such as HIV or hepatitis B virus. Your clinician may recommend vaccination for hepatitis A and B to prevent catching these viruses later.

Each HCV treatment regimen involves taking pills every day for 8 to 12 weeks. It is critical that the pills not be skipped during treatment, even for a single day. If the medicine is skipped or missed, it may not work and the virus could become resistant to that kind of medicine. Taking the medicine daily is the single most important thing you can do to increase the chance that HCV infection is successfully cured. Three months after completing treatment, a final blood test will be performed to make sure the virus is no longer present in your blood.

In the vast majority of cases, the virus will be completely eliminated. Rarely, a second course of HCV treatment may be required if the first one did not work. Even after the infection is treated, the HCV antibody test — a blood test that shows that your body has been exposed to the virus — will always remain positive, though the virus itself is gone.

Once HCV infection is cured, it cannot come back unless a person is exposed to HCV again. It is important to understand that people do not become immune to HCV, which means it is possible to become infected again after being cured.

WHY DOES HEPATITIS C MATTER TO WOMEN?

In addition to rising rates of HCV infection among women, HCV affects women's bodies differently from men's bodies. For example, women with chronic HCV infection are less likely than men with the infection to develop cirrhosis and liver cancer. Ultimately, women are less likely than men to die because of the virus. However, alcohol use changes this pattern. Alcohol seems to cause more liver damage among women infected with HCV than among men infected with HCV, increasing women's rate of death. Fortunately, HCV treatment is equally effective in both women and men.

Having HCV is an important consideration for women who could become

Symptoms of acute HCV

Symptoms of long-term liver damage from HCV

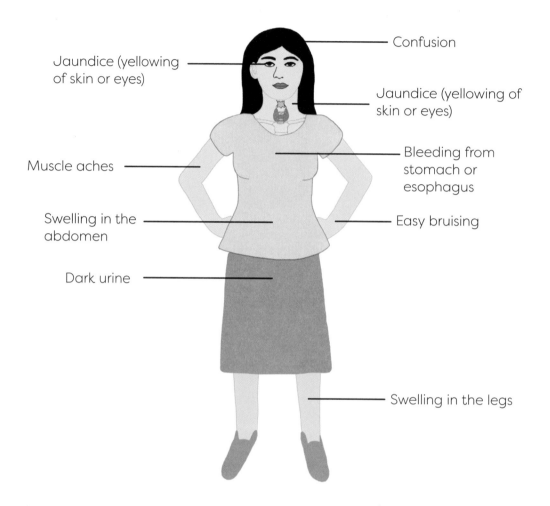

Jaundice (yellowing of skin or eyes)

Muscle aches

Swelling in the abdomen

Dark urine

Confusion

Jaundice (yellowing of skin or eyes)

Bleeding from stomach or esophagus

Easy bruising

Swelling in the legs

pregnant. If you're taking birth control pills, be aware that certain HCV medications can interact with the pills. Your clinician will be able to choose an effective and safe HCV medicine after reviewing your medications. If you are interested in becoming pregnant, there are several things you need to know. First, having an HCV infection does not change the chance of becoming pregnant. Since none of the medication options for HCV infection are proven safe during pregnancy and breastfeeding, women infected with HCV should consider treatment before becoming pregnant to avoid the risk of transmitting HCV to their babies. HCV infection in itself has not been shown to cause birth defects or pregnancy-related complications such as premature delivery. As noted, there is a small risk of passing the infection from mother to child during pregnancy.

QUESTIONS TO ASK YOUR HEALTH CARE TEAM ABOUT HEPATITIS C

For everyone
- Have I have been tested for HCV?
  - › Everyone should be screened for HCV at least once during their lifetime.
- Do I have any risk factors that mean I should be screened more frequently?

For people who have tested positive
- Has the virus caused any liver damage?
  - › If so, how much?
- Should I have other specialists on my treatment team, like a nutritionist, mental health provider, or a specialist in alcohol or drug treatment?

For people who will undergo treatment for HCV
- When is the right time for me to start treatment?
- What can I do to protect my liver after treatment is over?

PEARLS OF WISDOM

HCV infection is highly treatable. Treatment reduces the risk of long-term consequences from HCV, such as cirrhosis, liver failure, liver cancer and death. During treatment, taking the HCV medication every day is the biggest step you can take toward successfully getting cured.

"Providing health care is 20% offering information, 80% understanding women's intrinsic knowledge of themselves."

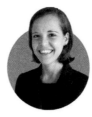

Mary Davies, M.D. - she/her
Mary is an addiction medicine fellow at the University of Washington in Seattle, with a focus on treating substance use disorders in primary care.

"All women deserve health care that respects their unique individuality and supports well-informed decision making."

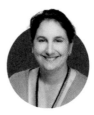

Lauren A. Beste, M.D., M.S., FACP - she/her
Dr. Beste is the Deputy Director of General Medicine at the Veterans Affairs (VA) Puget Sound Health Care System and is an Associate Professor at the University of Washington School of Medicine in Seattle, Washington. She is a board-certified General Internist practicing in the Women's Health Clinic and the Hepatology Clinic at the VA Puget Sound. She directs the data and analytics group for the national VA HIV, Hepatitis, and Related Conditions Program Office.

34
High blood pressure

Shawna D. Nesbitt, M.D., M.S.

WHAT IS HIGH BLOOD PRESSURE?

High blood pressure, also called hypertension, is when your blood pressure, which is the long-term force of blood flowing through your blood vessels, is consistently too high. High blood pressure damages the inside of the blood vessels that supply blood to your organs. This can have a number of significant negative effects on your organs, such as:

- **Eyes** Small bleeding and inflammation spots that may compromise your vision.
- **Kidneys** Leakage of protein into the urine, which leads to kidney failure over time.
- **Heart** The left side of the heart may have to work a lot harder to pump blood, and this results in the enlargement of the heart muscle, a condition called left ventricular hypertrophy (LVH). The enlarged heart muscle can lead to heart failure, such as heart disease or heart attack.
- **Brain** Small areas of bleeding or clots may appear, which lead to strokes.

However, most people with high blood pressure have no signs or symptoms and are unaware that they have the condition. Those who do have symptoms, usually have severely elevated blood pressure.

Symptoms of severe hypertension

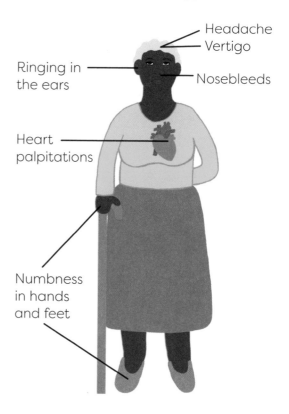

Headache
Vertigo
Ringing in the ears
Nosebleeds
Heart palpitations
Numbness in hands and feet

Stage	Systolic mm Hg (top number; indicates pressure when heart is pumping blood)		Diastolic mm Hg (bottom number; indicates pressure when heart is resting)	Follow-up
Normal	Less than 120	And	Less than 80	1 year
Elevated	120-129	And	Less than 80	3-6 months
Stage 1	130-139	Or	80-89	3-6 months
Stage 2	More than 140	Or	More than 90	1 month
Crisis	More than 180	Or	More than 110	Seek care immediately

Source: ACC/AHA 2017 Hypertension Guidelines

Thus, it is important to regularly make sure that your blood pressure measurements are normal. We measure blood pressure in millimeters of mercury (mmHg).

- Systolic blood pressure, the top number, is the pressure in blood vessels when the heart is contracting and pumping blood out to the body.
- Diastolic blood pressure, the bottom number, is the pressure when the heart is resting between beats.

A blood pressure measurement greater than 130/80 mmHg denotes high blood pressure.

Blood pressure must be elevated on at least two different clinic visits to make a diagnosis of high blood pressure. However, taking blood pressure measurements at home is helpful in confirming a diagnosis of high blood pressure. The following are some tips to help you take blood pressure accurately:

1. Avoid caffeine and smoking for at least 30 minutes prior to blood pressure measurement, as these substances will affect your blood pressure.

2. You should be in a seated position with your feet on the floor and your back supported.
3. Rest quietly in this position for at least 5 minutes.
4. Then wrap the cuff comfortably around your nondominant upper arm. (A cuff that is too tight will give incorrect measurements.)
5. Place your arm at heart level on a nearby table.
6. Take your blood pressure measurement.
7. Rest for 1 minute.
8. Now take a second measurement. An average of the two measurements will give you a more accurate reading.

Poor measurements can be misleading. For example, if your blood pressure at home is less than 130/80 mmHg and your blood pressure in your clinician's office is 130/80 mmHg to 160/100 mmHg, you may be experiencing what's called "white coat hypertension," in which your blood pressure goes up because you are nervous about the medical visit. About 10% to 35% of people experience white coat hypertension, and it is more common in women than in men. White coat hypertension can be confirmed by monitoring blood pressure over 24 hours with a take-home device.

Additionally, experiencing intense pain, emotional upset, anxiety, smoking, and some medications and supplements can temporarily raise blood pressure.

CAN HIGH BLOOD PRESSURE BE PREVENTED?

Risk factors for high blood pressure include:

- A high-salt diet
- Overweight and obesity
- Genetics
- Stress
- Sleep apnea
- Excess of hormones, particularly aldosterone and renin
- Excess alcohol
- Kidney disease and irregular blood vessels to the kidneys
- Thyroid disease (less common factor)
- Irregularities in chest/abdomen blood vessels, such as the aorta (less common factor)
- Excess adrenaline hormone from the adrenal glands (less common factor)
- Excess growth hormone from the brain (less common factor)

While we cannot change all of these factors, early interventions can prevent high blood pressure and/or help prevent blood pressure from rising. For example, eating a healthy diet and exercising also can help you lose excess weight. Losing even 2 pounds of weight leads to approximately 1 mmHg of blood pressure decline.

Diet
The Dietary Approaches to Stop Hypertension (DASH diet) is known to reduce blood pressure a few points in just two weeks and can reduce blood pressure by about 11 points over time. The DASH diet emphasizes foods that are low in fat and sodium — limiting sodium to 1500 milligrams (mg) a day — and rich in fruits, vegetables, and nutrients such as potassium, calcium and magnesium that help lower blood pressure. In particular, a potassium-rich diet (3500 to 5000 mg a day), facilitates blood pressure reduction.

Exercise
Physical exercise has a prominent effect on reducing blood pressure, regardless of the specific type of exercise. At least three exercise sessions a week will reduce blood pressure by 3 to 5 mmHg. It is also possible to treat elevated blood pressure with low-dose medication for a short time, reducing progression of the disease.

Caffeine and dietary supplements
Too much caffeine — from coffee, tea, energy drinks or diet pills — can elevate blood pressure for a short time after intake. Limit caffeine intake to less than 400 mg a day. An average cup of coffee has 96 mg of caffeine. Some dietary supplements can raise blood pressure and should be used with caution. Ask your clinician about use of these supplements:
- Licorice
- Bitter orange
- Ephedra
- Yohimbine
- Ma Huang
- St. John's Wort
- Siberian ginseng

Medications

Certain medications also can increase blood pressure and should be used sparingly. Talk to your clinician about using any of these medications:

- Nonsteroidal anti-inflammatory drugs (NSAIDs), such as ibuprofen or high-dose aspirin
- Decongestants or cold medicines
- Stimulant medications such as dextro-amphetamine-amphetamine (Adderall, Mydavis) and methylphenidate (Ritalin, Concerta, others)
- Prescription weight loss drugs
- Steroids such as prednisone, fludrocorti-sone, dexamethasone or hydrocortisone
- Antidepressant medications such as venlafaxine (Effexor)
- Estrogen hormone therapy
- Some birth control pills
    › Birth control pills that contain proges-tin with lower estrogen amounts are less likely to raise blood pressure than birth control pills that contain both progestin and higher estrogen amounts. Progestin-only birth control pills are least likely to elevate blood pressure.

Alcohol and drugs

The recommended limit for women is less than one drink a day. This is less than the recommended amount for men (two drinks a day) because women metabolize alcohol differently than men do. In addition to alcohol, recreational drugs such as cocaine, methamphetamine or bath salts raise blood pressure to dangerous levels and should be avoided.

HOW IS HIGH BLOOD PRESSURE TREATED?

Treatment of high blood pressure at a blood pressure of 130/80 mmHg starts with diet and exercise changes. Medication is added to the treatment plan if blood pressure reaches more than 140/90 mmHg, with the goal of keeping blood pressure below 130/80 mmHg. There are multiple classes of medications to lower blood pressure.

Treatment usually starts with the first-line options listed in the table on pages 208 and 209. If blood pressure is higher than 150/90 mmHg, two medications may be started together. Sometimes combination pills — two different medications in one pill — are prescribed; this is often an advantage in terms of cost and simplicity of use.

Dietary supplements

Some dietary supplements may lower blood pressure.

- **Fish Oil** Taking 1 gram of fish oil three days a week has been shown to reduce blood pressure. Fish oil contains two omega-3s called docosahexaenoic acid (DHA) and eicosapentaenoic acid (EPA), which are essential nutrients for heart health.
- **Coenzyme Q10 (CoQ10)** is an antioxidant that your body produces naturally, and your cells use for growth and maintenance. Levels of CoQ10 in your body decrease as you age. CoQ10 supplements have shown some positive effects on blood pressure, but larger studies are needed to confirm the results.
- **Garlic** has also been shown to lower blood pressure, but garlic supplements are difficult to standardize and have

Medication class	Most common examples	
First-line options		
Angiotensin-converting enzyme (ACE) inhibitors	lisinopril, benazepril, enalapril, quinapril, captopril, ramipril, fosinopril, perindopril	
Angiotensin II receptor blockers (ARBs)	candesartan, valsartan, losartan, azilsartan, telmisartan, irbesartan, olmesartan, eprosartan	
Calcium channel blockers (CCBs)	amlodipine, diltiazem, felodipine, isradipine, nifedipine, nisoldipine, verapamil	
Thiazide diuretics	chlorthalidone, hydrochlorothiazide, indapamide, metolazone	
Second-line options		
Loop diuretics	furosemide, bumetanide, torsemide	
Potassium sparing diuretics	triamterene, amiloride	
Aldosterone blockers	spironolactone, eplerenone	
Beta blockers	nebivolol, metoprolol, nadolol, atenolol, bisoprolol, propranolol	
Alpha-beta blockers	labetalol, carvedilol	
Direct renin inhibitors	aliskiren	
Alpha-1 blockers	doxazosin, prazosin, terazosin	
Central-acting agents	clonidine, guanfacine, methyldopa	
Direct vasodilators	Hydralazine, Minoxidil	
Combination pills	losartan/HCT, lisinopril/HCT, amlodipine/benazepril, amlodipine/valsartan	

inconsistent effects, making it difficult to give clear recommendations on their use.

One popular myth is that apple cider vinegar lowers blood pressure, but there is no evidence that it lowers blood pressure in humans.

Alternative therapies
When used consistently, alternative therapies such as biofeedback techniques, meditation and even music therapy have been shown to reduce blood pressure to varying degrees. Slow breathing with the guidance of a portable electronic device

May cause dry cough. Allergic reaction is more common in Black women. Avoid in pregnancy, especially in the 2nd trimester.
Avoid in pregnancy, especially in the 2nd trimester.
May cause mild leg or ankle swelling. Talk to your provider, who may adjust the dose, add a complimentary drug or discontinue the CCB.
May cause low potassium. You may need a potassium supplement. Add fruits and vegetables to your diet.
May cause low potassium. You may need a potassium supplement. Add fruits and vegetables to your diet.
Increases your potassium level. Very useful if your potassium is low. Low potassium is more common in Black women.
Increases your potassium level. Very useful if your potassium is low. Especially useful for women with polycystic ovarian syndrome (PCOS).
May cause some fatigue.
Avoid in pregnancy.
Can cause brief dizziness after the dose. Best taken at bedtime.
May cause fatigue, sleepiness and dry mouth.
Very effective in lowering blood pressure. May cause leg swelling. Minoxidil causes hair growth.

called Resperate (which uses musical tones to help you regulate your breathing), has also shown positive effects on blood pressure. Taking slow deep breaths — six breaths over 30 seconds — for 15 minutes three or four times a week has been shown to lower systolic blood pressure by 4 mmHg and diastolic pressure by 3 mmHg. Yoga also may help, but the extent of its positive impact is less measurable. Sometimes acupuncture is used to treat blood pressure, but the skill of the practitioner makes it difficult to assure consistency and effect, so it is not currently recommended as a high blood pressure treatment.

WHY DOES HIGH BLOOD PRESSURE MATTER TO WOMEN?

High blood pressure is often called the "silent killer" because it produces few signs or symptoms, if any. Women may not know that they have high blood pressure until harm has occurred. Although the absolute level of blood pressure in women tends to be lower than that of men, the effect of elevated blood pressure is more devastating for women, especially when it comes to cardiovascular disease. This is troubling and suggests that achieving ideal blood pressure goals is even more critical for women. In 2018, women made up 43% of high blood pressure cases but 51% of high blood pressure-related deaths.

The risk of developing high blood pressure in women increases most around age 45, which is also close to the time of menopause. However, the rate of pre-pregnancy high blood pressure in mothers, regardless of age, has nearly doubled over the past decade, suggesting a concerning trend. Women who have high blood pressure during pregnancy (preeclampsia) are at greater risk of complications with delivery, which increases both infant and maternal mortality. Women with high blood pressure in pregnancy are also more likely to have high blood pressure in the future.

The burden of high blood pressure is even greater in minority women. While 55% of Mexican American women, 64% of white women and 70% of African American women are aware of high blood pressure, with African American women being most aware, high blood pressure is well-managed in only 22% of African American women and 20% of Mexican American women. Furthermore, the risk of pre-pregnancy high blood pressure is double for African American women compared with white and Hispanic women. The combination of high blood pressure and other risk factors, such as obesity and diabetes, leads to heart disease, heart attack and stroke.

QUESTIONS TO ASK YOUR HEALTH CARE TEAM ABOUT HIGH BLOOD PRESSURE

- What is my blood pressure goal?
- What is my risk of a heart attack or stroke in the next 10 years?
- What are my other risk factors?
  › Be sure to ask about the following tests: cholesterol profile, serum creatinine, urine microalbumin, electrolytes, HgbA1C (diabetes) or glucose, TSH (thyroid function), EKG and possibly echocardiogram.
- If my legs or ankles are swelling, do you think this is due to my heart, my kidneys or my medication?
- If I'm under age 30 with newly diagnosed high blood pressure, are there hormonal elevations such as aldosterone levels or blood vessel abnormalities such as renal artery stenosis that are affecting my blood pressure?
- If I'm unable to reach my blood pressure goals with five medications that I have taken consistently, could I have a

hormonal elevation that causes high blood pressure?

- If I have low potassium, is my aldosterone level elevated?
  › This could suggest that you have an uncommon form of high blood pressure that develops from an adrenal cause.

To guide your treatment further, also be sure to bring up the following with your clinician:

- If anyone in your immediate family had an unusual kind of high blood pressure
- If you have panic attacks or anxiety episodes
  › Anxiety can elevate blood pressure and is treated separately from blood pressure, with or without medications.
- If you have chest pain, severe fatigue, left arm pain, shortness of breath or jaw pain with activity
  › This could be due to heart disease.
- If you have diabetes
  › Your high blood pressure may need to be treated more aggressively with an ACE inhibitor or ARB.

PEARLS OF WISDOM

High blood pressure can develop because of several factors. Treating high blood pressure is incredibly important to your health. Practicing healthy habits, such as eating a balanced diet and exercising regularly, is important for all women, but especially for those with high blood pressure.

If you have high blood pressure, measure and keep track of your blood pressure at home. Try to achieve and maintain a blood pressure goal of less than 130/80 mmHg. Alert your clinicians if your blood pressure is frequently higher than 140/90 mmHg. If you are taking medications for your blood pressure, take them consistently and see your clinician as instructed. Don't let high blood pressure be a "silent killer."

"Women's health is at the heart of excellent care for the whole family."

Shawna D. Nesbitt, M.D., M.S. - she/her

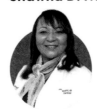 Dr. Nesbitt is a Professor in the Department of Internal Medicine at the University of Texas at Southwestern Medical Center, Dallas, Texas, where she is the Medical Director of the Hypertension Clinic at Parkland Hospital and Associate Dean of Student Affairs in the Office of Student Diversity and Inclusion. She is a certified Hypertension Specialist and a national leader in hypertension clinical trials with a special focus on prehypertension, hypertension in African Americans and health care disparities.

35
High cholesterol

Ellen K. Brinza, M.S., M.P.H., and Khendi White Solaru, M.D.

WHAT IS HIGH CHOLESTEROL?

Cholesterol is a waxy substance, similar to fat, that your body uses to make cells, vitamins and some hormones. Cholesterol comes from two sources: your liver, which makes all the cholesterol you need, and food from animals. For example, meat, poultry and dairy products all contain dietary cholesterol. Cholesterol is required for your body to function properly. However, too much cholesterol can lead to heart and blood vessel (cardiovascular) disease and stroke.

Cholesterol and dietary energy-storing fats called triglycerides serve as building blocks for plaque. When cholesterol and triglyceride levels are too high, plaque buildup (atherosclerosis) can develop in arteries, blocking blood flow and preventing nutrients and oxygen from reaching the body. Plaque buildup in the arteries of the heart can lead to heart attack, and plaque blockages in the arteries of the neck or brain can cause stroke. When plaque develops in the arteries, it is referred to as atherosclerotic cardiovascular disease — heart disease that involves plaque.

Since it takes time for high cholesterol to cause damage, most people with high cholesterol do not experience symptoms right away. Thus, it is very important that you discuss routine monitoring of your cholesterol levels with your clinician. When monitoring cholesterol laboratory values, there are a few key things to know. First, there are markers for both "good" and "bad" cholesterols.

- **Good** High-density lipoprotein (HDL) helps carry cholesterol out of the bloodstream and back to the liver, preventing buildup of plaque in arteries.
- **Bad** Low-density lipoprotein (LDL) is a marker for bad cholesterol. It carries cholesterol out into the bloodstream from the liver, where it can then build up to form plaque.

Healthy cholesterol levels are associated with a low likelihood of developing atherosclerotic cardiovascular disease. It is important that you discuss other risk factors for atherosclerotic cardiovascular disease (such as high blood pressure, smoking and diabetes) with your clinician when determining the best target cholesterol levels for you.

The total cholesterol level takes into account the amount carried in HDL, LDL, and other non-HDL lipoproteins. Ideally, you want

Healthy blood flow

High cholesterol

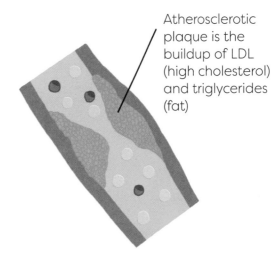

Atherosclerotic plaque is the buildup of LDL (high cholesterol) and triglycerides (fat)

"Good" HDL carries cholesterol out of blood and into the liver

"Bad" LDL carries cholesterol out of liver and into blood where it can form plaques

higher levels of good HDL cholesterol and lower levels of triglycerides and bad LDL cholesterol.

Cholesterol levels can be obtained through fasting or non-fasting blood tests. These numbers represent healthy cholesterol levels (measured in milligrams per deciliter or mg/dL):
- Total cholesterol levels of 200 mg/dL or less
- LDL cholesterol levels of 100 mg/dL or less

Similarly, triglycerides of less than 175mg/dL are associated with lower cardiovascular risk.

CAN HIGH CHOLESTEROL BE PREVENTED?

There are several modifiable risk factors for high cholesterol and atherosclerotic cardio-vascular disease that can be targeted through prevention strategies, such as:
- Eating a healthy and balanced diet
- Engaging in regular physical activity (at least 150 minutes a week)
- Losing excess weight
- Quitting smoking
- Maintaining healthy blood pressure and blood sugar levels

In some cases, another underlying condition or medication may cause elevated cholester-ol levels, and treatment of the condition will help lower cholesterol.

HOW IS HIGH CHOLESTEROL TREATED?

There are a few different treatment options for people with high cholesterol, and the decision to start medications depends on a person's age, risk of atherosclerotic cardio-vascular disease and the presence of other conditions, such as diabetes.

Lifestyle changes

If you do not have atherosclerotic cardiovascular disease, the first step to lower your cholesterol is to focus on lifestyle changes, primarily increasing aerobic exercise and switching to a heart-healthy diet that is:

- Low in added sugar
- Low in saturated fat (such as red meats)
- High in fiber-rich vegetables and fruits
- High in whole grains
- High in plant-based proteins
- High in healthy fats (from olive oil, fish and nuts)

Statins

If lifestyle changes are not enough or you already have atherosclerosis, medications may be needed to lower cholesterol. Statins are the first-line class of medications used to treat high cholesterol. While statins have been around for a long time and there is a lot of data to support their effectiveness and safety, some people do experience side effects with statins. The main side effect to watch for is muscle pain and cramping (myopathy). If you experience muscle pain at any point after starting a statin, talk to your clinician about next steps. It is also important to note that statins are unsafe to use during pregnancy.

Other medications

Other less commonly used medications to lower cholesterol include ezetimibe, bile acid resins, bempedoic acid and a newer class of injectable medications called PC-SK9-inhibitors. Fibrates and certain formulations of omega-3 fatty acids are medications used to treat high triglycerides and can help lower LDL levels as well. Some medications, such as niacin, raise HDL levels. However, it is not recommended to take medications solely for the purpose of raising HDL, as there is no evidence that this leads to improved outcomes. Work with your clinician to decide whether to start a cholesterol-lowering medication and which medication or medications may be the best choice.

Dietary supplements

Natural cholesterol-lowering therapies do exist, but data on these treatment options is limited. Some evidence suggests that certain dietary supplements may help lower either total cholesterol or LDL levels. These include stanols and sterols, flaxseed, soy, green tea, garlic, oats and oat bran. Red yeast rice has been found to contain a chemical called monacolin K that is used in one type of statin medication. However, dietary supplements with red yeast rice do not contain levels high enough to have an effect on cholesterol levels.

Dietary supplements are generally not recommended as a replacement for cholesterol-lowering medications, and there are several side effects that can occur from using these dietary supplements. If you are interested in trying these natural therapies, discuss their safety with your health clinician.

WHY DOES HIGH CHOLESTEROL MATTER FOR WOMEN?

Although women generally have higher levels of good HDL cholesterol at younger ages, they can develop high cholesterol later in life or have worsening disease at older ages. These changes may result from the decline of estrogen after menopause; estrogen is thought to protect against high cholesterol. Premature menopause increases the risk of high cholesterol and atherosclerotic cardiovascular disease.

There are also conditions associated with pregnancy that increase risk of atherosclerotic cardiovascular disease, including high blood pressure or elevated blood sugar during pregnancy, preeclampsia (a combination of high blood pressure, swelling in the legs or feet, and protein in the urine), and preterm deliveries.

Unfortunately, clinicians have historically treated and prescribed medications differently for women than for men. Compared with men, women with high cholesterol are less likely to be treated and are less likely to achieve cholesterol goals after starting cholesterol-lowering medications. For all of these reasons, it is really important that you ask your clinician about your risk of atherosclerotic cardiovascular disease and engage in shared decision making to identify the best treatment strategy.

QUESTIONS TO ASK YOUR HEALTH CARE TEAM ABOUT HIGH CHOLESTEROL

- What lifestyle changes can I make to reduce my chances of developing high cholesterol?
- What is my risk of developing atherosclerotic cardiovascular disease?
- Based on my cholesterol levels and risk factors for cardiovascular disease, should I be taking a cholesterol-lowering medication?

If your clinician recommends taking a lipid-lowering medication
- What side effects should I look out for?
- How much should I expect my cholesterol levels to change after starting this medication?

PEARLS OF WISDOM

Women should feel empowered knowing that high cholesterol is most often preventable through healthy lifestyle choices. Making these healthier choices doesn't mean you have to completely restructure your life — you don't have to run marathons or eat only broccoli and carrots for every meal. Find ways to slightly modify recipes you love to cook so you can reduce the cholesterol content. Try different types of physical activity to get a few more steps into your daily routine. Start small! This will make you more successful in the long term, and over time these choices will become easier.

If you find out that you have high cholesterol, don't panic! The treatments for high cholesterol have been around for a long time and are effective. Ask your health care team about which option is best for you based on your cholesterol levels and risk factors. Following your health care team's recommendations and incorporating healthy choices into your everyday life will keep you healthy and reduce your risk of heart disease.

"Health care providers must take an active role in reducing gender-based health inequities; it starts with empowering women with accurate information about their health."

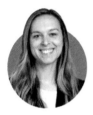

Ellen K. Brinza, M.S., M.P.H. - she/her
Ellen is a medical student at Cleveland Clinic Lerner College of Medicine of Case Western Reserve University. She is currently applying to internal medicine residency programs, with an interest in global health and mitigation of health disparities.

"As women, we often put the need of others before our own, but self-care when it comes to our health is the most important means of preservation and empowerment."

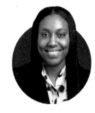

Khendi White Solaru, M.D. - she/her
Dr. White Solaru is a board-certified cardiologist and vascular medicine specialist at University Hospitals in Cleveland, Ohio, and an assistant professor of medicine at Case Western Reserve University School of Medicine. Her academic interest is in preventive cardiology, vascular disease, women's health, and health care disparities.

36

Hip osteoarthritis

Christina Liu, M.D., and Antonia F. Chen, M.D., M.B.A.

WHAT IS HIP OSTEOARTHRITIS?

Osteoarthritis, sometimes called "wear-and-tear arthritis," is a very common condition many people develop as they age, usually over the age of 60. In fact, of the 100-plus types of arthritis, osteoarthritis is the most common. Different types of arthritis are caused by different things, but overall the term arthritis refers to pain and stiffness in joints — the areas of the body where two or more bones meet to allow movement.

Osteoarthritis is the wear and tear of joints caused by physical overuse or injury, which results in pain and stiffness. Osteoarthritis can occur in any joint in the body, but the hip is the second-most impacted joint due to osteoarthritis (the first is the knee; see Chapter 39). The hip is a ball-and-socket joint that usually moves easily due to cartilage, a natural cushion that absorbs shock and protects our bones against impact. Cartilage is not as flexible as muscle but is less rigid than bone. Its placement in the hip joint enables movement by allowing the femoral head (the ball at the top portion of your thigh bone) to roll easily within the acetabulum (the socket, located in your pelvis). As the cartilage starts to wear down or get damaged over many years, bone-on-bone friction develops, causing the joint to become inflamed, swollen and scarred.

Hip osteoarthritis is a chronic disease that usually develops slowly and worsens over a period of months or years, although sudden onset is also possible. In hip osteoarthritis the most common symptom is pain, particularly in your groin or thigh and radiating to your buttocks or your knee. The pain can make it hard to do everyday activities, such as bending over to tie a shoe, rising from a chair or taking a short walk. Pain and stiffness may be worse in the morning or after sitting or resting. Over time painful symptoms may occur more frequently, including during rest or at night. Additional symptoms may include "locking" or "sticking" of the joint, a grinding noise (crepitus) during movement, and decreased range of motion in the hip that affects the ability to walk and may cause a limp.

CAN HIP OSTEOARTHRITIS BE PREVENTED?

Sometimes. There are some risk factors for hip osteoarthritis that you can't control. But there also are changes you can make to reduce your risk.

Healthy hip joint vs. osteoarthritis

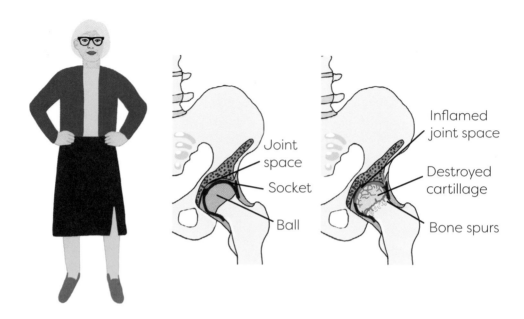

Joint space

Socket

Ball

Inflamed joint space

Destroyed cartillage

Bone spurs

Risk factors you can't control

Certain factors that increase your risk of developing hip osteoarthritis cannot be modified, reversed or halted, including the following.

Hip dysplasia This condition occurs when someone is born with abnormal hip alignment, meaning that the ball is not perfectly centered in the socket. Females are more likely to be affected by this condition, which is often identified at birth during the newborn physical exam. However, for some women, the diagnosis is made later in life on an X-ray of the hip. Over many decades, this malalignment can cause early erosion of the cartilage in the hip, leading to hip osteoarthritis.

Avascular necrosis This condition, also called osteonecrosis, occurs when the blood supply to the ball part of the hip joint is interrupted and the cartilage slowly suffocates and dies.

This can happen randomly, after a traumatic event that damages the hip, due to other medical conditions or, rarely, due to medications such as steroids.

STEPS TO REDUCE YOUR RISK

Fortunately, you can take the following steps to reduce your risk of developing hip osteoarthritis.

Exercise Many studies have demonstrated that loss of muscle strength is related to the development of hip and knee osteoarthritis. Strong gluteus (butt) and quadriceps (thigh) muscles help absorb some of the stress passing through your hip joint. As women age and go through menopause, we lose both muscle tone and bone density, which predisposes us to osteoarthritis, fractures and cardiovascular disease.

Maintain a healthy weight and body mass index While many of the studies looking at osteoarthritis and weight in women have been performed in the knee, some studies suggest that weight is also a factor in the development of hip osteoarthritis. The effect of obesity on hip osteoarthritis is not nearly as strong as it is on the development or prevention of knee osteoarthritis. However, fat cells in the body contribute to inflammation, which can speed up cartilage destruction and thus contribute to hip arthritis.

Eat a healthy diet Nutrition and food play a significant role in how our bodies respond to stress. Proteins, calcium and vitamins provide the building blocks to fight infection and build stronger muscles and bones. In contrast, excess fats are associated with creating more inflammation.

HOW IS HIP OSTEOARTHRITIS TREATED?

Osteoarthritis is usually diagnosed with an X-ray of the hip and pelvis. Occasionally an MRI scan is required. The X-ray helps the physician evaluate the amount of joint damage, such as the amount of joint space remaining or the amount of bone being formed or resorbed by the body in response to irritation. Taking into account a person's symptoms, and the severity of pain, osteoarthritis is classified as mild, moderate or severe. If you're diagnosed with hip osteoarthritis, your doctor may recommend one or more of several types of treatments.

Mild to moderate hip osteoarthritis

For mild to moderate hip osteoarthritis, the following steps may help.

Ice or heat Hip osteoarthritis commonly affects the surrounding muscles. Ice can help reduce muscle swelling, and heat can help relax the muscles and provide some pain relief. Often, however, ice and heat alone are not sufficient to treat the symptoms of hip osteoarthritis.

Activity modification Your doctor may recommend reducing activity that aggravates your hip or avoiding motions that increase hip arthritis pain, such as squatting and lunging. Taking time to rest your hip also can help decrease hip pain. Your doctor may recommend using assistive walking devices, such as a cane. Recent data has shown that using a cane in the hand opposite of the arthritic hip can help redistribute body weight back to the center of the body rather than completely transmitting stress through the arthritic hip when taking a step. For example, if the left hip is affected, the cane would go in the right hand and be used when the left leg takes a step.

Oral pain medication Nonprescription pain medication, including nonsteroidal anti-inflammatory medications (NSAIDs) such as ibuprofen (Advil, others) and naproxen (Aleve) can help reduce joint inflammation. These medications require good kidney function and should be taken with food to minimize stomach irritation. Around-the-clock NSAIDs for two weeks can be helpful in reducing joint inflammation and pain. Although acetaminophen (Tylenol) can help reduce pain, it is not an anti-inflammatory medication. Your clinician may recommend alternating use of acetaminophen and NSAIDs if NSAIDs alone don't provide sufficient pain relief.

Exercise Strengthening and stretching the gluteal and leg muscles and practicing tai chi have been shown to help alleviate some of the pain from hip osteoarthritis. Muscle training and physical therapy prior to hip replacement surgery is often encouraged to help speed up post-surgical recovery. These activities can also help with weight loss.

Injections A doctor can inject corticosteroids (a category of prescribed drugs that reduce inflammation) into the hip to offer temporary relief of symptoms. Injections can be a great option for someone who wants to delay surgery and can serve as a diagnostic tool to help confirm that the hip is the true source of pain. Injections can also help predict the amount of pain relief you can expect after full recovery from a total hip replacement surgery, though this can be imprecise. However, injections too close to the time of hip replacement can increase the risk of infection after surgery. While injections can help with pain management, they do not cure or reverse the underlying arthritis.

Severe hip osteoarthritis

Women with severe hip osteoarthritis often benefit from total hip replacement, also called total hip arthroplasty. While there are few risks with this surgery, rare complications, such as fractures (breaks in the bone), infections and dislocations (the ball coming out of the socket) can be severe. There is no scientific way to predict the right time to have a hip replacement surgery. The decision is personal and should only be made after you have tried nonoperative treatments, have found the right orthopedic surgeon and have had all your questions answered.

Unlike knee replacements, which are mostly performed through the same type of incision, hip replacement can be done through several types of incisions (front, side, back), each of which is each associated with its own risks and benefits. It's important that your surgeon be experienced and comfortable with the specific approach to the hip replacement surgery being used and that you understand the risks and benefits of that approach. It's also important for you to find a surgeon who listens to you.

Research has shown that, overall, people do well after total hip replacement and can expect to return to work and physical activity after three to six months. In general, people with stronger muscles and a lower body mass index (a measure of obesity) prior to surgery return to activities faster after surgery compared to those who have weaker muscles and a higher body mass index.

WHY DOES HIP OSTEOARTHRITIS MATTER TO WOMEN?

Recent research has shown that women are more likely to have arthritis than men are, and more women undergo joint replacement surgery. In fact, almost twice as many women undergo both hip and knee replacements compared to men. Women are also more likely to have higher risk factors for developing hip arthritis, including hip dysplasia, which affects more newborn females than males. In addition, women have more rheumatoid and inflammatory arthritis compared to men, at a rate of 9 to 1. Moreover, men and women have different bone quality, size and anatomy, which needs to be considered when performing a total hip replacement.

Despite the fact that women are more likely to be predisposed to conditions affecting hip function, they are less likely to be referred to an orthopedic surgeon and less likely to be offered hip replacement surgery. Furthermore, women are often primary caretakers of other family members and often delay their own treatment — particularly surgeries requiring long recovery — to care for others. Unfortunately, delaying surgery often means that women have lost more muscle mass at the time of surgery because they have been unable to exercise for longer periods of time due to hip pain. Thus, it's important to see your clinician if you're having difficulties with your hips to maximize your quality of life and long-term health.

QUESTIONS TO ASK YOUR HEALTH CARE TEAM ABOUT HIP OSTEOARTHRITIS

- Can I do something to help prevent my hip arthritis from getting worse?
- How safe is it for me to take NSAIDs?
- Will you screen me for depression?
  › *Depression is associated with less favorable treatment outcomes after total hip replacement surgery. Please make sure you are screened, as not everyone recognizes when they're depressed, and seek treatment for depression if appropriate.*
- Could my pain be coming from my knee or back (spine)?
- If you are overweight or experience obesity:
  › Can you help me with weight loss?

› Should I see a dietitian?
› Would I benefit from seeing a behavioral therapist to help me understand (and overcome) barriers to adopting healthier behaviors?
› Can you help me set goals and stay with me on this journey?

For mild to moderate disease
- If a hip joint injection is recommended, how beneficial might it be?
- What is the next step(s) if the injection doesn't help?

For moderately severe and severe disease
- Is my pain and joint damage bad enough to undergo surgery?
- Are there options other than surgery?
- Can we use a shared decision-making tool to help me understand if my personal goals support proceeding with surgery?

If the decision is to not have surgery
- Do you think I will eventually need surgery?
- If I delay surgery, how will that impact me later?

If the decision is to have surgery
- What can I do to decrease my risks of complications?
- Should I take iron or vitamin supplements prior to surgery?
- Will exercises prior to surgery help?
- What strategies should I use to minimize my risk of infection?
- How many hip replacements have you (the surgeon) done?
- Are there differences in risks or length of recovery with how you (the surgeon)

perform hip replacements versus how your colleagues perform them?

- How will my pain be managed after the surgery?
- Will I go home the same day, or stay in the hospital?
- Is it safe for me to go home the same day?
- How will I contact the surgical team if I have concerns after the operation and before my next scheduled visit?
  - › *This is particularly important because patients are increasingly going home the same day of surgery or only spending one night in the hospital.*

PEARLS OF WISDOM

Hip arthritis and pain can drastically affect your quality of life and overall health. Joint pain leads to decreased physical activity and increased weight gain, which then perpetuates a vicious cycle of reduced activity and further weight gain, ultimately resulting in severe hip and knee osteoarthritis. Furthermore, pain itself can be a risk factor for depression. Immobility and weight gain can lead to diabetes, heart disease and hypertension. Thus, it is critical to address joint arthritis and pain early on to maximize health, happiness and overall quality of life.

"A family is only as strong as the health of the women."

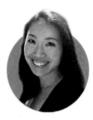

Christina Liu, M.D. - she/her
Dr. Liu is currently a third-year resident at the Harvard Combined Ortho-paedic Residency Program in Boston, Massachusetts.

"Women need to take care of their health, as they are always taking care of others."

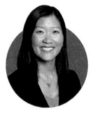

Antonia F. Chen, M.D., M.B.A. - she/her
Dr. Chen is currently an Associate Professor at Harvard Medical School and the Director of Arthro-plasty Research at Brigham and Women's Hospital. She specializes in total hip and knee arthroplasty.

36
Hip labral tear

Margaret L. Wright, M.D., and Sommer Hammoud, M.D.

WHAT IS A HIP LABRAL TEAR?

The hip is a ball and socket joint that consists of the ball (femoral head) and the socket (acetabulum). The ball remains securely in the socket because it is a deep bony socket. Additionally, there is a ring of tissue around the edge of the socket, called the labrum, which deepens the socket and creates a suction effect around the ball, holding it more securely in the socket.

Sometimes extra bone tissue that grows in the ball and socket joint causes a hip labral tear. The extra bone can develop because of repetitive activity, or it can just be a part of someone's normal anatomy. The extra bone may cause the labrum to get pinched when the hip is brought into positions associated with more inward rotation and flexion. Repeated pinching can lead to the degeneration and fraying of the labrum, causing it to

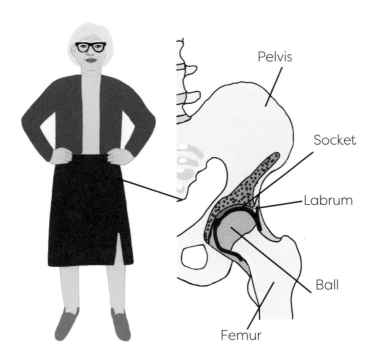

Pelvis

Socket

Labrum

Ball

Femur

Extra bone growth leading to hip impingement

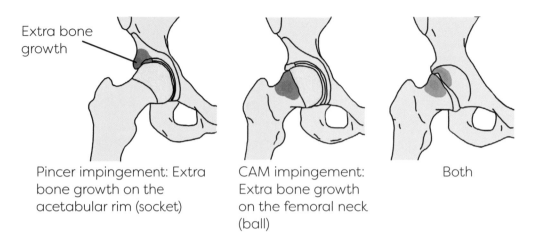

Extra bone growth

Pincer impingement: Extra bone growth on the acetabular rim (socket)

CAM impingement: Extra bone growth on the femoral neck (ball)

Both

tear away from the bone underneath it. The result is a hip labral tear. The pinching itself is called femoroacetabular impingement (FAI).

When the extra bone growth causing FAI occurs on the ball, it is called cam impingement. When the extra bone occurs on the socket rim, it is called pincer impingement. When it occurs on both the ball and socket, it is called combined or mixed impingement.

Another reason that hip labral tears occur is because a person's hip socket is too shallow (hip dysplasia). When the socket is shallower than usual, it does not hold the ball as securely in the joint. When the hip moves into positions that stress it, the labrum must work harder to hold the ball in the socket to prevent the hip joint from becoming unstable. Over time, this strain can cause the labrum to tear.

CAN A HIP LABRAL TEAR BE PREVENTED?

Hip labral tears are not easily prevented. One way to potentially prevent them is to avoid activities that repeatedly place the hip in extreme inward rotation and flexion, such as yoga, ballet, hockey and rowing. However, not all tears result from these activities, and not all people who do these activities will develop a hip labral tear. Everyone can benefit from exercises that stretch and strengthen the muscles around the hips, thighs, core and lower back. Your clinician can recommend exercises or direct you to a physical therapist who can help you strengthen these muscles and keep your hips healthy.

HOW IS A HIP LABRAL TEAR TREATED?

Before treating a hip labral tear, your clinician will want to make sure that a hip labral tear is what's causing your pain. A hip labral tear is not necessarily the main reason someone might have hip pain. Studies have shown that many people who have hip labral tears are completely pain-free. The diagnosis of a hip labral tear as the main cause of hip pain can be very challenging. There are many potential causes of pain around the hip that can mimic a labral tear. In addition, FAI sometimes leads to pain in the lower back or other areas near the hip, symptoms that are associated with many other conditions.

To help determine if the hip labral tear is the main source of your hip pain, your clinician will perform a history and physical exam, as well as order X-rays, and maybe also an ultrasound or MRI. If the hip labral tear is the primary source of pain, it can be treated without surgery or with surgery.

Nonsurgical treatment

Two or more of these nonsurgical treatments are usually used at the same time, as they can work together to improve symptoms in the hip.

Rest and activity modification Often the first course of treatment for a person with FAI and a hip labral tear is rest, with activity modifications (when possible) to avoid placing the hip in positions that worsen the pain. Rest allows the inflammation in the hip to improve while the tear is not being frequently pinched and aggravated.

Anti-inflammatory medications Nonsteroidal anti-inflammatory drugs (NSAIDs) such as ibuprofen (Motrin, Advil) and naproxen (Aleve) can help reduce inflammation and relieve pain in the hip joint. However, these are not long-term treatment solutions but just short-term fixes to use during activities such as exercise. Anti-inflammatory medications can help in the short term, while other treatment options, such as physical therapy and injections, are starting to work.

Physical therapy Physical therapy is an important part of any treatment regimen for FAI that is associated with a hip labral tear. Physical therapy targets the muscles around the hip, as well as the core and lower back muscles, improving the mobility, strength and balance of these muscles. This in turn improves the biomechanics of the joint and protects the hip labrum and cartilage. Physical therapy is important even if you're expecting to have surgery to treat the tear. It's also important for preventing pain even after symptoms improve.

Injections Injections are a useful treatment for hip labral tears because they can help diagnose the specific source of pain. Injections can also help predict how well certain surgical treatments might work. Usually ultrasound or X-ray is used to make sure that the injection is going into the hip joint. In younger people, lidocaine, a numbing medicine, is often injected alone. In older adults, lidocaine is injected with cortisone, an anti-inflammatory medication that works over the course of a few weeks and provides longer pain relief. Other therapies, such as platelet-rich plasma and stem cell injections, which are quite costly, have not proven to be effective for people with a hip labral tear. We typically do not recommend them as a treatment for hip labral tears.

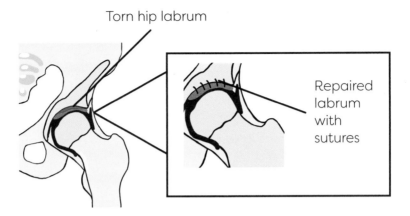

Torn hip labrum

Repaired labrum with sutures

Surgical treatment

There are several surgical options that may be considered for treatment of a hip labral tear.

Hip arthroscopy with labral repair Hip arthroscopy involves inserting a camera through a small incision into the hip joint. Two other small incisions are made to place instruments into the hip to perform the labral repair surgery. The camera is used to examine the labrum and determine the size of the tear and the quality of the remaining labral tissue. In most cases, particularly in younger people, the labrum is partially torn away from the underlying bone in the area where it is being pinched. In this case, the area (either on the femoral neck, acetabular rim or both) where the bone is overgrown is shaved down with a burr. This procedure is called an osteoplasty. Typically, X-ray imaging is used in the operating room so that the surgeon can see when enough bone has been removed. The labrum is then repaired back to the acetabular rim using anchors in the bone, with stitches (sutures) going around the labrum and holding the labrum tightly onto the bone, where it heals.

Hip arthroscopy with labral debridement For people with a degenerative labral tear that is too small or unlikely to heal after a repair, the labrum can be debrided, or trimmed down, so that there are no loose flaps that can catch and cause pain as the hip moves. This problem is relatively uncommon but can sometimes happen in hips with early arthritis.

For younger people without arthritis who have a labrum that cannot be repaired, the treatment is sometimes debridement with a labral reconstruction, which involves using cadaver labral tissue to make a new labrum. This is a challenging procedure and is only done when your own labrum is not functioning well and labral repair is not possible.

Open surgery There are a few scenarios in which traditional open surgery, which involves a larger incision, is needed to address a labral tear. One such scenario occurs when the tear or bone overgrowth involves a larger portion of the acetabular rim or femoral neck that cannot be reached with an arthroscopic procedure.

The other scenario occurs when a person has acetabular dysplasia, or a shallow acetabulum. Many people with a labral tear have what is considered borderline dysplasia, with findings of both FAI and dysplasia. For these individuals, treatment is not straightforward and may include either arthroscopic or open surgery. Open surgery may be the best option if arthroscopic surgery has already been attempted and pain recurs.

For people with more significant dysplasia, repairing the labrum arthroscopically does not fix the underlying problem of dysplasia, and an open surgery called periacetabular osteotomy (PAO) is performed. During this surgery, the surgeon cuts the pelvic bone around the acetabulum and redirects the acetabulum to provide more coverage of the femoral head and essentially create a deeper socket. If needed, a labral tear or extra bone on the femoral neck can be treated through the same incision.

Hip replacement The procedures already mentioned only relieve pain effectively in people without significant arthritis. When significant hip arthritis is also present, total hip replacement may be a consideration.

WHY DOES A HIP LABRAL TEAR MATTER TO WOMEN?

Women more commonly have the pincer type of impingement, which results from extra bone on the rim of the acetabular socket alone. Women are also more likely to have loose joints caused by flexibility of the soft tissues surrounding the hip and other joints in the body, a characteristic known as ligamentous laxity. People with ligamentous laxity and a labral tear are more likely to require a tightening of the hip capsule as part of their surgical treatment. A recent study found that with appropriate labral and capsular treatment, people with ligamentous laxity do just as well after surgery as people without ligamentous laxity and can have good surgical outcomes. The cam type of impingement that results from extra bone on the femoral head (the ball), as well as the mixed type of impingement with extra bone on the femoral head and acetabulum, occur at similar rates in men and women.

Outcomes after hip labral repair surgery are most closely associated with a person's age at the time of surgery. Younger people tend to get back to their sports and usual activities after surgery, but adults older than 40 to 50 are more likely to have underlying arthritis and have less satisfactory results after hip arthroscopy. Older adults are also more likely than younger people to undergo a total hip replacement within 5 to 10 years of their hip arthroscopic surgery.

Some studies have shown that women may have worse outcomes after arthroscopic hip surgery than men do, but women also tend to seek care for hip labral tears at an older age than men. Because studies more consistently demonstrate that age at surgery correlates with outcomes, it is likely that age is a much more important factor than sex when thinking about the results of hip arthroscopy.

QUESTIONS TO ASK YOUR HEALTH CARE TEAM ABOUT HIP LABRAL TEARS

If you have a hip labral tear
- Is the labral tear the primary source of my hip pain?
- Do I have arthritis that may be contributing to my pain?
- What types of exercises can I do to strengthen the muscles around my hip and improve my symptoms?
- What types of activities should I avoid in order to prevent my pain from worsening?

If surgery is chosen to treat the hip labral tear
- How often do you (the surgeon) do this type of surgery?
- What types of outcomes are typical for someone like me?
- How quickly should I expect to be back to my usual activities?

PEARLS OF WISDOM

Labral tears of the hip usually result from a larger process in the hip, most commonly femoroacetabular impingement (FAI). This occurs when the labrum is pinched between extra bone on the femur or the acetabular rim during hip motion, which causes tearing over time.

There are many causes of hip pain, and not all labral tears identified on MRI are the source of hip pain. Your doctor will consider your symptoms and physical exam, as well as imaging and a possible injection, to help decide if the labral tear is causing your pain and how well it might respond to surgical treatment. Even when the surgery is minimally invasive, it should not be taken lightly, as it is not the correct treatment for every person with a hip labral tear.

Physical therapy to develop strong core, back, thigh and hip muscles is very important to help prevent and treat pain from a labral tear.

"Women should feel empowered to play an active role in their health and health care."

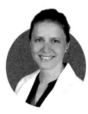

Margaret L. Wright, M.D. - she/her
Dr. Wright is a pediatric orthopedic surgeon at the Nicklaus Children's Hospital in Miami, Florida. She specializes in the treatment of fractures and sports injuries in children and young adults.

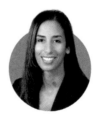

Sommer Hammoud, M.D. - she/her
Dr. Hammoud is an orthopedic surgeon at Rothman Orthopaedics and an associate professor of orthopedic surgery at Thomas Jefferson University Hospital in Philadelphia, Pennsylvania.

38
Irritable bowel syndrome

Asma Khapra, M.D., FAGA

WHAT IS IRRITABLE BOWEL SYNDROME?

Irritable bowel syndrome (IBS) is a functional disorder, which means the disorder affects how your gut functions but doesn't result in any physical irregularities of the gastrointestinal (GI) tract. IBS is a very common condition, estimated to affect 10% to 15% of the population in the United States. While IBS does not result in long-term medical complications, its symptoms can significantly impact your quality of life.

The symptoms of IBS include abdominal pain or bloating as well as bowel difficulties. The bowel difficulties can range from constipation to diarrhea or in some cases mixed diarrhea and constipation. Other symptoms include urgency (a sudden, strong urge to empty the bowels), incomplete emptying of the bowels and passage of mucus during bowel movements. These symptoms are long-term, lasting at least six months. IBS is diagnosed when your symptoms meet these criteria without any other alarm signs, such as GI bleeding, weight loss or anemia, which may need further evaluation.

CAN IRRITABLE BOWEL SYNDROME BE PREVENTED?

No. Unfortunately, there is currently no method for preventing IBS.

IBS is often viewed as a multifactorial disorder, meaning that many factors contribute to the development of the condition. Medical researchers and doctors know that there is a "brain-gut axis," which describes how chemical changes in the brain can cause symptoms in the GI tract, such as abdominal pain and bowel changes. Often these brain chemical changes result from stress or anxiety. Researchers currently believe that someone who has a genetic predisposition for IBS may develop the condition after experiencing a triggering event, such as a period of emotional stress or an infection. This event triggers the nerves in the gut to become more sensitive, leading to IBS.

Although there is no prevention strategy, there are lifestyle changes you can make to promote good digestive health, which can improve the likelihood of your gut feeling better. These include eating lots of fruits, vegetables and other healthy foods; exercising regularly; drinking plenty of water; and reducing stress. Some people with IBS feel better when they avoid certain foods. However, there's no clear evidence yet that specific foods or the gut microbiome (the microorganisms, including bacteria, that live in the digestive tract) are directly linked to the development of IBS. Study of the gut microbiome is an exciting area of research, and more information is becoming available every day.

HOW IS IBS TREATED?

If you're diagnosed with IBS, your doctor or clinician may recommend one or more of these treatment options.

Diet

Two-thirds of people with IBS feel that their symptoms are triggered by food. Therefore, dietary modifications are a major mainstay of treatment. The traditional wisdom of avoiding dairy, sugary foods, fried foods, spicy foods, caffeine and alcohol has been a longstanding recommendation for IBS. However, many people find that avoiding certain foods is not enough on its own to improve their symptoms. Thus, adding high-fiber foods to your diet or taking a fiber supplement may be beneficial. For example, studies show that taking the fiber supplement psyllium greatly improves IBS symptoms.

Aim for a fiber intake of about 25 grams per day. Foods such as fruits, vegetables, whole grains and legumes are examples of fiber-rich foods that can help you attain that goal. Keep in mind that if you add large quantities of fiber too quickly, you can develop side effects of bloating and cramping. Increasing fiber very gradually is a key strategy. It's also important to realize that fiber works best when there is adequate water, so be sure to also increase your water intake.

If you have difficulty tolerating a high-fiber diet or your symptoms persist, your clinician may recommend a low FODMAP diet. The term FODMAP is an acronym for Fermentable Oligosaccharides, Disaccharides, Monosaccharides, And Polyols. FODMAPs are complex carbohydrates that are not completely digested in the gut. Foods that contain FODMAPs may contribute to IBS symptoms by causing abdominal gas, pain, bloating and diarrhea.

A low FODMAP diet starts with a six-week elimination of FODMAPs to see if there is an improvement in symptoms. If you don't see a benefit, the diet should be stopped. If you experience symptom relief on the low FODMAP diet, you then slowly reintroduce individual foods to your diet, noticing which foods contribute to your symptoms. This strategy allows you to design a diet best suitable for you. One caution regarding elimination diets: Be careful to avoid creating severe and long-term food restrictions. An overly restrictive diet can lead to other problems, such as eating disorders or malnutrition, as well as changes to the gut microbiome. It's always helpful to undertake this type of diet with the help of a knowledgeable dietician.

FODMAP Diet

Food type	Avoid	Choose
Fruits	Apples	Bananas
	Apricots	Blueberries
	Avocado	Cantaloupe
	Blackberries	Cranberries
	Cherries	Grapes
	Canned fruit	Grapefruit
	Dried fruit	Honeydew
	Fruit juice	Kiwi
	Peaches	Lemons
	Pears	Limes
	Plums	Mandarins
	Lychee	Oranges
	Mangos	Passionfruit
	Watermelon	Raspberries
		Strawberries
		Pineapple
Vegetables	Asparagus	Artichokes
	Beetroot	Bamboo shoots
	Broccoli	Bok choy
	Brussel sprouts	Carrots
	Cabbage	Celery
	Eggplant	Ginger
	Okra	Green beans
	Mushrooms	Lettuce
	Rhubarb	Olives
	Garlic	Parsnips
	Onion	Potatoes
		Pumpkin
		Spinach
		Squash (yellow)
		Sweet potatoes
		Tomatoes
		Turnips
		Zucchini
		Cucumbers

FODMAP Diet, continued

Food type	Avoid	Choose
Dairy	Milk with lactose	Lactose-free milk
	Yogurt	Lactose-free yogurt
	Ice cream	Sorbet
	Soft cheeses	Hard cheeses
Starch	Popcorn	Gluten-free bread
	Tortilla chips	Rice
		Oats
		Quinoa
		Muffins
Proteins	Beans	Almonds
	Chickpeas	Peanuts
	Lentils	Salmon
	Sausages	Eggs
	Fried fish	Chicken
	Breaded meat	Tofu

Medications

In the past we have solely relied on diet, but over the last decade we have seen great progress in available medications and therapies for IBS. The goal of medications is to improve your symptoms and therefore quality of life. Nonprescription options for treatment include anti-diarrheal medications to reduce diarrhea, and laxatives to relieve constipation. If you experience abdominal pain, your clinician may recommend a prescription antispasmodic medication, which decreases cramping of the gut. Recent research suggests that peppermint oil, in doses of 200 mg taken three times per day, can be another effective option. At times, probiotics can also be helpful in symptom relief, particularly with bloating.

If these treatments fail to provide relief, other prescription drugs may be an option. Your clinician may prescribe antibiotic medications for a short period of time, directed at altering the gut microbiome. Alternatively, some medications, including antidepressants, are directed at the "brain-gut axis" and help decrease hormonal surges related to IBS. Antidepressants can improve abdominal pain and regulate bowel habits to correct either diarrhea or constipation. Another helpful treatment may be prescription medications that change how quickly or slowly food moves through the GI tract, with multiple options available for both constipation and diarrhea.

Complementary and alternative medicine (CAM)

CAM options have been used widely for IBS. If you're not satisfied with the pharmacologic options above or prefer to use a more holistic approach, CAM may be a great fit. These treatments include:

- Herbal remedies (such as aloe vera)
- Dietary supplements (such as curcumin)
- Mind-body-based interventions (GI-focused psychological therapies, such as cognitive behavioral therapy and hypnosis)
- Body-based interventions (massage-type therapies)
- Energy-healing therapies (acupuncture)

Current research into the benefits of all CAM options for IBS shows mixed results. However, studies suggests that all of the methods in the preceding list have characteristics that may promote improvement in general IBS symptoms and quality of life. Interestingly, these therapies may benefit you even if you don't respond to medications, and relief can last up to 12 months or more. In particular, mind-body treatments,

including cognitive behavioral therapy and hypnosis, have been shown to relieve abdominal pain and improve general well-being.

If you're interested in pursuing these treatment strategies, consult your clinician to discuss which CAM options would be a good fit for you.

WHY DOES IBS MATTER TO WOMEN?

As you've read, IBS is very common in the United States, but it is twice as prevalent in women versus men. The condition most often develops in women between the ages of 20 and 40, which are the key times for women to bear children.

Symptoms can adversely affect quality of life, sometimes to a severe degree. As a result, women with IBS may experience both a financial and a health care burden. But more notably, studies show that IBS can cause problems with sexual intercourse, difficulty leaving the house and traveling, and difficulty coping and concentrating. Women with IBS are also more likely to experience depression and anxiety, reproductive medical conditions (such as endometriosis), bladder problems, sleep disorders, fibromyalgia and chronic fatigue syndrome. As you can see, the burden of IBS symptoms in women can be quite significant. Fortunately, an increasing number of treatment options are available to relieve or reduce the symptoms of IBS and improve quality of life.

QUESTIONS TO ASK YOUR HEALTH CARE TEAM ABOUT IBS

- How do I know I have IBS?
- What are the most effective dietary changes for IBS?
  - › How should I approach them?
- How safe are the medications for IBS and how long can I take them?
  - › Are there alternatives to medication that I may try?
- Should I see someone who specializes in gastrointestinal (GI) psychology to find ways to cope with IBS?
- Are there other conditions I have that have contributed to or been impacted by my IBS?
  - › Will these conditions improve if my IBS improves?
- What lifestyle changes can I make to prevent my IBS symptoms from becoming worse?

PEARLS OF WISDOM

IBS is very common in women and can affect many aspects of life. It's important to seek medical attention from a knowledgeable and patient clinician who will explain the condition, review options and reassure you that this can get better. Establish a diagnosis with your clinician and work on improving your symptoms for a better quality of life. Remember to eat well, avoid your dietary triggers, work on reducing stress and, finally, exercise!

"Women have unique needs in their health care, and understanding these can go a long way in establishing the best care for women."

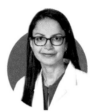

Asma Khapra, M.D., FAGA - she/her
Dr. Khapra is a practicing Gastroenterologist at Gastrohealth in Fairfax, Virginia, and is an Assistant Professor for Clinical Medicine at the University of Virginia School of Medicine. She specializes in women's digestive health and inflammatory bowel disease.

39
Knee osteoarthritis

Mary I. O'Connor, M.D.

WHAT IS KNEE OSTEOARTHRITIS?

Osteoarthritis is the most common form of arthritis, often referred to as a type of "wear-and-tear" arthritis. Osteoarthritis is typically isolated to a specific joint, most commonly impacting large weight-bearing joints, including the knee. In knee osteoarthritis, the normal cushioning tissue (cartilage) in the knee joint gradually wears away.

Cartilage wear can occur as older joints get worn down, if there is added pressure to the joint or if you have experienced a knee injury. As the cartilage erodes away, it becomes rough and frayed, losing elasticity and becoming stiff. When this happens the cartilage can no longer provide adequate cushioning to the bones, which can lead to bone-on-bone rubbing (resulting in bony growths called bone spurs) and the stretching of tendons and ligaments (all resulting in pain).

The thick liquid in joints (synovial fluid) also changes with osteoarthritis. Synovial fluid provides nourishment and lubrication to the cartilage. With osteoarthritis the synovial fluid becomes thinner and less effective. This change in synovial fluid also contributes to cartilage loss and to the symptoms of osteoarthritis, such as pain, stiffness and swelling.

CAN KNEE OSTEOARTHRITIS BE PREVENTED?

Yes, sometimes. If osteoarthritis runs in your family, you are at higher risk of developing the condition. While you can't select your parents, there are things you can do to keep your knee healthy.

Maintain a healthy weight
Obesity is the single biggest factor under our control to change our risk of developing knee osteoarthritis. Every 10 extra pounds of weight puts an additional 30 to 60 pounds of pressure on your knee joint. Moreover, obesity increases inflammation in your body, which can also damage your cartilage. (See Chapter 48.)

Avoid injury
A knee injury can directly damage your cartilage. For example, a torn knee ligament, such as your anterior cruciate ligament (ACL) (see Chapter 10), makes the joint less stable and results in increased stress to the cartilage. More common injuries are tears to the menisci, C-shaped structures between

Healthy knee joint vs. knee with osteoarthritis

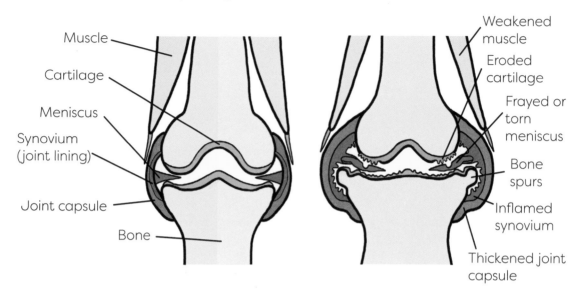

the shinbone and thighbone that help distribute body weight across the cartilage. A meniscus tear puts more stress on your knee joint. Since many meniscal tears cannot be repaired, a common treatment is arthroscopic surgery to trim back the tear. Although this procedure addresses the immediate pain from the torn meniscus, it results in less meniscal tissue and more stress being transferred to your cartilage, increasing the likelihood of developing osteoarthritis. Of course, it may not be possible to avoid all injury to your knee, especially if you're active in sports, but strategies such as neuromuscular training (see Chapter 10), wearing supportive shoes and stretching can help.

Stay active and keep your muscles strong

Motion is lotion for your joints. Your knee joint needs motion to keep it healthy. Strong muscles in your legs, especially your thighs, help protect your knee by promoting joint stability and absorbing some of the stress to the joint. As we age, we have a decline in muscle strength. This is especially common for women after menopause. When the muscles are weak, more stress is transferred to the cartilage, menisci and ligaments.

Eat a healthy diet

We are what we eat. Food impacts our immune system, which influences how much inflammation we have in our body and therefore in our joints. Inflammation in the joints leads to a release of chemicals that damage the cartilage, increasing your risk of developing osteoarthritis. To reduce inflammation, try to minimize your intake of sugar, salt, white flour, saturated fats, egg yolks, red meat and fried foods. Eat more fruits and vegetables and (unsalted) nuts.

Be cautious about nutritional supplements

Many supplemental products claim to help prevent knee osteoarthritis or lessen symptoms by decreasing inflammation. Examples include methylsulfonylmethane (MSM),

S-Adenosyl-L-methionine (SAMe), curcumin, avocado-soybean unsaponifiables (ASUs), glucosamine, chondroitin and fish oil. Unfortunately, the quality of medical research regarding these supplements is limited and often weak. What's more, some supplements may interact negatively with medications you're currently taking. Before trying any new supplement, please remember to always first discuss it with your clinician.

HOW IS KNEE OSTEOARTHRITIS TREATED?

Treatment for knee osteoarthritis can vary depending on the severity of your condition.

Mild to moderate knee osteoarthritis

You can help prevent or slow the progression of knee osteoarthritis by employing the preventive measures discussed in the previous section. Your clinician may also recommend one or more additional measures.

Activity modification Avoiding activities that aggravate your knee pain is commonsense advice. In general, avoiding activities such as running, jumping and other high-impact movements are appropriate. But remember, exercise is medicine. Your knee pain can improve with low-impact exercises like walking, swimming or using an elliptical machine. Modifying your activities does not mean more sitting!

Medications If your pain is preventing you from doing your normal activities or sleeping well at night, the first line of medicines to try are nonprescription drugs such as acetaminophen (Tylenol) and nonsteroidal

anti-inflammatory medications (NSAIDs) such as ibuprofen (Motrin) and naproxen (Aleve). If nonprescription medications are not effective, your clinician may give you a prescription NSAID. But be aware that the risk of side effects with NSAIDs increases with long-term use, including kidney failure, stroke and heart attack. Unfortunately, there is no clear guidance on exactly what "long-term" means. The best recommendation is that NSAIDS should be used at the lowest effective dose for the shortest period of time possible.

Injections Joint injection involves placing a needle into the knee joint to deliver a medication. This procedure is done in your clinician's office. The most common medication injected is cortisone, a powerful anti-inflammatory medication. Newer medications include a time-released type of cortisone, which may provide longer pain relief, and a lubricant medication (a type of hyaluronic acid), which has been shown to help some women. Injections may or may not help, and if they help, the relief may be temporary. If the injection doesn't help, your clinician may recommend focusing on other ways to improve knee pain, such as weight loss, strengthening muscles or other lifestyle measures. New research shows that having prior joint injections increases the risk of infection after knee replacement surgery, so experts generally recommend against receiving multiple knee injections.

Regenerative medicine treatments Regenerative medicine therapies for knee osteoarthritis seek to help the body slow down or stop damage to cartilage and potentially regenerate cartilage. These newer therapies include stem cell injections and platelet-rich plasma injections. Research into their effectiveness is promising but currently inconclusive. Injections of such products may help your pain, but there's no evidence to date that they will result in regeneration of your cartilage.

Acupuncture While acupuncture may decrease your knee symptoms, there is unfortunately no evidence that it slows progression of your knee osteoarthritis.

Severe knee osteoarthritis Women with severe osteoarthritis typically benefit from knee replacement surgery. However, this is a major operation with very uncommon, but not insignificant, risks. Moreover, a knee joint replacement is not as good as the healthy knee joint you had in prior years. So, it's best to try to prevent osteoarthritis. If you require joint replacement, this surgery can really help decrease your pain and improve your function, as advances in surgical care and technique as well as implant designs have improved outcomes.

The most important decision for you is who you select as your surgeon. Find someone who is experienced and, most important, listens to you. You need a surgeon you trust. If you have a problem after the operation, you want to know that your concerns will be heard and not brushed aside.

WHY DOES KNEE OSTEOARTHRITIS MATTER TO WOMEN?

Women experience knee osteoarthritis more often than men do. The condition is more common among Black women than white women. A rise in obesity and sedentary lifestyles has contributed to younger and younger women developing knee osteoarthritis. Young women are also more likely to tear their anterior cruciate ligament (ACL) compared to young men, setting them up for a lifetime risk of knee osteoarthritis. Finally, estrogen may play a role, as arthritis often develops or progresses more significantly after menopause.

Women's bodies are different from men's in ways that lie beyond the differences in reproductive organs. For example, research has revealed biological differences in tissues of women with severe osteoarthritis compared to men with the condition. However, effective therapies targeted toward women with osteoarthritis have not yet been developed. Research has also shown that women have a lower volume of cartilage compared to men — we simply have less cushioning in our knees. Moreover, women develop arthritis in the joint between the kneecap and thigh bone (patellofemoral joint) more than men; differ in how they respond to pain compared to men; and are at higher risk of experiencing chronic pain.

Differences between genders related to knee replacement surgery are also important. Women tend to wait longer than men to have knee replacement surgery and, for that reason, often have more severe osteoarthritis at the time of surgery. Such delays may be related to a woman's challenges in prioritizing her health needs. It's also possible that a woman may not be offered surgery at the same stage of disease as a man. Even with delays, women benefit from surgery — but they typically do not reach the same postoperative level of improvement in pain and physical function as men. Putting off appropriate knee replacement surgery may therefore not be in your best interest.

QUESTIONS TO ASK YOUR HEALTH CARE TEAM ABOUT KNEE OSTEOARTHRITIS

- Can I do something to help prevent my knee arthritis from getting worse?
- How safe is it for me to take NSAIDS?
- Will you screen me for depression?
  - › *Depression is associated with less favorable treatment outcomes among people with knee osteoarthritis, and not everyone recognizes when they're depressed. Please make sure you are screened!*
- If you are overweight or experience obesity:
  - › Can you help me with weight loss?
  - › Should I see a dietician?
  - › Would I benefit from seeing a behavioral therapist to help me understand, and overcome, barriers to adopting healthier behaviors?
  - › Can you help me set goals and stay with me on this journey?

For mild to moderate disease
- If a knee joint injection is recommended, how beneficial might it be?
- What is the next step(s) if the injection doesn't help?

For moderately severe and severe disease
- Is my knee osteoarthritis severe enough for surgery?
- Are there options other than surgery?
- Can we use a shared decision making

tool to help me understand if my personal goals support proceeding with the surgery?

If you decide to not have surgery
- Do you think I will eventually need surgery?
- If I delay surgery, how will that impact me later?

If you decide to have surgery
- What can I do to decrease my risks of complications?
  - › Should I take an iron or vitamin supplement prior to surgery?
  - › Will exercises prior to surgery help?
  - › What do you (the surgeon) do to minimize my risk of complications, especially infection?
  - › What can I do to minimize my risk of complications?
- How many knee replacements have you (the surgeon) done?
- How will my pain be managed after the surgery?
- How will I contact the surgical team if I have concerns after the operation and before my next scheduled visit?
  - › *This is particularly important because people are increasingly going home the same day of surgery or only spending one night in the hospital.*

PEARLS OF WISDOM

It's important to understand the profound impact that knee pain can have on your overall health. Knee pain leads to less physical activity, which promotes obesity. The extra pounds, in turn, put more stress on the knee joint, leading to even less activity and more weight gain. Thus, a vicious cycle is created (see Chapter 77), ultimately resulting in severe knee osteoarthritis. Obesity and immobility also lead to the development of diabetes, heart disease, hypertension and depression; all of these conditions compromise the length and quality of a woman's life. To avoid getting trapped in this vicious cycle, keep moving. Movement is the key — movement is life!

"New research shows that women who are operated on by a male surgeon are more likely to have an adverse outcome than women who are operated on by a female surgeon. While the reasons for this are not clear, I believe female surgeons listen to their female patients better than male surgeons and this improves outcomes for women. If you need a surgeon, make sure your surgeon really listens to you."

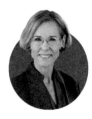

Mary I. O'Connor, M.D. - she/her
Dr. O'Connor is co-founder and Chief Medical Officer at Vori Health, an innovative health care enterprise with a mission to empower all people to lead their healthiest lives. She serves as Chair of Movement is Life, a national non-profit coalition committed to health equity. Dr. O'Connor is a past chair of the Department of Orthopedic Surgery at Mayo Clinic in Jacksonville, Florida, and Professor Emerita of Orthopedics at Mayo Clinic. She specialized in bone and soft tissue tumor surgery and hip and knee replacement surgery.

40

Knee meniscus injury

Arianna L. Gianakos, D.O., and Mary K. Mulcahey, M.D.

WHAT IS A MENISCAL INJURY?

Meniscal injuries are common knee injuries in women. The meniscus is a C-shaped, rubbery cartilage structure that cushions the knee joint. The menisci are located between the two bones of the knee joint, the thighbone (femur) and the shinbone (tibia). Each knee has two menisci, one on the outside (lateral) and one on the inner (medial) side of the knee.

Injury to the meniscus typically results from a twisting or turning type of motion. This can occur during a sporting activity involving running and changing directions. It can also occur with movements involved in getting out of a chair or something as simple as tripping over a curb. These are considered acute (sudden) injuries. The meniscus can also be injured by chronic wear and tear that can occur over a period of years. As women get older, the repetitive movements that are part of normal daily activities can lead to degeneration of the meniscus, causing it to fray or tear.

If you have a meniscus tear, you may notice intermittent swelling and pain in the knee. Pain frequently occurs when bearing weight on a bent knee, and you may feel as if the knee is "grinding." You may also have increased pain with range of motion and walking. Certain movements, such as squatting or walking up or down stairs, can become increasingly difficult. In addition, you may experience a sense of locking, catching or clicking as the knee moves. Many people with meniscal injuries often complain of pain on the inside or outside of the knee at the level of the joint line.

Your primary care clinician will perform a thorough physical exam to help determine the cause of your knee pain and may refer you to an orthopedic surgeon for further evaluation. Physical exam findings often include pain when touching the inside and outside of the knee at the level of the joint. You may also experience a click or sharp pain with certain exam maneuvers that are performed by an orthopedic surgeon.

X-rays of the knee help to assess the bone and the joint. Your doctor may ultimately order an MRI scan to better evaluate the bone and soft tissue structures of the knee. MRI allows your doctor to determine if there is a meniscus tear and if so, where it is located.

Knee meniscal tears

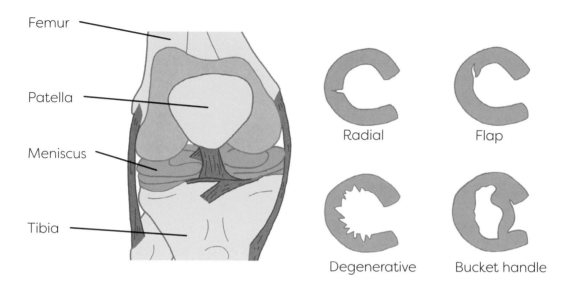

Femur

Patella

Meniscus

Tibia

Radial

Flap

Degenerative

Bucket handle

CAN MENISCAL INJURIES BE PREVENTED?

Yes, to an extent. Most meniscal injuries are either acute, due to a traumatic event, or chronic, due to overuse and degeneration over many years of activities. There are several things that you can do to help protect yourself from a meniscus injury:

- Maintain a healthy weight.
- Exercise with good form and biomechanics.
- Practice proper warm-up and stretching.
- If you feel pain, rest and see if the pain goes away with activity modification, such as limiting twisting movements and high-impact exercises like running and jumping.

HOW ARE MENISCAL TEARS TREATED?

There are several options for treating meniscal tears.

Nonsurgical therapies
Meniscal injuries can often be treated successfully with nonsurgical therapies.

RICE Pain can often be relieved with the RICE method (rest, ice, compress and elevate).

Anti-inflammatory medications Either oral or topical anti-inflammatory medications such as nonsteroidal anti-inflammatory drugs (NSAIDs) can help reduce swelling within your knee joint and improve pain.

Physical therapy Physical therapy can help reduce pain and improve day-to-day function. Physical therapy consists of exercises that help improve range of motion and strength.

Intra-articular steroid injections Steroid injections are frequently used to decrease pain and swelling in the knee joint. Usually, a single injection is performed, often at the first or second visit with your orthopedic surgeon.

Surgical options

If you still have pain after trying various nonsurgical treatment strategies, MRI is often ordered to better evaluate and diagnose your injury. If a meniscus tear is present, surgery may be recommended. Surgery typically involves a knee arthroscopy, in which the surgeon inserts surgical instruments and a small camera through small incisions (portals) to see the area inside the knee. Most people can be treated either by removing the damaged part of the meniscus or repairing the meniscus. The type of procedure is often determined by the tear pattern and tear location, both of which affect whether and how the meniscus will be able to heal following surgery.

There are two main types of meniscal surgery.

Partial meniscectomy This procedure involves removing the frayed edges of the meniscal tear, so that the edges are smooth, thereby limiting pain. If you undergo this procedure, you will be able to put full weight on your leg immediately following the procedure and start early range-of-motion exercises with physical therapy within a week of surgery.

Meniscal repair This procedure can be performed with a variety of techniques, which involve stitching up the two parts of the tear. Rehabilitation following this procedure is more intensive, as range of motion will be restricted for the first six weeks while the meniscus heals. You will likely be able to bear weight in a knee immobilizer or a hinged brace locked in extension (so the leg stays completely straight) following the procedure.

WHY DO MENISCAL TEARS MATTER TO WOMEN?

Evidence shows that women are more prone to knee injuries, particularly those that involve the ACL (see Chapter 10). Studies also show that knee injuries, including meniscal injuries, can predispose people to developing osteoarthritis in the knee joint (see Chapter 39).

QUESTIONS TO ASK YOUR HEALTH CARE TEAM ABOUT MENISCAL TEARS

- What are the best exercises for me?
  › Are there any activities I should avoid?
- What are the negative impacts of NSAIDs?
  › What is the difference between oral and topical anti-inflammatory medications?
- What are the side effects of an intra-articular steroid injection?
  › What should I expect after the injection?

- Am I a candidate for surgery?
- How long does surgery take?
- What is the recovery for partial meniscectomy versus meniscus repair?
- When will I be able to return to walking?
  › To running?
- What are complications of the surgery?
- What type of anesthesia is required?
- Will I need another surgery in the future?
- Am I at risk of developing osteoarthritis?

PEARLS OF WISDOM

Meniscus tears are a common injury experienced by women of all ages. Many tears can be successfully treated without surgery. If symptoms persist, surgery can be performed, typically allowing you to return to your regular daily activities. However, surgery to remove a torn meniscus increases the risk of developing osteoarthritis in your knee joint in later years. Taking measures to lower your risk of a meniscal tear is important. Maintain a healthy body weight, exercise with good form and practice proper warm-up and stretching!

"Gender- and sex-based differences exist in injury patterns between men and women; therefore, it is important to be cognizant of these differences in order to better individualize our management and treatment strategies."

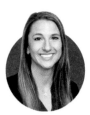

Arianna L. Gianakos, D.O. - she/her
Dr. Gianakos is a Clinical Orthopaedic Foot and Ankle Fellow at Harvard-Massachusetts General Hospital. She is currently completing her Ph.D. at the University of Amsterdam with her area of focus on Gender Studies in Orthopaedic Surgery.

"As orthopaedic surgeons, it is very important for us to be aware of the musculoskeletal issues that are unique and/or more common in women and use our expertise to treat these early and effectively."

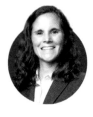

Mary K. Mulcahey, M.D. - she/her
Dr. Mulcahey is an Associate Professor, Assistant Program Director, and Director of Women's Sports Medicine at Tulane University School of Medicine. She specializes in sports medicine and shoulder and knee arthroscopy.

41
Low back pain

Leigh F. Hanke, M.D., M.S.

WHAT IS LOW BACK PAIN?

If you have experienced low back pain, you are certainly not alone. It is one of the most common reasons people go to the doctor or miss work — and even children get low back pain. The lower spine is more mobile than the upper spine, which allows for more bending and twisting, but also more risk of injury. Most people are familiar with low back pain, but not all low back pain is created equally.

Low back pain is a symptom caused by a wide variety of underlying problems. The cause of low back pain is important to determine because it can help guide proper prevention and treatment. Low back pain is often mechanical in nature, triggered by one (or a combination) of the following factors:

- Strained muscles
- Injured intervertebral discs (the layers of cartilage that act as cushions between the bones in the spine)
- Nerves pinched by bones, discs or ligaments as they branch off the spine
- Arthritis in the joints in the spine

The spine can be injured by heavy lifting, trauma and repetitive positions or movements that place stress on the back, such as poor sitting posture and frequent bending forward. Additionally, with aging comes the development of degenerative conditions, such as the loss of normal structure and function in the spine.

It is important to remember that symptoms of back pain can also stem from factors related to female reproductive anatomy, such as menstrual cramps or endometriosis. Less frequently, back pain may be due to an underlying medical condition, such as kidney stones or stomach ulcers. However, the focus of this chapter will be on musculoskeletal back pain, meaning that it is related to the joints, ligaments and cushioning discs in the spine.

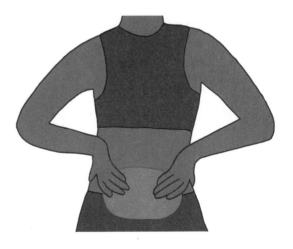

Low back pain can be further characterized based on the duration of symptoms:

- **Acute** back pain lasts for less than 4 weeks. It is the most common form of low back pain and typically gets better on its own regardless of whether you have seen a doctor, physical therapist or other clinicians.
- **Subacute** back pain lasts between 4 and 12 weeks.
- **Chronic** back pain refers to pain lasting 12 weeks or longer. Roughly 20% of people with low back pain experience chronic back pain. Even if pain persists for a long time, it doesn't necessarily mean there is a serious or unfixable underlying cause. In some cases, it's a matter of seeking help from a health care team to find the appropriate diagnosis and treatment plan for you.

CAN LOW BACK PAIN BE PREVENTED?

There are many ways to prevent low back pain, even if you have a family history of conditions associated with it. While 80% of people will likely experience at least one episode of low back pain at some point in their lives, the severity, frequency and duration of such pain can be minimized with proper preventive measures. Taking the following steps can help maintain or improve your posture, prevent injury and keep your back healthy.

Exercise regularly
Aerobic activity, stretching and strengthening keeps muscles strong and flexible. This helps avoid injury and prevent recurrence of back pain.

Eat nutritious meals
Well-balanced meals ensure that you're receiving adequate levels of calcium, phosphorus and vitamin D to promote healthy bones. Recommended amounts of each of these nutrients vary based on age, gender and other factors.

In general, the Institute of Medicine recommendations for women are:
- 19-50 years: 1000 milligrams (mg) calcium and 800 international units (IU) vitamin D
- 51-70 years: 1200 mg calcium and 600 IU vitamin D
- 71+ years: 1200 mg calcium and 800 IU vitamin D

Quit smoking
Smoking can reduce blood flow to the spine and contribute to chronic degenerative conditions. It can also increase risk of osteoporosis. Heavy smoking can lead to chronic coughing, which may trigger acute back pain or worsen chronic pain.

Optimize your environment
When sitting, use lumbar support or a small stool for your feet. Additionally, break up prolonged sitting periods with walk breaks or by gently stretching your muscles. This can promote good posture and relieve tension.

Use correct lifting mechanics
Good lifting mechanics can prevent injury. Lift from your knees, engage your core muscles, keep your back straight and avoid twisting when lifting heavy objects.

Keep an eye on overall well-being
Staying hydrated, maintaining good sleep

hygiene and managing stress have all been shown to play an important role in pain prevention.

HOW IS LOW BACK PAIN TREATED?

Most acute back pain gets better on its own, with simple self-care. This may include a short period of relative rest, heat or cold therapy, gentle stretching and nonprescription pain medication. Bed rest, high-intensity activity and surgery are typically not recommended for acute back pain.

When self-care measures don't work, treating back pain successfully and effectively means understanding what is causing the pain. The length of time you have experienced low back pain — whether it be two weeks or two years — is an integral part of determining the best treatment plan. In the acute phase of back pain, treatment is initially directed at reducing pain, decreasing inflammation and preventing deconditioning. For subacute or chronic pain, treatment is focused more on returning to pain-free, normal activity with a combination of the most effective approaches for your situation.

The vast majority of low back pain is musculoskeletal in nature. The foundation of low back pain management is typically a combination of lifestyle changes (behavioral modification), including exercises and medication. Sometimes injections, surgery or complementary and alternative medicine (CAM) are needed too. The following are some of the methods used to treat low back pain.

Behavioral modification

These are lifestyle changes that can help optimize how your back and whole body function. Behavioral modification might include implementing a home exercise routine to strengthen your core (the muscles in your abdomen and back); starting physical therapy to improve the way your body moves (kinematics) and to learn proper lifting mechanics; or improving the ergonomic setup in your car or at work. It can also include cognitive therapy, biofeedback, relaxation methods and other coping techniques to ease back pain. Optimizing daily behavior and exercise routines can not only treat back pain at any stage (acute or chronic) but prevent it from recurring.

Medications

Medications used for back pain are meant to decrease pain and inflammation. First-line treatments include nonprescription pain relievers such as acetaminophen (Tylenol) and nonsteroidal anti-inflammatory drugs (NSAIDs) such as ibuprofen. If these aren't effective, ask your clinician about other prescription medications that may help. These might include muscle relaxers; topical pain relievers, which come in the form of creams, gels and patches; nerve stabilizers, such as gabapentin or pregabalin; or antidepressants, which are often prescribed for chronic low back pain. Opioid drugs are sometimes used for severe pain, but they can be addictive and have numerous side effects. Opioids should only be tried for short periods under close medical supervision.

Injections and other nonsurgical procedures

Injections can be used with behavior modification and medications to decrease pain or improve your ability to participate in physical therapy. Injections target different structures — muscles, joints or nerves — and use different kinds of medications, such as numbing medications or cortisone, a strong anti-inflammatory drug. Here are common injections for low back pain:

- Trigger point injections target tight, painful back muscles by placing medication into them to promote relaxation, which can often decrease pain.
- Epidural steroid injections involve placing cortisone into the space where the nerve is located in the spinal canal. These injections can ease pain going down from your back into your leg (sciatic pain), which is often caused by inflamed nerves. These injections can also help decrease nerve pain caused by bulging or herniated discs that irritate nerve roots.
- Procedures for arthritic pain target the bony joints of the spine (facet joints). These procedures include facet joint injections, nerve block injections or radiofrequency ablations. Radiofrequency ablation procedures involve inserting a thin needle into the area causing pain and then heating the needle to destroy nerve fibers that relay pain signals to the brain.
- Injections using regenerative medicine, such as platelet-rich plasma and mesenchymal stem cells, are a promising new area of medicine. These injections are not often covered by insurance, but they may provide a way to decrease pain. More research is needed to understand if regenerative medicine injections stimulate healing of degenerative or injured structures of the spine.

Complementary and alternative medicine (CAM)

Although not widely adopted in mainstream Western medicine, research is starting to support incorporation of CAM to treat back pain. Mindfulness-based stress reduction has been shown to have moderate benefit in reducing chronic pain and improving function. Other nondrug therapies that have good supporting evidence include acupuncture, tai chi, exercise therapy, yoga and progressive relaxation. Additional CAM approaches that have been tried for low back pain include aromatherapy, biofeedback, chiropractic medicine, diet therapy and spinal manipulation.

Surgery

Surgery is typically considered when nonoperative therapies have failed and severe low back pain persists. Surgery may also be recommended for serious injuries or nerve compressions that limit the ability to do daily activities. Some surgical options include:

- Reinforcing the vertebral bone with bone cement (vertebroplasty) for fractured vertebra
- Removal of some of the bone (spinal laminectomy), also called decompression, to alleviate narrowing of the spinal canal, a condition that can cause pain, numbness or weakness
- Removal of part of the disc cushion (discectomy) for herniated discs
- Bridging spinal segments together (spinal fusion) to stabilize the spine if there is instability (spondylolisthesis) or slippage of the spine bones onto each other

An additional procedure includes surgically implanting a nerve stimulator, a device that uses low-voltage electrical impulses to block pain signals to the brain.

Know that surgery doesn't always guarantee pain relief and may require months of rehabilitation before you can return to prior levels of function.

WHY DOES LOW BACK PAIN MATTER TO WOMEN?

Low back pain is one of the most common musculoskeletal issues women face. Research suggests that it is slightly more frequent in females than in males of all ages, but the frequency of low back pain in females increases with age. The condition is especially common during and after menopause, and increasing menopausal signs and symptoms often correlate with chronic back pain symptoms. This suggests that back pain is an important condition for women of all ages to understand so that they can take preventive measures and seek help with treatment as needed.

Reproductive organ disorders, such as dysmenorrhea or endometriosis, can also predispose women to back pain. Although reproductive anatomy can sometimes factor into back pain symptoms, it is the degenerative conditions that become more common as women go through reproductive changes that often lead to increased pain. For example, postmenopausal women are at greater risk of osteoporosis, which is a common cause of vertebral compression fracture (VCF).

QUESTIONS TO ASK YOUR HEALTH CARE TEAM ABOUT LOW BACK PAIN

- What is causing my low back pain? In other words, what is the diagnosis?
  - › *It is important to rule out any other medical problems before focusing treatment on the spinal condition that may be causing the pain.*
- Would I benefit from physical therapy, or can I do my own exercises at home?
  - › *Physical therapy can target spinal problems, and it can also target the pelvic floor, which may help with gynecological or pregnancy-related back pain. A physical therapist will typically also give you a personalized home exercise program, which will specifically help your back pain.*
- What medications or injections can help if pain gets severe and I can't tolerate stretching or physical therapy?
  - › *Sometimes pain can limit you from participating in the activities you need to do to get better. In these cases, medications or injections can help decrease pain so you can participate in your physical therapy or home exercise program.*
- Do I need surgery? If not, what things should I look for that may indicate surgery is necessary?
  - › *It is important to understand which symptoms — such as loss of control of your bladder or of the muscles in your legs — might warrant more aggressive medical intervention such as surgery.*
- What is the best way to contact you if my condition urgently changes?

PEARLS OF WISDOM

Prevention of low back pain is key, even if you already have symptoms or are at high risk of developing low back pain. Behavior modification plays a large role in reducing back pain among women of all ages, so don't forget about the little things that you have the power to change. Correcting your posture throughout the day and avoiding prolonged sitting are good places to start. Find a way to make time for your back every day with a regular short home exercise program — combining stretching and strengthening — to maintain good spinal health.

Above all, be mindful of improving your overall health with regard to nutrition, weight, sleep and stress levels, which are aspects of back health that are often overlooked. This can make a big difference not only in preventing low back pain but also in helping relieve both acute and chronic back pain.

"Women must learn to take care of themselves so they can continue to care for others."

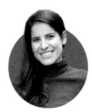

Leigh F. Hanke, M.D., M.S. - she/her
Dr. Hanke is assistant professor of clinical orthopedics and rehabilitation at Yale University School of Medicine and practices at Yale Medicine in Stamford, Connecticut. She specializes in interventional spine and sports medicine with research interests in regenerative medicine.

42
Lung cancer

Anjali T. Sibley, M.D., M.P.H

WHAT IS LUNG CANCER?

Cancer refers to an abnormal growth of cells. When that growth starts in the lungs, it is called lung cancer. In cancer a cell undergoes some type of abnormal change, or mutation, which results in the cancer cell multiplying far more rapidly than normal.

These cancer cells can come together to form a large mass (tumor), which can then spread (metastasize) to other parts of the body. Certain other types of cancer can affect the lungs, including mesothelioma. Lung cancer starts in the lung itself. Mesothelioma develops in the lining of the lung.

Four stages of non-small cell lung cancer

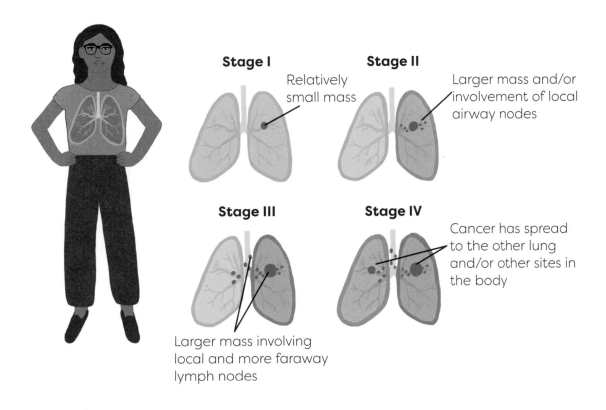

Stage I — Relatively small mass

Stage II — Larger mass and/or involvement of local airway nodes

Stage III — Larger mass involving local and more faraway lymph nodes

Stage IV — Cancer has spread to the other lung and/or other sites in the body

CAN LUNG CANCER BE PREVENTED?

While not all cases of lung cancer can be prevented, there are certainly things you can do to lower your risk of lung cancer.

Stop tobacco use
Tobacco use is the biggest risk factor and contributes to around 85% of cases of lung cancer. Tobacco contains tar and hundreds of other cancer-causing chemicals (carcinogens) that are directly toxic to the cells in your lungs. The risk of lung cancer increases with the extent and duration of tobacco use. This risk is measured by something called the pack-year measure. This is the number of packs of cigarettes smoked per day multiplied by the number of years smoked. For example, if you smoked one pack per day for 30 years, your pack-year history is 30 pack-years.

Occasionally puffing on a cigarette, using e-cigarettes, vaping or smoking cigars also increases the risk of lung cancer, but the extent of the risk has not been determined. Secondhand smoke can increase the risk of lung cancer by 20% to 30%. According to the Centers for Disease Control and Prevention (CDC), nearly 13% of women in the United States currently smoke. Let's get those numbers down!

Avoid or limit kerosene use if possible
Humankind has been using biofuels (such as wood), coal and kerosene in cooking for many years. Multiple studies have shown that various lung (pulmonary) diseases are related to poor use of biofuels and kerosene exposure. While we suspect that there is an increased risk of lung cancer with this exposure, the risk has not been definitively proven. When cooking with biofuels or kerosene, make sure to use proper ventilation. Also consider wearing a durable mask.

Avoid or limit the use of wood-burning stoves if possible
These stoves can cause lung cancer, among many other diseases, by producing additional levels of carbon monoxide, carbon dioxide, methane, nitrogen oxides and other dangerous and polluting particles. To protect your lungs, consider wearing a mask when using a wood-burning stove. Please also have your home carbon monoxide levels measured regularly by your gas company or another reliable source.

Be aware of home and building materials
Some older homes were built with dangerous materials, such as lead paint, or with materials that decay and expose us to dangerous chemicals, such as nickel, cadmium, asbestos, vinyl chloride, chromium and polycyclic aromatic hydrocarbons. In addition, radon (a radioactive gas that has no smell, color or taste) can be present in homes. It's important to have your home tested for radon levels because it causes about 10% of lung cancers in the United States.

Be aware of occupation exposure
People who work in mines, shipyards, factories, construction sites or kitchens can have occupational chemical exposure that can increase their risk of lung cancer. These chemicals include asbestos, cadmium, beryllium and inhalational smoke. As in other situations with chemical exposure,

wearing a mask can help protect your lungs and reduce your risk of lung cancer.

Pay attention to air pollution
Research indicates that people who live in congested, urban areas are at possibly higher risk of lung cancer, when other factors are controlled, compared with those in rural areas. Studies are underway to determine how much the exposure increases risk, but early data suggest that 1% to 2% of lung cancers are related to air pollution. Consider wearing a mask when walking outside during times of increased traffic. Try not to run outside in large urban areas.

Avoid or limit marijuana use
Marijuana use has become more common in the United States, as some states have lifted legal restrictions on use. Marijuana smoke contains many dangerous compounds, including nitrosamines, reactive oxygen species and vinyl chloride. Researchers have not definitively determined marijuana's contribution to lung cancer risk but in one long-term study, people who used marijuana more than 50 times over their lifetimes had a nearly double risk of developing lung cancer.

Consume alcohol wisely
Research on whether alcohol consumption increases the risk of lung cancer has been inconclusive. It's difficult to assess what risk can be attributed to alcohol alone in populations, as people often use alcohol with tobacco. Some studies have shown no association of lung cancer with alcohol intake. Some studies have shown a slightly lower risk of lung cancer with alcohol consumption, especially in smokers. Other studies are trying to determine which types of lung cancer will be more affected by alcohol. More research is needed to determine the exact relationship between alcohol and lung cancer risk.

Use caution with vitamin and mineral supplements
Many high-quality studies have examined the benefits of nutritional supplementation for cancer prevention. High doses of beta-carotene supplementation have been found to increase the risk of lung cancer development. Selenium supplementation, which had generated interest as a preventive for lung cancer, has not been shown to lower the risk of cancer development. Before considering any new supplement, talk to your primary care clinician.

HOW IS LUNG CANCER TREATED?

There are three main types of lung cancer. Doctors define the different types based on how the cancer cells look under the microscope. The major categories of lung cancer include:
- Non-small cell lung cancer (around 50% of cases)
  › Subcategories include squamous cell carcinoma, large cell carcinoma and adenocarcinoma (the type of lung cancer that nonsmokers often develop and can be associated with particular gene mutations)
- Small cell lung cancer (25% of cases)
- Neuroendocrine tumors (10% of cases)

Different types of lung cancer grow differently, so sometimes treatment is different. Treatment is also influenced by the stage of cancer.

Non-small cell lung cancer

This type of cancer has four stages, with stage I being the least advanced, or earliest, stage and stage IV being the most advanced form of lung cancer.

- Stage I cancer involves a relatively small mass in one part of the lung.
- Stage II involves a larger mass in one part of the lung, the spread of cancer to nearby airway lymph nodes, or both.
- Stage III is when the lung cancer mass is large and the cancer has spread to both nearby and more distant lymph nodes.
- Stage IV is defined by cancer that has spread from one lung to the other lung, to sites in the body other than the lungs or nearby lymph nodes, or to both the other lung and other parts of the body. This stage is considered incurable.

Doctors usually treat lung cancer with surgery, radiation therapy, chemotherapy or a combination of these options. Common treatments of non-small cell lung cancer are based on stage.

Stage I and II cancers These stages, usually considered early stage lung cancer, are commonly treated with surgery or radiation therapy in an attempt to cure the body of cancer. Surgery for early stage lung cancer involves the removal of a part or lobe of the lung. People who aren't candidates for surgery or who don't want an invasive procedure can sometimes be treated with radiation therapy. There are different forms of radiation therapy, including stereotactic body radiation therapy (SBRT) among others. Chemotherapy is sometimes added to treatment for early stage lung cancer.

Stage III cancer Treatment involves a combination of several strategies, including surgery, chemotherapy and radiation therapy.

Stage IV cancer Although stage IV lung cancer is considered incurable, treatment may help relieve symptoms and extend a person's life. Stage IV lung cancers are usually treated with chemotherapy, immunotherapy or a combination of both. In some cases of stage IV cancer, there is limited spread of the disease to another part of the body. In those situations, a doctor may recommend surgery or radiation therapy. Targeted therapies, which target the abnormal mutation driving the cancer, are increasingly used in stage IV lung cancer.

If you're diagnosed with advanced stage IV cancer, other considerations become important. One consideration is comfort (palliative) care. Palliative care can help with pain and symptom control. It's also important to

Lung cancer risk factors

Second-hand smoke

Chemical exposure

Tobacco use

Air pollution

Radon gas
Lead paint
Kerosene
Wood-burning stove

decide on your code status, meaning whether doctors should medically intervene if your heart stops or if your breathing fails. Getting your personal and financial affairs in order is another step you can take to help not only yourself but also your loved ones. For terminal cancers, in which treatment is not desired or is no longer effective, hospice may be an appropriate option.

Small cell lung cancer

This type of cancer is categorized as either limited or extensive, depending on how advanced the cancer is. Small cell lung cancer is treated with chemotherapy and radiation therapy, and sometimes surgery or immunotherapy.

Neuroendocrine tumors

These rarer tumors are categorized by stage and treated in a manner similar to that of other types of lung cancer.

Survival rates for lung cancer are better in early stages of the disease than in late stages. New, targeted therapies are making revolutionary progress in helping fight lung cancer and managing advanced lung cancer. However, survival rates are low compared to similar stages of other cancers. The five-year survival rate for treated stage I lung cancer varies from 73% to 90% depending on the extensiveness of disease, while it is less than 15% for treated stage IV disease. Unfortunately, over 65% of lung cancer cases are diagnosed in later stages. Survival rates for neuroendocrine tumors of the lung tend to be much better than those for non-small cell lung cancers such as adenocarcinoma or squamous cell carcinoma.

WHY DOES LUNG CANCER MATTER TO WOMEN?

Lung cancer is the third most common cancer in women in the United States, after localized skin cancer and breast cancer. Lung cancer accounts for over 118,000 cases of cancer per year in women and is the leading cause of cancer deaths in women. While treatments are improving and extending the length of time that people with lung cancer can live, the disease is responsible for more deaths than any other cancer around the world, including in the United States.

Unfortunately, disparities among different populations exist when it comes to lung cancer. Mortality rates are higher for African American men but are around the same for African American women and white women. However, cancer is sometimes diagnosed at later stages in Black populations, which can make outcomes worse for Black women. This difference is not due to biological factors but rather to issues related to access to treatment, supportive services and other social factors that determine health. For example, programs to encourage tobacco cessation may not reach all communities equally. Additional studies on other disparities in lung cancer are underway.

QUESTIONS TO ASK YOUR HEALTH CARE TEAM ABOUT LUNG CANCER

- What treatment options have been shown to improve outcomes for lung cancer?
- Are there any long-term side effects on my heart and body from my therapy for lung cancer?

- What can I do to lower my odds of the cancer returning?
- With any stage, what should I know about my lifespan?
- Are there things I should do about my future now (such as planning for my family or genetic testing)?

PEARLS OF WISDOM

Please do not smoke! Don't ever start — nicotine causes upregulation of nicotine receptors in the brain, leading to greater dependence on the product. If you smoke now, please stop! The damage from tobacco use is greatly improved around 15 years after stopping smoking. Try to avoid people who smoke, as secondhand tobacco exposure increases your risk of lung cancer. Additionally, pay attention to your environment. Watch out for chemicals in your environment and workplace that can damage your lungs, and monitor radon levels in your home.

If you're diagnosed with lung cancer and are undergoing treatment, it's important to take good care of yourself. Consider these tips:
- Eat nutritious, healthy foods, including five or more servings of vegetables and fruits per day, whole-grain foods and foods low in saturated fats (aim for those fats comprising less than 10% of your total calories per day).
- Drink around 64 to 72 ounces of water per day.
- Consume supplement drinks such as Ensure, Boost or Carnation Breakfast Essentials to help maintain calories. Specifically, taking two supplements for

each missed meal can help replenish calories.
- Avoid beta-carotene supplementation.
- Get adequate rest and strive to manage stress.

Exercise as regularly as you can safely tolerate. Exercise has been shown to improve outcomes during cancer therapy, including mobility. Exercise also helps you cope with stress and improves depression and anxiety.

Engage in activities that make you feel good, improve your outlook and don't cause you harm. Examples include:
- Journaling
- Socializing with supportive and positive people and avoiding negative people and attitudes
- Engaging in hobbies that don't involve chemical exposure
- Practicing meditation

"Education about health risk factors is a human right and basic need, to maintain a thriving population."

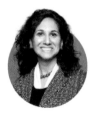

Anjali T. Sibley M.D., M.P.H. - she/her
Dr. Sibley is a board-certified hematologist and medical oncologist at Stanford Healthcare in California. She is the Medical Director of the Stanford Emeryville Cancer Center. She is part of the Thoracic Cancer CCP at Stanford. She is passionate about interactive health education, promotion and screening for patients, especially around topics relating to cancer.

43

Lupus

Vaidehi R. Chowdhary, M.D.

WHAT IS LUPUS?

Lupus is an autoimmune disease in which the body's immune system mistakenly attacks healthy tissue, causing chronic inflammation and affecting multiple organs of the body.

Often when we use the term "lupus," we are referring to systemic lupus erythematosus, or SLE. In this chapter we will primarily be discussing SLE because it's the most common form of the disease.

SLE is called systemic lupus because it affects many different parts of the body. Joint pains, fever, skin rashes and low blood counts are the most frequent complaints. But SLE can also seriously affect internal organs, such as the kidneys, heart, nervous system, lungs, etc. When the primary symptom is skin rash, the condition is called cutaneous lupus erythematosus. Experts estimate that 20% of people with cutaneous lupus may develop SLE over 20 years.

The exact reason why people develop lupus is not known, but the illness is likely caused by a combination of genetic factors and an improperly functioning immune system. Environmental factors such as infections or ultraviolet light may trigger the disease or cause flares (a worsening of symptoms). Studies of large populations have shown that lupus tends to occur in young women and nonwhite people, but children, older adults, men and white people are susceptible, too. The reason for the predominance in women is not exactly known, but may be related to female hormones or genetics.

Some medications cause lupus (called drug-induced lupus), and symptoms may decrease when the medications are no longer taken.

CAN LUPUS BE PREVENTED?

No, SLE cannot be prevented. However, there are several things you can do to prevent flares, improve your overall health and prevent damage from the disease. These include:
• Taking your medications regularly
• Wearing a wide-brimmed hat to protect yourself from the sun
• Using sunscreen
• Wearing ultraviolet protection factor (UPF) coated clothing to minimize risk of flares from ultraviolet light

Lupus signs and symptoms

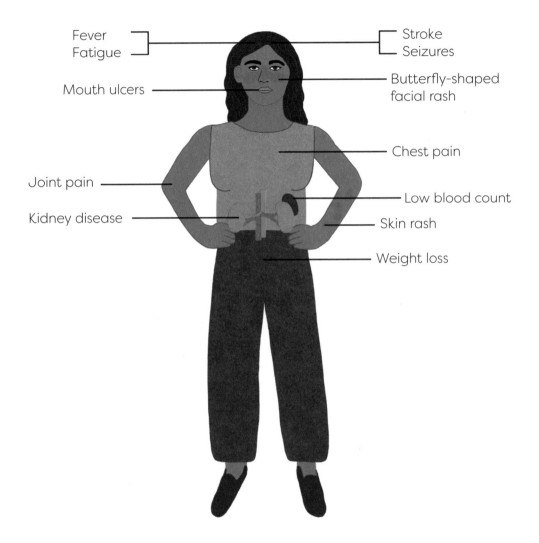

Fever
Fatigue

Mouth ulcers

Joint pain

Kidney disease

Stroke
Seizures

Butterfly-shaped
facial rash

Chest pain

Low blood count

Skin rash

Weight loss

Obesity is common in SLE patients and is associated with greater severity of symptoms and heart disease. A Mediterranean diet, rich in olive oil, nuts, legumes and polyunsaturated fatty acid, promotes weight loss, helps lower disease activity and has beneficial effects on reducing risk of hypertension (high blood pressure), diabetes and heart disease in people with lupus.

HOW IS LUPUS TREATED?

If you're diagnosed with SLE, your treatment will depend on your symptoms and the organs that are affected. Your physician will do a series of laboratory and imaging tests to determine the extent of the disease and to help determine the best course of treatment. There are common treatments for various symptoms and complications of SLE.

Medications and creams

A variety of medications can help relieve symptoms and treat other conditions common in people with lupus, including these.

Joint pain and swelling These symptoms are treated with nonsteroidal anti-inflammatory medications (NSAIDs), steroids and antimalarial medications like hydroxychloroquine. Hydroxychloroquine has numerous other benefits. It prevents disease flares, decreases risk of blood clot formation and may prevent lupus from affecting internal organs.

Skin rashes Rashes are directly treated with steroid skin creams and also benefit from hydroxychloroquine. Lupus rashes are quite sensitive to sun, and the ultraviolet light in sun rays can cause lupus flares. Avoid going out in the sun during peak UV hours of 10 am to 4 pm, wear a wide-brimmed hat and sunscreen and use UPF-coated clothing. For persistent joint pains and rashes, your clinician may recommend additional immunosuppressive medications such as methotrexate or azathioprine. Beta-carotene can also help treat skin rashes.

Lupus-related diseases Some people with SLE develop lupus nephritis (kidney disease), central nervous system lupus or lupus-related cardiopulmonary (heart and lung) disease. In these situations, a doctor may recommend a steroid medication like prednisone and other prescription medications, such as mycophenolate mofetil or cyclophosphamide. Other medications used for treatment are belimumab (Benlysta) for resistant disease. Rituximab may also be beneficial for people with low blood counts and lupus nephritis. Voclosporin (Lupkynis)

and Anifrolumab (Saphnelo) are two drugs recently approved by the FDA for treatment of lupus.

Other conditions People with SLE may be prescribed medications to treat other common medical conditions, including hypertension and hyperlipidemia (high cholesterol). Anxiety and depression are also common in people with SLE and can contribute to fatigue, pain and problems with thinking and memory. Medications can help.

Psychotherapy Along with medication, psychotherapy (talk therapy) can help treat mood disorders such as depression and anxiety. It can also help you manage chronic stress, which can cause flares of SLE symptoms and high disease activity. Psychotherapy methods such as cognitive behavioral therapy have been shown to improve quality of life and physical symptoms in people with lupus.

Exercise Aerobic exercises and strength training can help improve your mood, reduce stress and manage fatigue. Exercising regularly can also help you manage conditions such as high blood pressure and fibromyalgia, which you may be more likely to experience if you have SLE.

Supplements Depending on your symptoms, your clinician may recommend certain dietary supplements:
- Vitamin D may help treat a vitamin D deficiency, which can affect the immune system.
- Fish oil, which contains high levels of omega-3 fatty acids, eicosapentanoeic acid (EPA) and docosahexaenoic acid

(DHA), may help reduce lupus activity, improve cholesterol levels and promote well-being.

- N-acetyl cysteine (an antioxidant), a high-fiber diet, curcumin supplements and flaxseed may help lower lupus activity.

Research shows that high doses of vitamins A, C and E do not help prevent the development of lupus. In particular, high doses of vitamin E (more than 400 IU per day) are not recommended because it may increase the risk of death. Before taking any supplement, it's important to discuss safety and effectiveness with your clinician.

WHY DOES LUPUS MATTER TO WOMEN?

For every man with lupus, there are nine women with the condition. Women are at greater risk of developing this disease, especially during childbearing years. Mortality is higher in people with SLE compared to the general population. Black women with lupus are three times as likely to die prematurely compared to Black women in the general population. Pregnant women with lupus, especially Black and Hispanic women, have a higher risk of preterm labor, preeclampsia and gestational hypertension.

If you have lupus and are considering pregnancy, talk to your clinician. It's very important to understand and discuss contraception and pregnancy in relation to lupus. Ideally lupus should be inactive for four to six months prior to pregnancy. Be sure to also discuss with your clinician any medica-

tions you're taking. Certain medications, such as hydroxychloroquine, should be continued to help prevent lupus flares, which may increase during pregnancy. Other medications may need to be stopped, as they can cause birth defects. The switch should occur at least three to six months prior to pregnancy. Lupus can affect pregnancy, with a greater risk of premature births. Although rare, some people with lupus have factors that can increase the risk of pregnancy loss (antiphospholipid antibodies) or cause a rare complication of heart block in the baby (presence of anti-Ro/SS-A and La/Anti-SS-B).

Talk to your clinician to personalize your treatment plan for lupus, including potential changes to your physical appearance. Steroids, although very useful in treatment, can cause weight gain, stretch marks over the abdomen and changes in facial appearance. Lupus rashes can scar or cause hair loss. This can be very distressing, and discussing cosmetic strategies is important.

QUESTIONS TO ASK YOUR HEALTH CARE TEAM ABOUT LUPUS

- Can you refer me to a rheumatologist?
  › *Care of lupus is specialized and should be under the guidance of a rheumatologist. If you are not being treated by one, ask your primary care clinician for a referral.*
- Who is part of my health care team?
  › *Your health care team may include other specialists, such as a kidney doctor (nephrologist) or blood doctor (hematologist). It can be hard to keep track of all your clinicians, so ask about the specific role of each member of your subspecialist team.*

- What should I know about my medicines?
  - *Some lupus medicines require regular blood tests or a special eye exam to make sure that you are not experiencing any adverse side effects from the medicine. Ask your health care team about these tests and how many times these tests should be done in a year.*
- What can I do to prevent infections?
  - *Infections are common in lupus patients. Talk with your clinician to find out if you need any vaccines or antibiotics for prevention.*
- What contraceptive can I use?
  - *Choice of contraceptives is influenced by the severity of lupus, active versus inactive disease and risk of blood clotting, which is increased in some people with lupus. A discussion between your gynecologist and rheumatologist may be needed to arrive at the correct contraceptive choice for you. Estrogen-containing oral contraceptives may be used in people with mild and inactive disease, whereas progesterone-containing intrauterine devices (IUDs) are often recommended for people at high risk of blood clotting. Progesterone-containing IUDs also reduce the risk of bleeding and do not decrease bone density.*
- Can I get pregnant?
  - *It is advisable not to get pregnant while taking medications such as mycophenolate mofetil and methotrexate because they can cause serious birth defects. If you do get pregnant, you may experience flares of lupus. Your health care team will also check blood work and follow you more closely with ultrasound monitoring or additional medications throughout your pregnancy.*
- Do I need any blood tests for regular monitoring?
  - *Many medications used for lupus require regular checking of blood counts, as well as kidney and liver tests. The frequency of these tests depends on the type of medications you're taking. Hydroxychloroquine requires an eye exam every year. Special eye tests may be needed, and it's a good idea to check with your eye doctor to make sure she's aware that you're taking this medication.*
- Am I taking any medications that can cause lupus to flare?
  - *Certain medications can trigger lupus rashes or cause drug-induced lupus. People with lupus may have an increased risk of allergic reactions to some antibiotics.*
- Do I need a referral to a dietitian or nutritionist or a physical therapist?
  - *Maintaining a healthy body weight has many benefits, but it can be more challenging for people with lupus due to steroids prescribed to treat your condition. A dietitian or nutritionist can help you create a diet plan tailored to your needs and identify your potential barriers to weight loss. Exercise can also improve your health, but joint and muscle pains make it harder to exercise. A physical therapist can work with you to customize your exercise regimen. Aerobic exercise combined with strength training helps lessen fatigue and pain and improves wellness. Aquatic exercises promote fitness and wellness. Exercise does not flare disease.*
- Should I see a mental health professional?
  - *Stress in modern life is inevitable, and managing it gives a sense of control over challenges posed by disease. Depression can make pain and fatigue worse.*

PEARLS OF WISDOM

Educate yourself, your family and co-workers about this disease. It can be harder for others to appreciate the periods of incapacity caused by flares of pain and fatigue. People with lupus often hear comments like "but you look so well …," making it difficult to convey their situation. Give yourself time to feel better, and have patience, as medications do not work quickly. Modern treatments have greatly improved the outcome of lupus, and ongoing research promises to unlock new therapies for this condition.

"Know your health history and advocate for yourself."

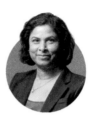

Vaidehi R. Chowdhary, M.D. - she/her
Dr. Chowdhary is Associate Professor and Clinical Chief, Section of Rheumatology, Allergy and Immunology at Yale School of Medicine. She specializes in rheumatic diseases, especially lupus.

44

Migraines

Saher Choudhary, M.D.

WHAT ARE MIGRAINES?

Migraines are the second most common type of recurring headache, after tension headaches. There are two main types of migraine — migraine with aura (classic migraine) and migraine without aura (common migraine). Migraine is not simply a bad headache but rather a complex neurologic process which affects about 12% of the population.

A migraine can consist of up to four phases, though not everyone will have all the phases. The four phases of migraine are as follows:

1. **Prodrome (preheadache)** Lasts several hours to days with symptoms of fatigue, irritability, depression, food cravings, yawning, sensitivity to light or sound or both, difficulty concentrating, and difficulty sleeping.
2. **Aura** Lasts a few minutes to an hour with a range of symptoms, the most common of which are visual disturbances, but may also include sensory changes such as numbness and tingling, or even motor and speech difficulties.
3. **Headache** Lasts 4 to 72 hours with symptoms of headache that get worse with movement; sensitivity to light, sound or smell; nausea and vomiting; and depressed mood.

4. **Postdrome (migraine hangover)** Lasts 24 to 48 hours with symptoms of fatigue, difficulty concentrating and depressed mood.

CAN MIGRAINES BE PREVENTED?

Like a lot of things relating to the brain, the exact cause of migraine headaches is not clearly understood yet. Migraines are thought to be related to activation, or possibly overactivation, of brain cells. This activation spreads signals through parts of the brain, causing inflammation and pain. Other factors thought to contribute to migraine include imbalances in brain chemicals, particularly serotonin, as well as genetic and environmental factors.

While there is no cure for migraine, there are things you can do to reduce the frequency and severity of migraine attacks. Identifying and avoiding migraine triggers is essential to preventive care. Significant variations in daily routine can trigger migraine attacks. A key step for people who have migraines (migraineurs) is to focus on building and maintaining a consistent and balanced daily routine.

There are several common triggers that may be modified to help prevent migraine.

Stress

Increased stress can trigger a migraine attack, but so can changing from a high-stress situation to a low-stress one (stress letdown), such as going on vacation. Stress is a part of life; everyone experiences stress at times. The key is using stress management and coping strategies to keep daily stress levels even and manageable. Stress management techniques include meditation, yoga, exercise, working on a hobby, walking or hiking in nature, and other relaxing activities. Even spending just 15 mins a day on such activities can have a positive effect on migraines. By learning to balance work, relationships, and relaxation, you can actually reduce the frequency of migraine significantly.

Sleep

Though sleep itself is considered a treatment for migraine, poor sleep and changes in sleep, including lack of sleep or too much sleep, can trigger a migraine attack. Maintaining a regular sleep schedule and practicing good sleep hygiene is important for migraineurs. Good sleep hygiene includes going to bed at the same time and waking up at the same time every day, as well as avoiding screens — such as TV, tablet, phone and so on — in bed.

Additionally, if you have difficulty sleeping, it could be related to an underlying sleep disorder, such as insomnia, sleep apnea or teeth grinding. Recognizing and treating underlying sleep disorders is vital for migraine prevention. Both behavior therapy for insomnia and continuous positive airway pressure (CPAP) for sleep apnea have been shown to decrease migraine frequency.

Diet

Poor eating habits, such as skipping meals and eating unhealthy foods, can trigger migraine. Maintaining a healthy, balanced eating pattern and avoiding food triggers is essential. Food triggers can vary from person to person, but some common ones include foods that contain nitrates, such as hot dogs and lunch meat; foods that contain monosodium glutamate (MSG); and foods that contain tyramine, an ingredient found in foods such as aged cheese, soy and red wine, for example. Changing your diet can be tough, but it is usually worth the effort.

Drinks

Common drink ingredients such as caffeine, alcohol and artificial sweeteners are also known to contribute to migraines. Even though caffeine can be beneficial during a migraine attack, too much caffeine or caffeine withdrawal also can cause a migraine attack. Stopping all caffeine for two to three months can help you determine whether caffeine is contributing to migraine frequency. Similarly, avoiding alcohol and artificial sweeteners such as aspartame, commonly found in sugar-free and diet drinks, can be beneficial. Keeping hydrated — plain water is almost always the best option — is crucial to preventing migraines.

Other triggers

Bright lights, loud noises, strong odors, weather changes and hormone changes are known to trigger migraines. Avoiding known trigger environments and preparing

Migraine triggers

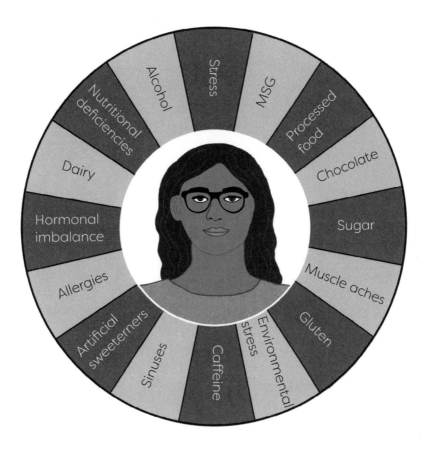

for unexpected triggers can also help reduce frequency and severity of migraine. Because there are so many potential triggers, and they vary from person to person, identifying what triggers your migraines can be difficult. Keeping a headache diary can help you identify your own migraine patterns and potential triggers for migraine attacks. A headache diary can also be helpful in keeping track of your body's response to migraine treatment. There are headache apps for smartphones and tablets to help you maintain a digital migraine diary.

HOW ARE MIGRAINES TREATED?

The approach to migraine treatment may be both preventive, to reduce migraine frequency, and abortive, to treat the migraine when it occurs.

Preventive therapies

These approaches are helpful when migraine frequency or severity has a significant impact on your life despite other steps you have taken, including lifestyle modifications, trigger avoidance and use of acute treatments.

Medications There are several prescription medications approved by the Food and Drug Administration (FDA) for migraine prevention. Common categories of medications include blood pressure and heart medications such as beta blockers, as well as antidepressants and seizure medications. These medications are taken daily, and the choice of medication depends on several factors including side effects, cost, and your preferences. Recently, several monoclonal antibodies, which are laboratory-made proteins that mimic the immune system's ability to fight off harmful pathogens, received FDA approval for migraine prevention through monthly injections. These monoclonal antibodies target a specific protein called calcitonin gene-related peptide (CGRP), which can cause inflammation and pain associated with migraine. Botox injections may be a treatment option for people who have 15 or more days of migraine a month. And yes, it's the same kind of Botox used for wrinkles, but the injection sites are targeted for migraine.

Neuromodulation devices Noninvasive devices with FDA approval for migraine prevention include transcranial magnetic stimulation (TMS), transcutaneous supraorbital nerve stimulation (tSNS) and external trigeminal nerve stimulation (eTNS). These devices are typically placed on the head. While they can cause side effects such as numbness, tingling sensations, lightheadedness, and sleep disturbance, they are considered generally safe. Some studies show that using these devices on a daily basis, for a few minutes, can help with both severity and frequency of migraine headaches. These devices are not currently considered first-line therapy, as more

studies are needed to better understand their benefits in migraine treatment.

Behavioral therapies These are valuable for all migraineurs but particularly for those who have migraines triggered by stress or behavior, and for those who cannot tolerate medications. Behavioral therapies such as relaxation training, biofeedback therapy and cognitive-behavioral therapy are proven to reduce migraine frequency. In combination with medication, behavioral therapy can be even more beneficial.

Alternative therapies Supplements such as coenzyme Q10, magnesium citrate and riboflavin may be recommended by some clinicians to help reduce migraine frequency. Some studies show that acupuncture may be effective in reducing migraine frequency, but the evidence is unclear and further studies are needed. However, given that acupuncture is a relatively safe practice, it is commonly used around the world as an alternative therapy for migraine prevention, particularly in Germany.

Abortive therapies

Abortive therapies are used to treat an acute migraine attack — a migraine attack that is in the process of happening. These therapies are more effective when used early in the migraine process. As with preventive medications, abortive therapy is tailored to each person based on side effects, cost, and preferences.

Nonprescription medications Medications such as acetaminophen (Tylenol), aspirin, ibuprofen (Advil, Motrin, others) and naproxen (Aleve), as well as combination medications such as those containing acetaminophen, aspirin and caffeine (Excedrin Migraine), are effective in treating migraine. Though these medications are generally safe, they do have side effects, and long-term use is not recommended. In fact, regularly using these medications over the long term can actually cause "rebound headaches" and complicate headache treatment.

Prescription medications Triptans are a class of drug that stimulate serotonin, a brain chemical, and reduce inflammation. Triptans are effective in treating acute migraine, particularly in combination with other drugs such as naproxen. However, because triptans affect both the brain and blood vessels, they are not recommended for people with history of stroke, heart attack, coronary artery disease, uncontrolled hypertension or peripheral vascular disease.

Ditans are like triptans in that they also stimulate serotonin, but they do not affect blood vessels. This makes ditans a possible alternative to triptans for those with vascular disease. To date, there is only one FDA-approved ditan available in the U.S., lamiditan (Reyvow).

Medications targeting the protein CGRP can help prevent migraine when given as a monthly injection. Recently, two oral medications in this class, ubrogepant (Ubrelvy) and Rimegepant (Nurtec), have been approved for acute migraine treatment, as well. Studies show that these medications are effective and well tolerated.

Nerve blocks Evidence to support the use of peripheral nerve block for acute migraine is limited. However, they are considered safe and may be an option in some cases.

Neurostimulation Noninvasive devices for external neurostimulation are used for migraine prevention and some may help acute migraine, as well. Cefaly, an eTNS device that is approved for preventive migraine treatment, became the first device approved for over-the-counter treatment of acute migraine treatment, as well. Though more studies are need, Cefaly may be a good option for people who cannot tolerate or want to avoid medications for acute migraine attacks.

Status migrainosus, a debilitating migraine lasting more than 72 hours, often requires a combination of medications such as a nonsteroidal anti-inflammatory (NSAID), antiemetics, steroids and fluids, which may be given intravenously. Status migrainosus may require treatment in urgent care or an emergency room.

WHY DO MIGRAINES MATTER TO WOMEN?

Migraine is three times more common in women than in men. Additionally, hormones, particularly estrogen, play a big role in migraine for women. Migraine commonly starts after the first period (menarche) and occurs more frequently during premenstrual and menstrual periods. Interestingly, the frequency and severity of migraine headaches often improves during pregnancy and menopause, further supporting the significance of hormones in migraine.

Because of the major role estrogen plays in migraines, certain hormonal therapies, including birth control, can help regulate hormonal fluctuations and reduce migraines in some women. In other women, certain types of birth control can worsen migraine severity and frequency. Hormonal therapy also may not be an option for some women, given the therapy's increased risk of blood clots, stroke, and other serious health complications.

QUESTIONS TO ASK YOUR HEALTH CARE TEAM ABOUT MIGRAINES

- What should I keep track of in a headache diary?
- What lifestyle changes can I make to prevent migraine headaches?
- Could any of the medications I take, including birth control pills, be making my migraine headaches worse?
- Could underlying medical conditions, such as sleep apnea, be contributing to my migraines?
- Would prescription medications or hormonal therapy be likely to help me?
  - › Are there other therapies that may help me?
- What are the side effects and drug interactions of the medications you have prescribed?
  - › What can I do to handle or prevent side effects or drug interactions?

PEARLS OF WISDOM

Migraine is often dismissed as just a bad headache. But it's important for women to understand that migraine is a disabling neurologic condition that requires appropriate treatment and management. The impact of migraine is profound for women, as it affects their health, relationships, work and quality of life. Migraine treatment is complex, and it often takes time to truly understand and manage migraine. It is important for women to find their triggers, implement lifestyle modifications and work closely with their doctors to reduce migraine frequency and severity.

"We must empower women to advocate for their health."

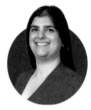

Saher Choudhary, M.D. - she/her
Dr. Choudhary is the Director of the Neurology Residency Program at Prisma Health/University of South Carolina School of Medicine Greenville. She is a neurohospitalist whose primary focus is the care of hospitalized patients and acute stroke care.

45

Multiple sclerosis

Patricia K. Coyle, M.D., and Nancy McLinskey, M.D.

WHAT IS MULTIPLE SCLEROSIS?

Multiple sclerosis (MS) is the most common central nervous system (CNS) disease affecting young adults. MS is an immune-mediated condition, meaning it is a condition in which a person's own immune system starts to attack body organs — in this case, the brain, spinal cord or optic nerve of the CNS. As immune cells move into the CNS from the blood instead of exiting as they should, they cause inflammation and subsequent damage of the CNS tissue. What exactly causes MS is unknown, but something triggers the immune system to act in this way. The result is ongoing, accumulating, permanent damage to the CNS that disrupts its ability to function. Depending on the area involved, a host of neurologic abnormalities may result.

In MS, a process called demyelination occurs, which means that the immune system attacks the protective coverings (myelin sheaths) that surround nerve fibers. Demyelination blocks the ability of nerves to send out electrical signals (nerve conduction) and damages the spaces where nerve cells connect (synapses). This results in damage to the brain, spinal cord and optic nerve (neurodegeneration), which can lead to injury or death of brain nerve cells (neurons) and the cells that make up the myelin sheaths (oligodendrocytes). Altogether, this contributes to the slow worsening of MS.

Types of multiple sclerosis

There are several types of MS.

Relapsing MS The most common form of MS is referred to as relapsing MS, which affects up to 85% to 90% of people with MS. The first time a person experiences an attack of MS symptoms is referred to as a clinically isolated syndrome. These people then experience acute attacks or relapses of neurologic symptoms that evolve over a period of days to weeks. Examples of a relapse include:

- Vision loss in one eye (optic neuritis)
- An inflammatory spot (lesion) affecting the spinal cord, with leg weakness or numbness in both legs from the waist down (transverse myelitis)
- Double vision or unsteady gait, due to brainstem or cerebellar syndrome

Relapses may also cause symptoms of fatigue, problems with mental processing (cognitive impairment), and bladder and bowel problems, such as urinary retention

Areas affected by multiple sclerosis

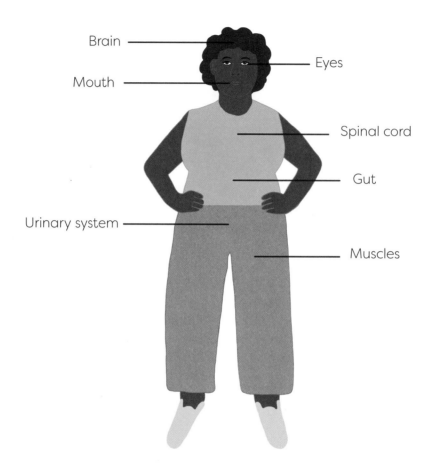

Brain

Eyes

Mouth

Spinal cord

Gut

Urinary system

Muscles

or constipation. In between attacks, people recover from relapses and symptoms typically subside.

People with relapsing MS are at risk of transitioning to a slowly worsening course of the disease called secondary progressive MS, which occurs on average within 20 years from the time symptoms start. In a small number of people, relapses may continue to occur on top of disease progression.

Primary Progressive MS (PPMS) This type of MS occurs in 10% to 15% of cases of MS. People with primary progressive MS

experience a slow, gradual worsening of symptoms. Symptoms typically affect the ability to walk, with leg weakness in both legs and imbalance that progresses over time. PPMS generally occurs at a later age of onset compared with relapsing MS and is the only form of MS to affect women and men equally.

CAN MS BE PREVENTED?

Currently, no. There is no cure for MS because its cause remains unclear.

The disease is not inherited. However, there are over 230 genes that slightly increase the risk of developing MS. In addition, there are genes being identified that likely provide protection from disease severity. Having a first-degree relative with MS increases disease risk from about 0.13% to 2% to 2.5%.

Certain environmental factors are known to increase the risk of MS:
- Epstein-Barr virus infection, especially if the infection is symptomatic with mononucleosis. Thus far, there has not been a single documented case of adult-onset MS in a person who has not been infected with the Epstein Barr virus.
- Smoking
- Adolescent obesity
- Low vitamin D levels
- Limited exposure to sunlight or ultraviolet light

HOW IS MS TREATED?

Treatment of MS can be divided into four broad areas, all of which are important to address.

Disease-modifying therapies (DMTs)
Early use of disease-modifying therapies (DMTs) likely reduces the degree and rate of progression over time. The Food and Drug Administration has approved a number of DMTs that decrease CNS damage and result in better outcomes. These drugs limit future disease damage, lower the risk of future relapses, decrease disease worsening on neurologic examination, and minimize development of CNS lesions that are detected on imaging, such as MRI.

DMTs do not improve MS symptoms or reverse existing damage. Instead, they try to prevent or slow down future damage to the CNS. Currently, all DMTs are approved for relapsing forms of MS, and one DMT is approved for primary progressive MS. Some are considered "high efficacy" treatments, which are more likely to reduce ongoing damage. Although none of the DMTs are considered cures, they can be very effective. Many people taking DMTs go for many years without experiencing new obvious neurologic issues. The earlier a DMT is started, the greater the advantage may be in minimizing later disability.

Management of relapses
Attacks in relapsing MS are often treated with a short course — three to seven days — of high-dose corticosteroids. Steroids are typically given by daily intravenous (IV) infusion, although high-dose oral daily steroids are another option. The goal is to speed up the time frame of recovery. Use of steroids is not believed to change the ultimate course of MS, and they are not guaranteed to work. They are often used, however, particularly during earlier phases of MS, due to their ability to reduce inflammation.

Management of symptoms
MS symptoms such as fatigue, muscle tightness (spasticity), cognitive impairment and problems with bladder function can interfere profoundly with quality of life. If you have MS, it is important to work with your doctor to identify MS symptoms, rank them in order of significance to your daily life, and create a management plan that works for you. Treatment may involve exercise programs, rehabilitation procedures and medications. In addition, assistive

devices such as a mobility aid, stimulation techniques such as percutaneous tibial nerve stimulation (PTNS), and implantable devices such as sacral nerve stimulators can help minimize symptoms, including urinary frequency, bladder and bowel incontinence, and foot drop.

General wellness practices

It is important to recognize and manage other conditions that may occur alongside MS, such as high blood pressure, diabetes and depression. Treating these conditions contributes to a better outcome.

If you have MS, following a healthy lifestyle also helps. This includes not smoking, maintaining a healthy weight, engaging in regular aerobic exercise, practicing good sleep hygiene, eating a healthy diet and maintaining intellectual and social stimulation. Participating in a wellness program has been shown to improve the central nervous system and optimize aging in the course of MS, potentially reducing accelerated brain shrinkage and ongoing deterioration of the CNS.

WHY DOES MS MATTER TO WOMEN?

MS affects females to males by a ratio of 3 to 1. Only primary-progressive MS does not show a female predominance.

A typical person with MS is a young woman of child-bearing age. MS is more likely to occur in females and generally before the age of 50. Nearly 90% of people with MS will experience initial symptoms between the ages of 15 and 50 years.

MS is more common in certain areas, such as Canada, northern United States, most of northern Europe, New Zealand, southeastern Australia, and Israel. Very little MS occurs at the equator, although frequency increases with higher degrees of latitude. The first 15 years of childhood spent in a geographic area seems to determine lifelong disease risk. However, this geographic restriction has diminished in the era of global travel.

Currently, MS affects an estimated 1,000,000 people in the United States. Diagnoses of relapsing MS, particularly among women, have increased in recent years. The explanation for this is not known. Women with MS generally have a more favorable prognosis than men do, and women with relapsing MS show an 18% higher relapse rate than the rate among men with relapsing MS. The disease is affected by race and ethnicity, and for unclear reasons may be more severe in people who are Black or Latino.

Pregnancy has marked effects on MS activity. Disease activity decreases during pregnancy, particularly the last trimester, and then temporarily rebounds in the first three months after childbirth before returning to prepregnancy levels. Breastfeeding exclusively, without supplementing formula, may have a protective effect in the postpartum period. Failed in vitro fertilization has been associated with a three-month period of increased disease activity. These observations suggest that hormonal or immune factors play a role in MS, and could provide insight into the development of new treatments for the disease.

Although some DMTs can be used safely during pregnancy and breastfeeding, there are others that should be avoided due to possible risk to the fetus. It is important to discuss family planning with your MS health care team to optimize pregnancy outcomes and reduce the risk of postpartum relapse.

QUESTIONS TO ASK YOUR HEALTH CARE TEAM ABOUT MS

- What type of MS do I have?
- How do I recognize an MS attack?
- Do I have features that suggest mild or severe MS?
- Do you think I need a high efficacy DMT?
- What do you think is the best DMT for me and why?
- Before I start my DMT, what is the best form of contraception to use?
- Once I give birth, how long should I breastfeed? When should I resume a DMT?
- Beside DMTs, what can I do to stay as healthy as possible?
- How does my treatment affect vaccinations?

PEARLS OF WISDOM

MS has become a very treatable disease, allowing people with MS to live a productive, engaged life. It is important to start an effective DMT as early as possible to reduce disease progression. It's also critical to maintain ongoing communication with your health care team and attend follow-up visits as recommended. Be sure to discuss family planning early on with your doctor.

"Women should seek a health care provider who is smart, who cares, and who considers women's health as a valued area."

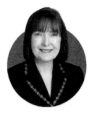

Patricia K. Coyle, M.D. - she/her
Dr. Coyle is a Professor and Vice Chair (clinical affairs) and Director of the MS Comprehensive Care Center, in the Department of Neurology at Stony Brook University, in Stony Brook, New York. She specializes in MS/neuroimmunology and neurologic infections/Lyme disease.

"It's important to address the many unique aspects of women's health that have been long overlooked."

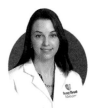

Nancy McLinskey, M.D. - she/her
Dr. McLinskey is an Assistant Clinical Professor of Neurology at Stony Brook University's Multiple Sclerosis Comprehensive Care Clinic in Stony Brook, NY. Her areas of expertise include Multiple Sclerosis, NMO spectrum disorders, and Memory Disorders.

46

Neck pain

Ellen Casey, M.D., and Heidi Prather, D.O.

WHAT IS NECK PAIN?

Neck pain often develops over time due to muscle overuse from the way we sit and move. Poor postures cause muscles to work inefficiently; over time, this inefficiency can result in pain. Neck pain can result from several structures:

- Muscle
- Fascia, the tissue that wraps around muscles
- Discs between vertebral bones
- Nerves
- Facet joints at the back of the neck. Facet joints are connections between the bones of the spine that allow the spine to bend and twist appropriately. Facet joints also serve as passageways for nerve roots as they go from the spinal cord to the arms, legs and other parts of the body.

As we age, it is also common to develop arthritis in the neck (cervical spine). This does not always result in neck pain but may be associated with stiffness and narrowing of the canals where the spinal cord and nerve roots travel in the spine. Over time, for some people, this can lead to pain and weakness that eventually requires treatment.

CAN NECK PAIN BE PREVENTED?

Neck pain can be prevented by paying attention to how you sit, stand, carry and lift items, and sleep. Since stress can inadvertently cause muscle tension in your neck, take time to breathe deeply and do gentle stretches as part of your routine. When conducting work that requires you to repeatedly move your arms or look up or down, or sit in front of a computer for long periods, be sure to change positions two to three times an hour.

Finding the ideal ergonomic setup for your workstation is another important step in both preventing and reducing pain. To follow general ergonomic guidelines:

- Keep your eyes level with the top portion of the computer screen.
- Pull your shoulders back and down.
- Keep your elbows bent, with your forearms resting on the desk parallel to the floor.
- Sit upright, with your pelvis tilted slightly forward toward the front of the chair.
- Keep your thighs parallel to the floor.
- Rest your feet flat on the floor.

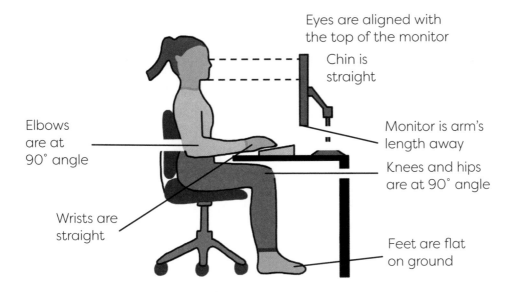

Eyes are aligned with the top of the monitor

Chin is straight

Elbows are at 90° angle

Monitor is arm's length away

Knees and hips are at 90° angle

Wrists are straight

Feet are flat on ground

However, even with ideal posture, the human body was not made for prolonged sitting. In fact, studies show that sitting for more than six hours per day is linked to neck pain. Movement is key!

HOW IS NECK PAIN TREATED?

Although there are many different causes of neck pain, common treatments can help address most of those causes.

Activity and behavior modifications
Pay attention to your daily activities to try to identify movements or positions that cause you pain so that you can avoid or limit them. There are several changes you can make to reduce neck pain.

Computer or workstation Prolonged sitting at a computer, especially if the monitor and keyboard are too high or too low, can cause neck pain. Thus, it is important to find and use the best ergonomic setup for you. Strategies to reduce neck pain with sitting include getting up every one to two hours, stretching, using a standing desk and having walking meetings.

Handheld devices When people use cell-phones and tablets, they tend to sit with their heads forward and shoulders rounded. This position increases stress on the neck muscles and deeper structures, which leads to pain. Strategies to reduce device-related neck pain include reducing time on devices and holding the device at eye level so that good posture is maintained.

Exercise Regular exercise — such as walking, cycling, swimming, jogging or yoga — can reduce neck pain. There is no evidence that running causes neck pain or neck damage, but some people find that running and other high-impact activities worsen their neck pain. If this is the case for you, you may need to modify how much and how often you perform certain exercises. Discuss ways to modify those exercises with your clinician.

Sleep The National Sleep Foundation recommends that adults get seven to nine hours of sleep each night. People who get less than the recommended amount of sleep are at increased risk of neck and other musculoskeletal pain. Adequate sleep is an important part of the treatment plan for neck pain. If neck pain is preventing you from falling asleep or staying asleep, discuss this further with your clinician.

Stress Stress, anxiety and fear can make the experience of pain worse or more prolonged. Therefore, another part of treating neck pain is reducing feelings of stress, anxiety and fear — not only about the neck pain itself, but in all areas of life.

Rehabilitation

An exercise program guided by a skilled physical therapist is a key part of the neck pain treatment plan. Ideally, programs are individualized, but most exercises will focus on:

- Improving strength and endurance of the muscles surrounding the neck, spine and shoulders
- Improving range of motion of the neck, spine and shoulders
- Improving posture
- Learning how to prevent future episodes of neck pain

Medications

Medications for neck pain can be used when pain is limiting your sleep or your ability to participate in rehabilitation or daily activities.

Nonprescription medications Choices include acetaminophen (Tylenol) and nonsteroidal anti-inflammatory drugs (NSAIDs), such as ibuprofen (Advil, Motrin, others) or naproxen (Aleve). Several topical treatments that can be applied to your skin in the area of your neck pain are also available, such as NSAID diclofenac; lidocaine, a numbing medication; heat wraps, such as Thermacare; and capsaicin, which reduces a chemical released by pain nerves.

Prescription medications Your clinician may prescribe prescription medications if you're having severe pain that is interfering with your daily activities despite using nonprescription medications. There are several choices available, and your clinician can discuss with you the risks and benefits of each option.

Injections and other nonsurgical procedures Injections do not cure neck pain but may be helpful when pain is severe despite rehabilitation, medications and activity modification. Typical injections used for neck pain are:

- **Epidural steroid injections** These injections reduce swelling and pain related to a pinched nerve (cervical radiculopathy).
- **Facet joint steroid injections** This type of injection reduces swelling and pain related to arthritis in the facet joints.
- **Nerve-numbing injections (nerve blocks) and radiofrequency ablation procedures** Nerve blocks numb the nerves that are causing neck pain. Radiofrequency ablation procedures involve inserting a thin needle into the area causing pain and then heating the needle to destroy nerve fibers that relay pain signals to the brain.

Surgery

Surgery is not necessary for most people with neck pain. It is considered when there is severe pain that has not improved with other treatments, or if there are signs of spinal cord or nerve injury that is getting worse despite treatment. Surgery is typically performed to protect the spine and nerves from further damage. The type of surgery required depends on the specific injury and can range from the removal of a portion of bone or soft tissue to a fusion of the bones in the neck.

Alternative treatments

Alternative treatments that have been shown to be effective in reducing neck pain include acupuncture, massage, meditation and exercise such as yoga and tai chi. Often, these treatments are used in combination with other medical treatments as part of a comprehensive program.

WHY DOES NECK PAIN MATTER TO WOMEN?

Neck pain is common in both women and men, but some studies show that women are more likely to develop neck pain throughout their lives. It's not exactly clear why women are at greater risk of neck pain, but some of the possible reasons include differences in the shape and alignment of the spine. Women have smaller bones, discs and joints than men. This may lead to increased risk of injury with trauma, such as from a fall or motor vehicle collision, which might include whiplash. Women are more likely to develop sideways curvature of the spine (scoliosis) and forward curvature of the mid-back (kyphosis), which can lead to neck and back pain. However, even though women are more likely to develop neck pain, they are as likely as men to improve with the treatments described in this chapter.

QUESTIONS TO ASK YOUR HEALTH CARE TEAM ABOUT NECK PAIN

- What can I change in my daily routine to reduce neck pain?
- What type of exercise should I do, and what type should I avoid?
- What can I do to prevent my neck pain from getting worse?
- When do I need to see a clinician to prevent future episodes of neck pain?
- For any treatments, particularly injections or surgery, what are the benefits and potential risks?

PEARLS OF WISDOM

Being mindful of your posture and repetitive movements is key to avoiding and managing neck pain.

- Pain can radiate or move from the neck to the arm, head and down the upper back, especially along the shoulder blade.
- Radiation of pain is not directly associated with a more serious condition. But do talk to your clinician about any pain that is not getting better over time or has not responded to your attempts at making changes to improve your neck health.
- Seek urgent care if you're experiencing progressive weakness in your arms or problems with bowel and bladder control (incontinence), along with neck pain.

"Women's health is more than reproductive health. My goal is to enable women to be physically active throughout the lifespan."

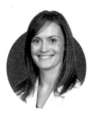

Ellen Casey, M.D. - she/her
Dr. Casey is an Associate Professor in Physiatry and Sports Medicine at the Hospital for Special Surgery in New York City and the USA Women's National Gymnastics Team Physician. She specializes in conservative management of sports and spine disorders.

"We still have a lot to learn through research and clinical outcomes regarding specific preventative and treatment needs for women to be and stay healthy. I hope to contribute to this knowledge."

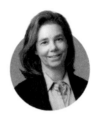

Heidi Prather, D.O. - she/her
Dr. Prather is an Attending Physician at the Hospital for Special Surgery and Weill Cornell Medical College, where she is the Medical Director of the Lifestyle Medicine Program and Clinical Lead of the Osteoarthritis Program. Dr. Prather specializes in musculoskeletal care with special interest in the hip-spine connection, gender-specific needs and the application of lifestyle medicine for patients with musculoskeletal conditions.

47

Nonalcoholic fatty liver disease

Shima Ghavimi, M.D.

WHAT IS NONALCOHOLIC FATTY LIVER DISEASE?

Nonalcoholic fatty liver disease (NAFLD) is a condition characterized by the accumulation of fat (lipids) in the liver. You may also hear it referred to as hepatic steatosis. Technically, NAFLD is defined as fat accumulation in more than 5% of liver cells in people who consume little or no alcohol.

NAFLD is set to become the next worldwide epidemic affecting people of all ages, ethnicities and races across the globe. The leading explanation for why some people develop NAFLD has to do with genetic differences involved in the way their bodies break down food for energy (lipid metabolism). The prevalence of this condition is increasing in women in the U.S., and Hispanics are disproportionately affected. NAFLD is most commonly associated with specific hormone imbalances, which are more likely to occur in women. Younger women, in their reproductive age, have lower rates of NAFLD when compared with men in the same age range. However, the prevalence of NAFLD in women of menopausal age exceeds that of men from the same age groups.

NAFLD can run in the family and usually is associated with high blood pressure (hypertension), unhealthy blood fat levels (hyperlipidemia), diabetes and obesity — although it can occur in people who are not overweight. Other conditions that may be associated with NAFLD include obstructive sleep apnea and hormone conditions such as polycystic ovary syndrome, decreased thyroid function (hypothyroidism), decreased sex glands function (hypogonadism) and growth hormone deficiency.

Fat accumulation in the liver can have causes other than NAFLD, such as excessive alcohol consumption, viral hepatitis, starvation, intravenous nutrition, certain medications (such as tamoxifen, amiodarone, methotrexate, corticosteroids, lomitapide and others), abnormal accumulation of fat in the body (lipodystrophy) or Wilson disease, a condition characterized by copper accumulation in body organs. Your clinician will likely want to rule out these other possibilities before making a diagnosis of NAFLD.

CAN NAFLD BE PREVENTED?

Yes, NAFLD can be prevented by exercising 30 to 45 minutes a day, eating a proper nutritional diet, maintaining a healthy body weight and maintaining healthy blood sugar and lipid levels.

While a loss of 10% to 15% of body weight is desirable if you are overweight, losing even 3% to 5% of excess body weight can improve the outcome of NAFLD. Decreasing your calorie intake by 500 to 1000 calories a day can support weight loss and improve NAFLD. This can be achieved by embracing a healthy plant-based diet rich in fruits, vegetables, whole grains and non-fat protein, and by decreasing your intake of processed foods, red meats, carbohydrates and alcohol (limit to a maximum of one glass of red wine, once a week).

It is important to understand your body and become an advocate for your own health. Make sure to get your annual health checkup and ask your health care team to create a personalized nutrition plan for you based on your age and health condition.

HOW IS NAFLD TREATED?

There are currently no treatments approved by the Food and Drug Administration (FDA) for NAFLD, but experimental treatments are under investigation. Your clinician will probably order blood tests and imaging studies to better understand the

Stages of fatty liver disease

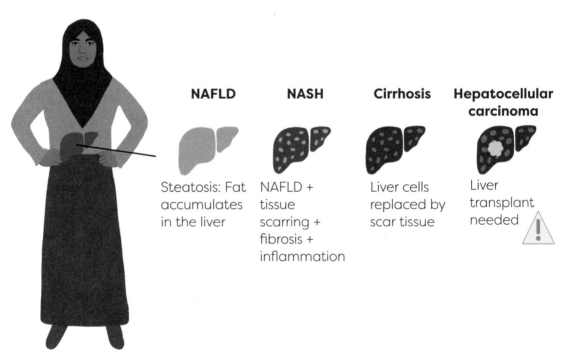

NAFLD

Steatosis: Fat accumulates in the liver

NASH

NAFLD + tissue scarring + fibrosis + inflammation

Cirrhosis

Liver cells replaced by scar tissue

Hepatocellular carcinoma

Liver transplant needed

severity of your disease and how well your liver is functioning. One test that may be ordered is transient elastography, an enhanced form of ultrasound that measures the stiffness of your liver; stiffness indicates scarring (fibrosis) of the liver from NAFLD.

Next, a small sample of liver cells (biopsy) may be obtained to further assess the disease's severity. If the biopsy shows inflammation in addition to fat accumulation, it indicates a condition called nonalcoholic steatohepatitis (NASH). NASH is more serious than NAFLD, as it can lead to liver cirrhosis and liver cancer. For those who have severe cirrhosis (late stage scarring of the liver) due to NASH, a liver transplant may be the only treatment option.

Healthy diet and exercise

The first line of treatment for NAFLD or NASH is usually weight loss through a combination of a healthy diet and exercise. If you do not already exercise regularly, talk with your primary care clinician or someone on your health care team about how you can start to get at least 30 to 45 minutes of exercise a day. If you are overweight, start reducing the number of calories you eat each day and increase your physical activity. Calorie reduction is the key to losing weight and managing this disease. Keep track of all of the calories you take in each day by creating your own personal dietary journal.

Weight-loss surgery

If you have tried to lose weight in the past and have been unsuccessful, ask your health care team for help. If diet and exercise aren't enough to help you lose weight, bariatric weight-loss surgery may be an option. If you think weight-loss surgery might be for you, talk with your clinician to find out if you meet the criteria for bariatric weight-loss surgery.

Other therapies

While no alternative medicine treatments have been shown to cure NAFLD, some studies suggest that coffee may be helpful for people with NAFLD. Research has shown less liver damage in people with NAFLD who drink two or more cups of coffee a day compared with those who drink little or no coffee. It is not clear how coffee may influence liver health, but findings suggest that coffee contains certain compounds that may play a role in fighting inflammation. If you don't already drink coffee, make sure to discuss the potential benefits of coffee with your health care team before starting to drink it.

Additionally, for women with NASH, a daily dose of 800 international units (IU) of vitamin E a day may improve liver tissue. However, vitamin E is not recommended if you have diabetes or cirrhosis. If you have diabetes, talk with your clinician about adjusting your diabetes medications, which can affect NASH. Your clinician may switch you to pioglitazone or exenatide, for example, if there is no contraindication for you to use one of these medications. If you have diabetes, follow your diabetes care team's instructions on how to manage your diabetes, take your medications as directed and closely monitor your blood sugar.

WHY DOES NAFLD MATTER TO WOMEN?

NAFLD is one of the most common causes of chronic liver disease, impacting women in many ways. Prevalence of NAFLD is 10% among females in their reproductive years. Pregnant women with NAFLD have a higher risk of cesarean section, preterm labor, low birth weight, high blood pressure (preeclampsia), impaired blood sugar metabolism (gestational diabetes) and bleeding after delivery.

NAFLD is linked to colorectal polyps, polycystic ovary syndrome, osteoporosis, obstructive sleep apnea, stroke, and various non-liver cancers, such as breast cancer. Women with NAFLD are at risk of cardiovascular diseases, including heart attack — one of the leading causes of death in the U.S. and many other countries. Managing cardiovascular risk factors such as blood sugar, cholesterol and triglycerides is strongly recommended in treating NAFLD.

QUESTIONS TO ASK YOUR HEALTH CARE TEAM

- If I have NAFLD, is the fat in my liver hurting my health?
- Will my fatty liver disease progress to a more serious form?
- What are my treatment options?
- What can I do to keep my liver healthy?
- I have other health conditions. How can I best manage them together?
- Are there any printed or digital materials that I can read on my own?
  - › What websites do you recommend?
- What is the typical outcome of NAFLD?
- If I am diagnosed with NAFLD, can I drink alcohol? How much?
- When is a liver transplant necessary?
- Am I at risk of liver cancer?

PEARLS OF WISDOM

NAFLD is a serious health condition for women of all ages. Lack of exercise, genetic predisposition, unhealthy diet and obesity contribute to the development of NAFLD. If NAFLD is not prevented, it may cause NASH or even cirrhosis of the liver.

If you are diagnosed with NAFLD, make sure your health care team involves a doctor who specializes in managing diseases of the digestive system (gastroenterologist) and a doctor who specializes in managing liver diseases (hepatologist) to better serve you. Work with your health care team to obtain guidance on nutrition, understanding your test results and learning how to prevent NAFLD from becoming more severe.

Create a journal to track your diet and exercise habits, previous test results and medications you are taking. In this journal, make a list of questions to ask your liver disease specialists and bring this journal with you when you visit your health care team. It is both acceptable and encouraged that you bring someone with you to your appointments. This family member or friend can help support you by writing down the information your liver disease specialist shares with you during your visit. Remember, after any tests are conducted, always plan a follow-up visit with your health care team so that you understand the results and know what to do going forward.

"Counties, Communities, Countries and the whole World are only as strong as the Health of their Women."

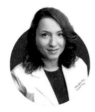

Shima Ghavimi, M.D. - she/her
Dr. Ghavimi is a member of the Women in GI committee of the American College of Gastroenterology, and Assistant Professor of Medicine at Marshall University Joan C. Edwards School of Medicine in Huntington, West Virginia. She specialized in gastroenterological, hepatological and functional GI disorders, and her focus is prevention of colorectal and liver cancer.

48

Obesity and metabolic syndrome

Chika Vera Anekwe, M.D., M.P.H., and
Fatima Cody Stanford, M.D., M.P.H., M.P.A., M.B.A., FAAP, FACP, FAHA, FAMWA, FTOS

WHAT ARE OBESITY AND METABOLIC SYNDROME?

Obesity is a chronic disease characterized by excess body fat, with the most common definition based on having a body mass index (BMI) of 30 or greater. BMI is calculated as the ratio of a person's weight in kilograms divided by height in square meters (square meters is equal to height in centimeters divided by 100). Being overweight (pre-obesity), means having a BMI greater than 25 but less than 30.

Obesity increases the risk of developing metabolic syndrome, which is defined as having three or more of these conditions:
- High blood pressure
- High blood sugar
- Elevated triglycerides
- Low HDL (or "good") cholesterol
- Excess fat around the waist

Obesity and metabolic syndrome are highly correlated. Both conditions raise your risk of heart disease, stroke and diabetes.

CAN OBESITY AND METABOLIC SYNDROME BE PREVENTED?

The short answer is, sometimes. There are many biologic, genetic and environmental factors that cannot be changed but that predispose some individuals to develop obesity or metabolic syndrome. Factors include having many family members with obesity, being born to a mother with obesity or having many social contacts who struggle with their weight.

Since losing weight and keeping it off is so difficult for so many people, it is critical to prevent weight gain in the first place. Here are some strategies:

Maintain a healthy dietary pattern
Although no single diet is recommended for preventing obesity, there are many dietary practices that can ensure healthy nutrition. These include eating plenty of fruits, vegetables, lean protein and whole grains, and reducing processed foods and foods high in added sugars, refined carbohydrates and saturated fat. In addition, keeping portions moderate is key for maintaining caloric and energy balance.

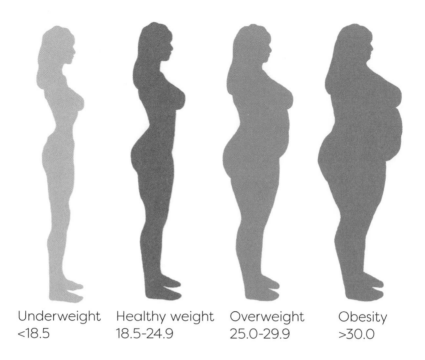

Underweight
<18.5

Healthy weight
18.5-24.9

Overweight
25.0-29.9

Obesity
>30.0

Engage in regular physical activity

National health guidelines recommend at least 150 minutes of moderate to vigorous physical activity a week for health and weight maintenance. A combination of both aerobic and resistance training will help you reap the most health benefits. Longer duration and higher-intensity activity are needed in order to promote weight loss.

Get adequate restful sleep

A minimum of seven hours of sleep is recommended for optimal health. Ensure high-quality sleep by keeping your bedroom quiet, dark and cool; keeping a consistent bedtime and wake time; avoiding large meals at least three hours prior to bedtime (a small snack prior to bed is OK) and caffeine and alcohol at least four hours prior to bedtime, as well as minimizing blue light exposure from electronics at least one hour before bedtime; and treating any underlying sleep disorders.

Reduce stress

Chronic stress increases cortisol levels, which can cause weight gain. Stress (and sleep deprivation) can increase the desire for unhealthy foods and reduce the willpower and judgment needed to avoid them. Many activities can reduce stress, such as exercising, meditating, engaging with others, listening to music or taking part in any activities that may bring you joy.

Address past traumas

Studies have found that childhood traumas, such as neglect and sexual or physical abuse, can raise a person's risk of binge eating disorder, post-traumatic stress disorder and body dissatisfaction, which subsequently increase the risk of developing obesity. While these past traumas cannot be reversed, it is important to recognize them and seek mental health support to reduce any ongoing negative impacts on your mental and physical health.

HOW ARE OBESITY AND METABOLIC SYNDROME TREATED?

Overweight, mild obesity, moderate obesity and metabolic syndrome can be treated by following the preventive measures discussed earlier in this chapter. Here are additional recommendations:

Diet

Consider establishing a habit of tracking or journaling your daily food intake. Although it is important to be mindful of total energy intake, you will achieve more consistent results by paying attention to diet quality versus diet quantity. Consider eating less processed food, as this appears to have a great impact on the body's desire to store energy in the form of fat. While many have relied on calorie counting, we know that calories are not all created equal.

Physical activity

As mentioned earlier, 150 minutes a week of physical activity can help prevent weight gain. But to lose weight, physical activity guidelines suggest a minimum of 300 minutes a week of physical activity. This means aiming for at least 60 minutes of exercise at least five days a week.

Treatment of related medical conditions

Seek treatment for any weight-related or metabolism-related medical conditions that can put you at added risk of poor health. These include obstructive sleep apnea, high blood pressure, unhealthy levels of blood fats (hyperlipidemia or dyslipidemia), polycystic ovary syndrome and diabetes.

Reduction of medications that cause weight gain

Many medications are known to cause weight gain as a side effect. Examples include steroids, beta-blockers, insulin, sleep medications, hormone replacement therapy and hormonal contraceptives, as well as many antidepressants, antipsychotics and anti-anxiety medications. Work with your clinician to adjust your medication regimen to minimize any potential weight gain associated with these medications.

Anti-obesity medications

There are medications that can reduce appetite and cravings and improve your body's metabolism and response to insulin, thereby promoting weight loss. These medications are approved for use in people with a BMI of 30 or higher, or a BMI of 27 with a weight-related medical condition. Talk to your clinician about medications which might be right for you, or ask your clinician to refer you to an obesity medicine and nutrition specialist.

Weight-loss surgery

Severe obesity is defined as BMI of 40 or greater. For people with severe obesity — or moderate obesity (BMI of 35) with another medical condition — who do not have an adequate response to other treatment measures, metabolic and bariatric surgery is an important option. It is a safe and effective treatment for obesity that can lead to significant long-term weight loss and weight maintenance, as well as resolution of metabolic syndrome and other weight-related medical conditions. The risks of the surgery are similar to those associated with any surgical approach requiring anesthesia. There are several different metabolic and bariatric surgical operations. The two most common are the Roux-en-Y gastric bypass and the sleeve gastrectomy. A bariatric surgeon will work with you to determine which type of surgery may be best for you. If you decide on a surgical approach, be sure to engage in follow-up care for careful monitoring of your weight and nutritional status after surgery.

WHY DO OBESITY AND METABOLIC SYNDROME MATTER TO WOMEN?

Obesity in adults has increased steadily over the past 20 years. Although obesity was just as common in men as in women in 2017 to 2018, the prevalence of severe obesity was higher in women than in men. Adults between ages 40 and 59 had the highest prevalence of severe obesity during this same time period. Obesity rates are highest for non-Hispanic African Americans, followed by Hispanic Americans and non-Hispanic white Americans.

Biologically, women have higher body fat and lower muscle mass percentages compared with men, thus setting them up for a metabolic disadvantage when it comes to weight loss and maintenance. Furthermore, certain issues related to obesity are relevant only for females, such as monthly hormonal shifts affecting hunger, cravings and weight, postmenopausal changes to the body affecting metabolism, and the inability to use anti-obesity medications or undergo bariatric surgery during or shortly after pregnancy. Obesity can also contribute to reduced fertility and pregnancy complications. For women who have had bariatric surgery, there are added concerns about increased risk of bone loss and fractures.

Because weight is visible to others, another concern faced by women with obesity is that of weight discrimination. Although men are by no means immune to weight discrimination, women tend to experience it a much higher rate and at much lower levels of excess body weight. This is particularly true for women who are middle-aged or have lower levels of education.

QUESTIONS TO ASK YOUR HEALTH CARE TEAM ABOUT OBESITY AND METABOLIC SYNDROME

- What is my BMI?
- Do I have any weight-related medical conditions?
- What dietary recommendations do you suggest for me?
- What physical activity goals should I aim to meet?
- Do I meet diagnostic criteria for depression, anxiety, binge eating disorder or post-traumatic stress disorder?
- Should I be tested for sleep apnea?

For overweight, mild and moderate obesity, and/or metabolic syndrome
- What lifestyle changes can I make to reduce my weight and risk factors?
- Should I consult with a registered dietitian for further guidance?
- Should I consult with a physical therapist, exercise physiologist or personal trainer?
- Should I consult with a psychologist or psychiatrist for further evaluation and management of any mental health disorders?

- Am I taking any medications that could be causing weight gain?
- Would I be a good candidate for weight-loss medications?

For severe obesity and metabolic syndrome

- Do I meet criteria for metabolic and bariatric surgery?
- What are the risks and benefits of metabolic and bariatric surgery?
- If I decide against surgery, what are my chances of achieving weight loss?
- How much weight can I expect to lose if I decide to have surgery?
- How do I prepare for surgery?
- How long should I expect to stay in the hospital after surgery? How much time should I take off from work after surgery?

- What is the recommended follow-up schedule after surgery?

PEARLS OF WISDOM

It's important for women to know that obesity and metabolic syndrome can cause serious problems such as heart disease, stroke, diabetes and even some cancers. Maintaining a healthy weight is also key to maintaining a good quality of life. Some important strategies for maintaining weight, health and well-being include following a healthy dietary pattern, engaging in regular physical activity, reducing stress, getting adequate restful sleep and treating any associated mental and physical health conditions.

"All women should be empowered to fully understand and take control of their own health and wellbeing."

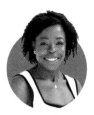

Chika Vera Anekwe, M.D., M.P.H. - she/her
Dr. Anekwe is an obesity medicine physician at Massachusetts General Hospital (MGH) and Medical Director of the Center for Weight Loss Surgery at Newton-Wellesley Hospital, one of the community hospitals affiliated with MGH. She practices at both the Boston and Newton, Massachusetts, locations. Dr. Anekwe is an Instructor in Medicine at Harvard Medical School and specializes in nutrition, obesity and related conditions, and non-surgical weight management.

"Women with intersectional identities (i.e., Black and woman) are often neglected and unheard, and I am committed to changing the status quo."

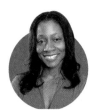

Fatima Cody Stanford, M.D., M.P.H., M.P.A., M.B.A., FAAP, FACP, FAHA, FAMWA, FTOS - she/her
Dr. Stanford is one of the first fellowship-trained obesity medicine physicians in the world. She is an obesity medicine physician scientist, educator, and policy maker at Massachusetts General Hospital and Harvard Medical School in Boston, Massachusetts. She is a nationally and internationally sought-after expert in obesity medicine who bridges the intersection of medicine, public health, policy, and disparities.

49
Osteoporosis

Elizabeth M. Haney, M.D.

WHAT IS OSTEOPOROSIS?

Osteoporosis is a condition that causes bone strength to decrease. When bone strength is decreased, bones are more likely to break (fracture). Osteoporotic fractures are those that result from mild trauma, such as falling from a standing height or less. Examples of osteoporotic fractures include fractures of the hip, wrist and spine. Some rib and upper arm (humerus) fractures are also included under osteoporotic fractures. These fractures are described as osteoporotic fractures because they impact life expectancy and quality of life. Experiencing one osteoporotic fracture indicates that you are likely at risk for another.

Bone is a living tissue made of cells, protein (collagen) and minerals (calcium phosphate). Collagen provides the framework for calcium phosphate, which gives strength to bones. Peak bone mass, or the amount of mineral in bone, for women is achieved around ages 28 to 30. Bone mass then declines with age, and there is a particularly quick period of bone loss in the first five years after menopause.

Healthy bone   **Osteoporosis**

Osteoporosis over time

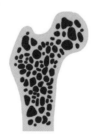
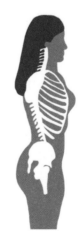
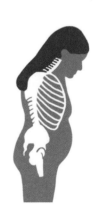

The inside of bone has small, honeycomb-like spaces. In healthy bone (left), these spaces are small. In osteoporotic bone (right), the spaces are larger, which makes the bone weak.

Bone strength is comprised of two components: bone quality and bone density. A useful analogy when thinking about bone density and bone strength is to compare the bone to a wooden train trestle. The interlacing wood of the trestle provides enough strength to support the train as it crosses a canyon; but if several of the wood pieces start to wear out — become thin or brittle, or even break entirely — then the trestle may be at risk of collapse. This is similar to what can happen with bone. With osteoporosis, the framework that provides bone strength can become weaker, less connected, less full and more likely to fracture.

Diagnosing osteoporosis

Of the two components of bone strength, bone density is the easiest to measure. To detect and prevent fractures, the U.S. Preventive Services Task Force, along with the national health organizations of many other countries and the World Health Organization (WHO), recommend screening for osteoporosis by measuring bone density. Typically this is done with a dual-X-ray absorptiometry (DXA) scan. DXA results are conveyed in terms of T-scores and FRAX scores.

T-score This test result provides a standard comparison between your bone density and that of a young woman who has healthy bone and a negligible risk of fracture. This comparison gives an estimate of how much additional risk of fracture you might have. Because bone density declines with age, a comparison of your bone density with the bone density of a young healthy woman offers a reliable insight into your fracture risk. The National Osteoporosis Foundation and the WHO define osteoporosis as a level of bone density that predicts future fracture. These organizations consider a T score of -2.5 or less an indicator of future fracture risk. Low bone mass (osteopenia) is another category of bone health. Osteopenia is effectively a "pre-osteoporosis" state and is characterized as a T score between -1.0 and -2.5.

FRAX score A FRAX score is a calculated estimate of a person's risk of fracture over the next 10 years. It is helpful because not all fractures happen in people with a T-score of -2.5 or below. Some fractures occur in people with low bone mass or a T-score -1.0 to -2.5. Determining which factors contribute to higher risk of fracture among people with low bone mass can identify who might benefit from treatment.

CAN OSTEOPOROSIS AND FRACTURES BE PREVENTED?

There are several things you can do to lower your risk of osteoporosis and prevent fractures. These include:

Eat a well-balanced diet

Maintaining a well-balanced diet ensures adequate intake of nutrients essential for bone health. Dairy foods provide the most reliable source of calcium. Milk intake across various cultures is associated with better bone health. Studies that randomly assign people to drink milk or not drink milk show that girls who drink milk develop more bone tissue, and postmenopausal women who drink milk have less bone loss compared with the groups that do not drink milk. The National Osteoporosis Foundation and the Institute of Medicine recommend 1200 milligrams (mg) a day of calcium for women aged 51 and older.

Get adequate vitamin D

Vitamin D is needed for your body to absorb calcium from the foods you eat. You can get vitamin D from certain foods, such as fatty fish, egg yolks and foods that are supplemented with vitamin D. You can also get the vitamin from a nutritional supplement and from sunlight on your skin. For sunlight to convert the vitamin D precursor just beneath your skin to its active form, the intensity of the sun's rays must be at a certain level. If you live in a part of the world that doesn't allow for adequate skin conversion of vitamin D, such as in the northern latitudes, consider talking to your doctor about taking a vitamin D supplement. Vitamin D is available over the counter and a typical dose is 600 to 1000 international units (IU) a day; this amount is included in many women's multivitamins and also in several calcium supplement formulations.

Low vitamin D levels can cause a condition called osteomalacia, which is similar to osteoporosis in that it makes bones more fragile. If you are diagnosed with osteoporosis, your clinician may recommend measuring your blood serum vitamin D level to make sure you don't have osteomalacia. If your vitamin D level is low, your clinician may suggest a supplement to help you maintain adequate vitamin D. For the purposes of bone health, the Institute of Medicine recommends a vitamin D blood serum concentration between 20 and 30 nanograms per milliliter (ng/mL). Currently there is no recommendation for measuring vitamin D levels in the general population of people without osteoporosis.

Exercise

Physical activity is essential for building and maintaining bone strength and bone density. With exercise, and indeed any movement, muscles put a healthy strain on bones, promoting bone formation and building bone strength. Weight-bearing exercise, such as dancing, low-impact aerobics and stair climbing, has been the traditional recommendation for osteoporosis; however, what is most important is that you find an exercise you enjoy and can do regularly. Walking is a wonderful weight-bearing exercise. If you can't walk in your neighborhood because of safety or weather, consider walking at an indoor mall or community center.

Avoid smoking and alcohol

Certain lifestyle choices, such as smoking and excess alcohol use, are harmful to bone. Not smoking and consuming alcohol in moderation, if at all, are important ways to optimize bone health.

Practice fall prevention strategies

Preventing fracture is, to a large degree, about preventing falls. The Centers for Disease Control and Prevention (CDC) recommends screening everyone over age 65 for falls, so you may encounter this evaluation in a routine health maintenance appointment. If you are at high risk for falls, or if you have experienced a fall recently, there are several things you can do to prevent future falls:

- **Choose the right shoes** Adequate footwear is important. Choose shoes that have a back and a secured top, with laced ties or Velcro. Avoid slip-on style shoes.

- **Get help from a physical therapist** Physical therapy for a gait and balance evaluation can be helpful to identify areas for improvement in strength, and to get a set of exercises specifically designed for you to improve your balance. Balance really is something that can improve with practice!
- **Address dizziness and balance issues** Adequate hydration can prevent you from getting dizzy when standing up quickly. Your clinician might evaluate whether your blood pressure drops when moving from a lying to standing position — this is called orthostatic hypotension and can be treated. Similarly, if you are getting up to use the bathroom at night, talk to your clinician about strategies to reduce the chances of a fall.
- **Go over medication side effects with your clinician** Some medications used for sleep or anxiety contribute to falls. If you're taking one of these medications, work with your clinician to reduce or stop these medications in order to reduce your risk of falls.
- **Make your home safe** Importantly, you can also do a safety check of your home to reduce the risk of falls. Pay attention to items that might cause you to trip and fall, such as placement of area rugs, cords and end tables.

Discuss prevention and treatment strategies with your clinician

Some factors that contribute to osteoporosis and falls are less amenable to intervention. For example, genetics play an important role in bone health. Some genetic conditions may impact how your body handles cal-

cium. If either of your parents suffered a hip fracture, you are at higher risk of osteoporosis and fracture.

Peak bone mass, which occurs around ages 28 to 30 for women, is genetically determined but also influenced by lifestyle during the adolescent and young adult years. Achieving a higher bone mass in the younger years helps prevent low bone mass and osteoporosis in the later years. Identifying which lifestyle factors contribute to osteoporosis or low bone mass and which contribute to fracture risk can help you and your clinician create strategies to address those issues directly and strategically.

In addition, medical conditions can sometimes contribute to osteoporosis. The ways in which these conditions impact bone and risk of fracture are varied. Some diseases, such as celiac disease, may affect absorption of vitamin D. Other diseases, such as rheumatoid arthritis and inflammatory bowel disease, may contribute to osteoporosis through inflammatory pathways, or because of medications that are used to treat these conditions. A careful conversation with your clinician can help you identify risk factors for osteoporosis and find ways to minimize their impact on your bone health.

HOW IS OSTEOPOROSIS TREATED?

The overarching goal of treating osteoporosis is to prevent fractures. Once osteoporosis has been identified, the next step is usually to do an evaluation that checks for treatable causes. This may include lab tests for thyroid function, serum calcium and vitamin D levels, and kidney function. Your clinician will likely also consider other conditions that might be contributing to bone loss.

There are several classes of medication available for treatment of osteoporosis. Common options are the bisphosphonates; examples include alendronate (Fosamax), risedronate (Actonel), ibandronate (Boniva) and zoledronic acid (Reclast). Bisphosphonates are very effective for preventing fractures. In fact, the fracture prevention benefit of bisphosphonates appears to continue even after the medication is stopped. Your doctor may recommend a drug "holiday" — stopping the bisphosphonate and continuing with just calcium, vitamin D and exercise for a period — or transitioning to another medication after being on a bisphosphonate for some years.

Other FDA-approved options include denosumab (Prolia), abaloparatide (Tymlos), teriparatide (Forteo), romosozumab (Evenity) and raloxifene. Estrogen is beneficial for bone health and prevents fractures while it is being taken. However, current guidance is to use the lowest dose of estrogen needed to control menopausal symptoms for the shortest period of time. This makes it a less optimal choice for treating osteoporosis in the long term. As a result, estrogen supplementation is not typically chosen as a primary treatment for osteoporosis.

Calcium, vitamin D and exercise are mainstays of osteoporosis treatment during periods of medication use as well as during medication holidays.

WHY DOES OSTEOPOROSIS MATTER TO WOMEN?

Osteoporosis is most common in postmenopausal women, though it can also occur in premenopausal women and in men. Osteoporosis is asymptomatic — that is, it does not cause symptoms. People may not know they have osteoporosis until they develop a fracture.

The goal of treating osteoporosis is to prevent fractures.

- **Hip fractures** contribute to significant disability. People who fracture a hip can develop short-term complications, such as pneumonia, infection or blood clots. They may also develop long-term complications: People who fracture a hip may lose their independence by having to move out of their home or rely on others for help with their activities of daily living, may have limitations in their ability to walk and may develop chronic pain.
- **Spine fractures** are also important because over time they contribute to curvature of the spine (kyphosis), height loss and chronic back pain. Spine fractures can also reduce the size of the chest and abdominal cavities. As a result, internal organs may become compressed, eventually affecting lung function and bowel function.

It is important for women to stay current with their routine health maintenance. Routine screening for osteoporosis is recommended starting at age 65. Once you have had the initial screening with DXA scan, ask your doctor how often the test should be repeated. Depending on the results of your first DXA scan at age 65, you may be asked to repeat the DXA in 2, 5 or 15 years.

QUESTIONS TO ASK YOUR HEALTH CARE TEAM ABOUT OSTEOPOROSIS

For all women
- When should I be screened for osteoporosis?
- What can I do now to prevent osteoporosis?

If you have low bone mass
- When should I have another DXA scan for monitoring my bone density?
- Should I take vitamin D? How can I make sure that I have adequate calcium in my diet?
- What kind of exercise is safest for me?

If you have had a fragility fracture
- Should I have a DXA scan?
  - *This is particularly relevant if you are under age 65 and would not otherwise be getting screened for osteoporosis.*
- Can we talk about medications to treat osteoporosis?
- Do I need to take calcium or vitamin D supplements or both supplements?
- What kind of exercises can I do now that I am at higher risk for another fracture?

PEARLS OF WISDOM

Adequate nutrition throughout life is important for building strong bones and preventing bone loss as you get older. Calcium is best obtained through diet. If you are taking medication for osteoporosis, your clinician may ask you to take a calcium supplement. Vitamin D is important for bone health and may be most easily obtained through a supplement. Exercise, in the form of both an aerobic activity such as walking and a balance activity such as tai chi, is essential for building strong bones, and for preventing falls and fractures.

"Women's health care can be complex, but always benefits from listening, collaboration, and a team-based approach."

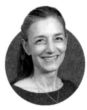

Elizabeth M. Haney, M.D. - she/her
Dr. Haney is Associate Professor in the Departments of Medicine and Medical Informatics & Clinical Epidemiology at Oregon Health & Science University in Portland, Oregon. She is a primary care clinician with focus on osteoporosis, chronic disease management, evidence-based medicine and resident teaching.

50
Ovarian cancer

Teresa P. Díaz-Montes, M.D., M.P.H., FACOG

WHAT IS OVARIAN CANCER?

Ovarian cancer is a type of cancer that arises from the ovaries. The ovaries and fallopian tubes are a pair of organs that are located deep in the pelvis and close to the uterus.

Ovaries contain the eggs a woman is born with. The ovaries release eggs during the menstrual cycle, and they produce hormones. An egg is released from the ovary into the fallopian tube, which connects the ovary to the uterus. Fertilization of the egg by the male sperm usually occurs in the fallopian tube, and the fertilized egg then implants in the uterus to grow into an embryo.

Ovarian cancer develops when the DNA in healthy ovarian cells is altered, causing the cells to grow and multiply rapidly. This rapid cell growth leads to the formation of a mass or tumor that crowds out healthy tissues. Cancerous cells may eventually spread (metastasize) to other parts of the body. An increasing amount of evidence suggests that ovarian cancer may actually originate in the fallopian tubes. Regardless of where the

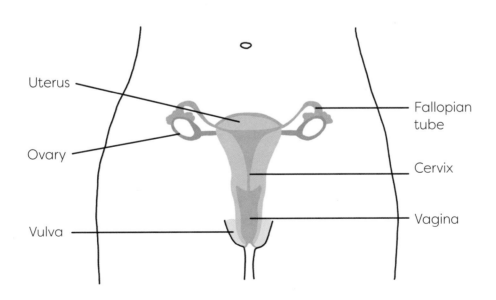

cancer starts, both ovarian and fallopian tube cancers are treated the same way.

CAN OVARIAN CANCER BE PREVENTED?

Unfortunately ovarian cancer often cannot be prevented, and currently no routine screening tests for this type of cancer are available. Some women with a family history of certain types of cancers have a higher risk compared with others and may benefit from genetic testing.

There are several steps that you can take to help you manage your risk.

Review your family history of breast, ovarian or fallopian tube cancer

About 5% to 10% of ovarian cancers are due to family cancer syndromes. A family cancer syndrome is a genetic disorder in which inheriting an altered (mutated) gene can increase your risk of cancer. People who carry the altered gene are at risk of developing cancer earlier in life. They can also pass those genes to their children.

It's important for women who are diagnosed with ovarian cancer to undergo genetic screening tests for specific gene variants. People diagnosed with pancreatic cancer or certain colon, prostate and breast cancers may need to be tested as well. Talk to your clinician about your need for genetic testing. Testing involves meeting with a genetic counselor. The test is usually done using a blood or saliva sample. Genetic testing is mostly covered by insurance, but check with your insurance provider to avoid any surprises.

Test results can help determine recommendations for treatment, screening for other types of cancers or even recommendations for other family members to be tested. The risk of ovarian cancer is higher for family members if the person with ovarian cancer is a first-degree relative (such as a mother, sister or daughter).

Genes more commonly known to increase the risk of ovarian cancer include BRCA 1 and BRCA 2, which are also known to increase the risk of breast cancer, and other genes.

- BRCA 1 mutation carriers may have an increased risk of up to 30% to 40% of developing ovarian cancer compared with average-risk women, who have a 1% to 2% risk of developing ovarian cancer.
- BRCA 2 mutation carriers have about 10% to 20% increased risk compared with average-risk women.
- Variations of other genes are known to increase ovarian cancer risk. These genes include TP53, STK11, PALB2, MLH2, MLH1 and CDH1.

Consider birth control pills

Using birth control pills for five or more years can lower the risk of developing ovarian cancer by 50% compared with people who don't use them.

Talk with your clinician about having ovaries and fallopian tubes removed

Women who are at high risk of ovarian cancer might consider having their ovaries and fallopian tubes removed to decrease their risk after they have completed childbearing. This can include women who discover from genetic tests that they are carriers of a gene variation linked to ovarian cancer but who have no signs or symptoms of that cancer. Removing the ovaries and fallopian tubes can reduce the risk of ovarian cancer by 70% to 90% and the risk of breast cancer by 40% to 70%.

HOW IS OVARIAN CANCER TREATED?

The treatment of ovarian cancer depends on how big the tumor is and how far the cancer has spread (the stage of the disease). Most ovarian cancers require a combination of surgery and chemotherapy. The sequence in which treatments are given depends on the individual circumstances of each person.

Surgery

Surgery is typically recommended at all stages of disease. Most women diagnosed with early-stage disease (stage I or II) require removal of the uterus, both ovaries and fallopian tubes, lymph nodes, and some additional tissue in the abdomen. For advanced-stage disease (stages III and IV), treatment involves what is commonly known as debulking or cytoreductive surgery. Cytoreductive surgery involves removing all visible tumor parts or lesions so that no visible disease remains at the completion of the surgery. These types of surgeries are complex and are best done at specialized centers. In addition to removing the uterus with the ovaries and fallopian tubes, it may also be necessary to remove part of the bowel (intestines), spleen and gallbladder.

Surgery results are an important factor in determining the outcome (prognosis) for women with ovarian or fallopian tube cancer. The prognosis for long-term survival is best if the tumor is completely removed with surgery, ideally prior to any chemotherapy.

Chemotherapy

Chemotherapy plays a big role in the treatment of ovarian cancer. When to initiate chemotherapy depends on a woman's specific circumstances.

Neoadjuvant chemotherapy This is chemotherapy that is given prior to surgery to reduce the size of the tumor. It is reserved for women in whom surgery is not a first choice because of the large size of the tumor. It may also be recommended for women in whom surgery may diminish an already impaired ability to engage in daily activities, such as walking or getting dressed without help. Tumors may be more successfully removed after they are reduced in size.

Adjuvant chemotherapy This is chemotherapy given after the surgery to remove the original tumor. Its purpose is to maximize the surgery's effectiveness. Adjuvant chemotherapy may be administered through a vein (intravenously, or IV) or directly into the abdomen (intraperitoneally, or IP).

Maintenance therapy This treatment option may involve the use of chemotherapy, targeted therapies or hormonal therapies to decrease the risk of cancer returning (recurring), control cancer growth or control symptoms caused by the cancer.

WHY DOES OVARIAN CANCER MATTER TO WOMEN?

Ovarian cancer is an aggressive type of cancer once diagnosed. About 50% of women diagnosed with ovarian cancer do not survive. This is because the cancer has usually metastasized outside of the ovaries at the time of diagnosis. Among those diagnosed and treated, 75% eventually experience a recurrence of the cancer. Recurrent disease is not considered curable.

Most women with ovarian cancer will need to be on some type of treatment for prolonged periods, which can impact quality of life. Quality of life may also be impacted by the location of the cancer. On occasion, ovarian cancer can cause a blockage of the intestines, leading to weight loss, nausea, vomiting and dehydration. Or the cancer can cause fluid to accumulate around the lungs or in the abdomen, causing difficulty in breathing as well as pain.

If you or a loved one develops ovarian cancer, don't hesitate to look for a female cancer specialist (gynecologic oncologist) who has experience treating ovarian cancer. Look for a specialist who is able to take your circumstances and preferences into account and whose team can help you manage the impact of the cancer on your life. Having a cancer care team you trust can make a big difference in your experience.

QUESTIONS TO ASK YOUR HEALTH CARE TEAM

At your first visit with your gynecologic oncologist
- What is the best option for management of my diagnosis?
- What type of blood work and imaging tests will I need?
  - › How soon do I need to get this done?
- Will I be referred for genetic testing?
- What can I eat to improve my nutrition prior to treatment?

If surgery is recommended
- How much experience do you have managing ovarian cancer?
- How many of these surgeries do you perform a year?
- How successful are you in removing all the cancer during surgery?
- What are potential complications from the surgery? What is your most common complication during this surgery?
- What can I do to improve my health in preparation for surgery?
- How soon will the surgery be scheduled?
- Are there any restrictions prior to or after surgery?

If chemotherapy is recommended
- What are the side effects of the chemotherapy you're recommending?
- What type of blood work will I need to have done and when?
- Will I get medications to prevent side effects from the chemotherapy?
- Do I need to follow a particular diet during chemotherapy?
- Are there any restrictions that I will have during chemotherapy?

After treatment is completed

- How frequently do I need to come back for visits and for how long?
- What testing will be done to detect if there is any cancer coming back (recurrence)?
- What symptoms do I look for?
- Who do I contact if I have any problems?

PEARLS OF WISDOM

Ovarian cancer is a very diverse disease. Each woman's experience is different. Surgery plays an important role in a woman's prognosis. Make sure that you seek care in centers that have expertise in ovarian cancer, as results are better in specialized centers. Make sure that you have genetic testing done after the diagnosis.

"All women should have access to the best health care."

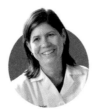

Teresa P. Díaz-Montes, M.D., M.P.H., FACOG - she/her
Dr. Díaz-Montes is a board-certified gynecologist oncologist and Associate Director of the Lya Segall Ovarian Cancer Institute at Mercy Medical Center in Baltimore, Maryland. She is an Adjunct Associate Professor at the Department of Obstetrics and Gynecology, University of Maryland. She specializes in ovarian cancer surgery and hyperthermic intraperitoneal chemotherapy (HIPEC) surgery.

51
Painful sex

Alexandra Dubinskaya, M.D., and Jennifer T. Anger, M.D., M.P.H.

WHAT IS VULVODYNIA?

Sexual activity, including vaginal penetration, should be pleasurable and not painful. Occasional discomfort may be normal. However, persistent or recurrent pain that creates personal discomfort often indicates a problem that can be treated. There are many potential reasons behind pain associated with sex: vaginal dryness, infections, skin conditions, uterine fibroids, pelvic floor muscles spasms and others. This chapter focuses on a common but underdiagnosed condition called vulvodynia.

Vulvodynia is a scientific term for pain around a woman's external genitalia. The exact cause of vulvodynia is unknown. The pain is most often described as a burning sensation that tends to persist and worsen while wearing tight clothes, sitting down or having sex. The pain can be generalized over an area or it can be localized and felt only at certain points along the vaginal opening. Vulvodynia can be triggered (provoked) by touch to the genital region or tampon placement, or it may occur without any trigger (unprovoked).

CAN VULVODYNIA BE PREVENTED?

Most of the time, vulvodynia occurs spontaneously and is not preventable. However, taking certain measures can help minimize some known causes of vulvodynia.

Maintain a healthy vaginal pH

Maintaining a vaginal pH in the more acidic range between 3.8 and 4.5 helps prevent overgrowth of harmful bacteria (bacterial vaginosis), which often causes discomfort and pain. A healthy vaginal pH can be maintained by avoiding actions that tend to increase the pH level, such as douching, cleaning the inside of the vagina with soap, leaving a tampon inside for too long or using vaginal lubricants containing ingredients that can cause harm to vaginal tissue (glycerin, nonoxynol-9, petroleum, propylene glycol, parabens, chlorhexidine gluconate).

Get tested for vaginal infections

Get tested and treated for sexually transmitted infections (STIs), including herpes if you have engaged in unprotected sexual activity. If you have a herpes infection with frequent outbreaks, ask your clinician about taking preventive (prophylactic) therapy, to avoid outbreaks and associated long-term

Generalized

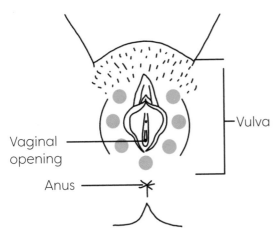

Pain is diffused in the external genitalia region and fairly constant

Localized

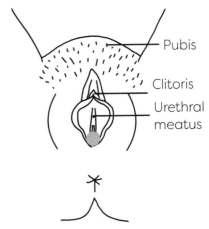

Pain is at the vaginal opening and occurs only with pressure or touch

lingering pain. Get tested and treated for a vaginal yeast infection, particularly if you have had prior vaginal yeast infections.

Consider factors affecting your hormones

Hormonal changes — such as those brought on by menopause, breastfeeding or hormonal treatments, including contraception — may play a role in vulvodynia. Contraceptives such as intrauterine devices (IUDs), which work locally, may cause fewer cases of vulvodynia compared with oral contraceptives. Make sure your method of contraception does not interfere with your vulvar health.

Practice vulvar self-care

It's important to prevent trauma to the nerves in your pelvis and vagina by avoiding improperly fitted seats, such as bicycle seats, stationary bike seats and horseback-riding saddles.

Rehab your pelvic floor muscles

Women tend to carry the weight of stress, anxiety, depression and emotional trauma not only on their shoulders, but also on their pelvic floor muscles. Those muscles can become stiff and tender, leading to alterations in bladder, bowel and sexual function. Pelvic floor therapy involves rehabilitation massage and stretching techniques done with the help of a physical therapist who specializes in the pelvic floor. Pelvic floor physical therapy helps relieve stress and normalize the function of the pelvic muscles. It is also an excellent way to help your muscles recover after childbirth, especially after vaginal delivery.

HOW IS VULVODYNIA TREATED?

There is no standardized treatment for vulvodynia. Usually, treatment is tailored to the suspected cause. When no specific cause is identified, you might have to try the various methods of treatment described in the rest of this section to find the ones that work for you. In some cases, vulvodynia cannot be completely cured. But in most cases, it can be managed and improved.

Avoiding irritants

Give preference to cotton underwear that is washed without detergent or with hypoallergenic soap. If tight clothing causes discomfort, consider wearing loose-fitting pants or skirts. Do not apply soap directly on the vulva or inside the vagina. Using a squirt bottle or bidet after urinating or having a bowel movement may be helpful in preventing irritation. Avoid wearing pantyliners and using feminine wipes.

Talk about sex

Talk to your partner about vulvodynia, what it means and what symptoms you experience. Remember that sex is not defined only by vaginal penetration and can still be enjoyable for both partners without it. Try to focus on the areas of the body that give you pleasurable sensations. Make sure you are not committing to activities that cause you pain and discomfort, as these will trigger your brain to anticipate the pain and fear having sex. Consider using a lubricant for internal and external foreplay. Regular use of vibrators on the vulva has demonstrated improvement in pain among women with vulvodynia. Consider getting one!

Try topical treatments

Some women find relief with topical numbing creams and gels. Use them with caution, since occasionally they can cause sensitivity and irritation. Topical use of tricyclic antidepressants (in a compounded formulation) may improve pain when used for intercourse-provoked vulvodynia. Vaginal estrogen and compounded estrogen and testosterone creams are helpful in the treatment of hormonally mediated vulvodynia. Pelvic physical therapy, intravaginal muscle relaxants such as vaginal diazepam, and injection of stiff pelvic muscles with numbing medicine (Lidocaine) and even onabotulinumtoxinA (Botox) can give relief to those whose pain is caused by a muscular component or pelvic trauma.

Oral treatments

Tricyclic antidepressants and anticonvulsants taken by mouth (orally) work for nerve-related (neuropathic) pain and may provide significant relief for women with vulvodynia. Be sure to also get treated for sexually transmitted infections. Your clinician will likely prescribe an oral antibiotic or antiviral drug to treat the STI.

Surgical treatment

Women who have localized vulvodynia and no response to other treatment measures might benefit from surgical removal of the painful area.

WHY DOES VULVODYNIA MATTER TO WOMEN?

Vulvodynia has a significant impact on a woman's quality of life, and there's no reason for it to go untreated. Unfortunately, the subject of vaginal pain has been under-recognized and under-researched. Sexual pleasure is a basic human right for both men and women. Vulvodynia can rob a woman of experiencing intimacy and being close to her partner. It is important to seek treatment, since the longer you wait, the more severe and difficult to treat the condition becomes.

Talk to your clinician about any vulvar pain or discomfort you may be experiencing. Not every clinician is able to recognize and treat vulvodynia. Frequently women see several clinicians before receiving the right diagnosis and treatment. Do not take no for an answer, and do not get discouraged! There are clinicians who will give you information and support, and will keep offering different treatment options until you find the right one for you.

Search the internet for gynecologists or urologists in your area who are familiar with vulvodynia. You can find information on treatments and clinicians by visiting the websites of these organizations: the International Society for the Study of Women's Sexual Health (**www.isswsh.org**) and the International Society for Sexual Medicine (**www.issm.info**).

QUESTIONS TO ASK YOUR HEALTH CARE TEAM

To find the right clinician, call the office and ask:
- Does this clinician treat women who have pelvic pain?
- Does this clinician treat women who have pain with sex?

At your appointment, explain your symptoms and don't be afraid to ask questions, such as:
- I have been experiencing pain with vaginal penetration (tampon insertion)

and when sitting down, and I am concerned about having vulvodynia. Would you do an exam to take a look?
- Are there medications that I am taking that could contribute to my condition?
  > *If you are taking multiple medications, bring a list of the medication names and doses with you to show to your clinician.*
- Would I benefit from pelvic physical therapy?
- Would I benefit from topical or oral muscle relaxants?
- Would I benefit from hormonal
- treatment?
- Can I have a referral to a sexual therapist?
- Do you perform surgeries for women who are not responding to medical treatments?

PEARLS OF WISDOM

Women have tremendous reserve and are able to tolerate a lot of pain. However, not every pain comes with gain. The pain of vulvodynia tends to multiply and trigger more pain. Vulvodynia also affects a woman's self-image, relationships and career. Talk to your female friends; you will likely be surprised to find out how many women around you are facing the same problem. Remember, constant recurrent pain is not normal, and it is not "in your head."

"Speak up for what matters to you. Every time you do, women are one step closer to being heard."

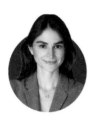

Alexandra Dubinskaya, M.D. - she/her

Dr. Alexandra Dubinskaya is a Beverly Hills-based gynecologist who is fellowship trained in female pelvic medicine and reconstructive surgery. She is specializing in urinary incontinence, pelvic organ prolapse, pelvic reconstruction, hormone replacement therapy, and sexual dysfunction.

"Women deserve high quality, evidenced-based care."

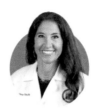

Jennifer T. Anger, M.D., M.P.H. - she/her

Dr. Anger is Vice Chair of Research in the UC San Diego Department of Urology. She is dual fellowship trained in urologic reconstruction and health services research. She currently leads the UC San Diego program in gender affirming pelvic ("bottom") surgery.

52
Pelvic inflammatory disease

Linda M. Nicoll, M.D.

WHAT IS PELVIC INFLAMMATORY DISEASE?

Pelvic inflammatory disease (PID) is an infection of the female upper reproductive tract, which includes the uterus (womb), fallopian tubes and ovaries. It can also involve other nearby organs and tissues. PID is caused by micro-organisms, most commonly bacteria, that invade these organs and tissues, causing inflammation and tissue damage. Most cases of PID are caused by sexually transmitted infections (STIs), such as gonorrhea or chlamydia, or by gardnerella, the bacteria associated with bacterial vaginosis.

Some cases of PID are associated with infections that occur during childbirth, during gynecologic surgery or other procedures, such as treatment of a miscarriage or insertion of an intrauterine device, or after injury or trauma to the reproductive tract. Less commonly, PID is caused by bacteria associated with the gastrointestinal tract, or by bacteria often linked with the respiratory tract, such as strep or staph species. Many infections are caused by a mixture of several bacteria species, and it is often impossible to find the initial cause of the infection.

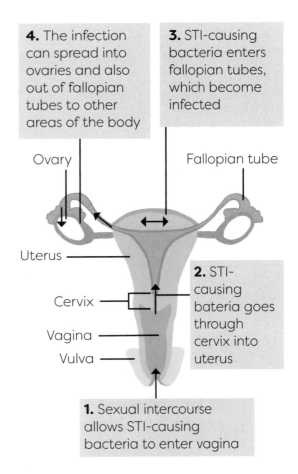

4. The infection can spread into ovaries and also out of fallopian tubes to other areas of the body

3. STI-causing bacteria enters fallopian tubes, which become infected

Ovary

Fallopian tube

Uterus

Cervix

Vagina

Vulva

2. STI-causing bateria goes through cervix into uterus

1. Sexual intercourse allows STI-causing bacteria to enter vagina

Pelvic inflammatory disease can come on suddenly with severe symptoms, or it can follow a longer, more chronic course, which can make it difficult to diagnose. Laboratory tests, including blood counts showing elevated white blood cells, and imaging, such as ultrasound or CT scan, can help support a diagnosis of PID. However, the diagnosis of PID is usually made based on these common signs and symptoms.

- Lower abdominal pain that's often:
  - › On both the left and right sides
  - › Worse with intercourse
  - › Lasting less than two weeks
- Abnormal uterine (vaginal) bleeding such as:
  - › Bleeding after intercourse
  - › Bleeding between periods
  - › Abnormally heavy menstrual bleeding
- More frequent urination
- Abnormal vaginal discharge
- Fever

Other conditions can cause pain and similar signs and symptoms. Before making a diagnosis of PID, it's important to rule out:

- Vaginal or cervical infections
- Urinary tract infection (UTI)
- Infection of the appendix (appendicitis)
- Endometriosis, a noncancerous condition in which uterine tissue grows outside the uterus
- Ectopic (tubal) pregnancy
- Uterine cancer

Most of these possibilities can be excluded with laboratory or imaging tests.

If severe enough, or left untreated, PID can damage or destroy the reproductive organs and cause infertility or other long-term complications, including chronic pelvic pain, painful intercourse (dyspareunia) and increased risk of ectopic pregnancy. In very severe cases, PID can cause an infection of the bloodstream (sepsis) and death.

CAN PELVIC INFLAMMATORY DISEASE BE PREVENTED?

The most effective ways of reducing your risk of PID are:

- Limiting your number of sexual partners
- Using barrier contraception, such as condoms
- Making sure both you and your partner are regularly screened for STIs

Pelvic inflammatory disease is more common among women with multiple sexual partners and among women who do not use a barrier contraceptive device. Women in monogamous relationships — those who have sex with one regular partner — are at lower risk. It's important for all women at risk of PID to use latex condoms whenever possible to prevent transmission of sexually transmitted infections.

If you are sexually active, get screened for STIs on a regular basis. Early detection of common STIs can prevent these infections from affecting the upper genital tract and developing into PID. If you experience fever and pelvic or lower abdominal pain or abnormal vaginal bleeding, promptly make an appointment with a clinician to check for the possibility of PID. Early treatment can help prevent complications.

HOW IS PELVIC INFLAMMATORY DISEASE TREATED?

Treatment of pelvic inflammatory disease focuses on restoring a woman's health and on preserving her fertility.

PID is usually treated with a combination of antibiotics that are typically taken by mouth (oral antibiotics). However, if PID is severe, or if there is concern that incomplete treatment may increase a woman's risk of infertility, she is often admitted to a hospital for treatment and given her medication through an IV line (intravenously). Pain medication is often needed and given.

Sometimes, abscesses — walled-off collections of bacteria and pus-like (purulent) fluid — develop in the pelvic area and may need to be drained. Drainage is sometimes done using a needle guided by an ultrasound or CT scan. Other times, surgical removal may be necessary. In rare cases, the reproductive organs have been so damaged by the infection that they need to be removed. This is a treatment of last resort and is usually only considered when a woman's life is in danger.

Antibiotics and drainage or removal of infected tissue are effective treatments for PID. Time spent pursuing herbal, alternative and complementary treatments may increase the risk that a delay in medical care will reduce the chances of full recovery.

WHY DOES PELVIC INFLAMMATORY DISEASE MATTER TO WOMEN?

Early treatment of PID can prevent complications such as infertility, future ectopic pregnancy and chronic pelvic pain.

Although the most common cause of PID is sexually transmitted infection, in rare cases it can occur in women who have never had sexual intercourse, girls who have not yet menstruated and women who are no longer menstruating (menopausal). PID in pregnancy is also rare but can occur in the first trimester. In such cases, it can cause pregnancy complications or miscarriage. The risk of developing PID after insertion of an IUD is very low.

Since women with multiple sexual partners and those who do not use barrier contraception are most at risk, PID is a significant risk to women who are sex workers, including those who are trafficked against their will. It is also a threat to transgender men who are at risk of violence or victimization on the basis of their gender identity or expression.

Pelvic inflammatory disease is most common in sexually active women of reproductive age. Young women are associated with a higher risk of PID compared with older women. Of the almost 1 million cases of pelvic inflammatory disease (PID) diagnosed annually in the United States, 20% are estimated to occur in adolescents. Studies also report rates of PID to be two to three times higher among Black women than among white women. Among the many factors that may relate to this disparity, it's important to note possible differences in access to health care or differences in attitudes of clinicians and systems toward women who are young, Black or both.

QUESTIONS TO ASK YOUR HEALTH CARE TEAM

- What are my risk factors for developing PID?
- What steps can I take to reduce my risk of PID?
- If I suspect I might have PID (I have a fever and abdominal or pelvic pain, or abnormal vaginal bleeding or discharge) should I see my clinician in the office, or should I go straight to an emergency room or urgent care center?
- How might my history of PID affect my plans to start or expand my family?

PEARLS OF WISDOM

- Remember, the most effective ways of reducing risk of PID are:
  - › Limiting your number of sexual partners
  - › Using barrier contraception, such as condoms
  - › Making sure both you and your partner are regularly screened for sexually transmitted infections
- If you think you may have PID, seek care as soon as possible. A delay in diagnosis and treatment may worsen your chances of a quick and complete recovery.
- Don't exclude PID as a possible diagnosis if you are not currently sexually active or if you are currently pregnant.
- Don't be embarrassed to talk about PID. There is no shame in taking your sexual and reproductive health seriously. You are and should be your own best advocate!

"A well-informed patient is an empowered patient."

Linda M. Nicoll, M.D. - she/her
Dr. Nicoll is an Assistant Professor at the NYU Grossman School of Medicine and practices at NYU Langone Hospital–Long Island in Mineola, New York. She specializes in minimally invasive and robotic gynecologic surgery.

53

Pelvic organ prolapse

Nia Thompson Jenkins, M.D., M.P.H., FACOG, and Stacey A. Scheib, M.D.

WHAT IS PELVIC ORGAN PROLAPSE?

Pelvic organ prolapse is a common problem for women — approximately 45% of women are affected by some degree of pelvic organ prolapse in their lifetimes. While prolapse can occur at any age, women are more likely to experience prolapse between the ages of 70 and 80. The term prolapse means "slipping out of place" and refers to the downward displacement of an organ. The uterus, vagina, rectum (the lowest part of the intestines just prior to the anus), bowel (the intestines) and bladder (the organ in the lower abdomen that stores urine) make up the pelvic organs.

There is a large network of ligaments and tissues that supports the pelvic structures and holds them in place. Prolapse occurs when the muscles of the pelvic floor and related connective tissues weaken. Damage to these supporting structures causes organs within the pelvis, such as the uterus, to fall into the vagina. Women may see or feel tissue coming out of the opening of their vagina. Different types of pelvic organ prolapse include:

- Bladder prolapse (cystocele)
- Rectum prolapse (rectocele)
- Bowel prolapse (enterocele)
- Uterine prolapse
- Vaginal vault (after a hysterectomy, the remaining tissue is referred to as the vaginal vault, which can also prolapse)

There are five different stages of pelvic organ prolapse, ranging from zero to four, with four being the most severe. Most women have some degree of uterine prolapse and have very few, if any, symptoms. With advancing degrees of prolapse, women are more likely to have symptoms that disrupt their quality of life.

There are a variety of symptoms associated with pelvic organ prolapse.

- **Common symptoms** can include feeling a lump inside or at the opening of the vagina, the feeling of sitting on an egg, a dragging sensation in the lower back, and pelvic pressure. Some women may complain of difficulty using a tampon, pain with intercourse, and vaginal irritation or dryness from rubbing against undergarments.
- **Bladder-related symptoms** include a slow urinary stream, incomplete emptying of the bladder, frequent urination, urgency to use the restroom, difficulty

passing urine, the need to strain and accidental leakage of urine (urinary incontinence; not directly caused by prolapse).

- **Bowel-related symptoms**, such as difficulty with bowel movements, incomplete emptying of the rectum and a need to press on the vagina to have a bowel movement.

Rarely, some women may experience vaginal bleeding or spotting from prolapse. This may occur when tissue from the vagina or uterus rubs against undergarments, causing tears and superficial scratching. If more than spotting occurs, tell a doctor or other clinician right away, because spotting could be a sign of a more serious condition.

In general, prolapse is not painful but rather uncomfortable. If you have a significant amount of pain with prolapse, you and your clinician may want to consider other possible conditions that might be causing the pain.

CAN PELVIC ORGAN PROLAPSE BE PREVENTED?

The truth is, there is no ideal way to prevent prolapse. There are many factors that lead to the weakening of the pelvic floor over a woman's lifetime, and they can increase the risk of prolapse.

Childbirth and pregnancy

By far the most common risk factor for uterine prolapse is childbirth and pregnancy. Approximately 33% of women who have had at least one child are affected. Vaginal deliveries cause more damage to the muscles and nerves and increase the risk of prolapse compared with a cesarean birth. Women who have had multiple babies vaginally or a large baby or who had forceps used at the time of delivery may be at an increased risk of prolapse. However, this does not mean that women who have had a cesarean birth cannot develop prolapse. Regardless of the type of delivery, the actual process of pregnancy and childbearing causes stretching of the ligaments and tissue in the pelvis. It is possible for prolapse to develop immediately after childbirth, but most commonly it develops years later.

Aging

With increased age comes menopause. Menopause is associated with decreased levels of the hormone estrogen. Many women often associate the decline in estrogen with hot flashes, vaginal dryness or mood swings, but it also causes weakening of the ligaments, muscles and tissues in the pelvic floor. Therefore, it's most common for women to experience prolapse symptoms after menopause.

Heavy lifting

Strength training that involves repeated heavy lifting or a job that demands a lot of heavy lifting can increase the risk of prolapse.

Genetics

The strength of your connective tissue and ligaments is somewhat linked to genetics. If your mother or sister had pelvic organ prolapse, there is a high likelihood that you may experience it as well.

Chronic health conditions

There are some health conditions that place

excessive force on the pelvic floor, such as chronic cough (due to tobacco use, for example) or asthma, as the diaphragm (the muscle at the base of the lung) moves abruptly down toward the abdomen, causing sudden increased pressure on the pelvic floor. Other conditions include obesity and chronic constipation. Over time these forces cause damage to the pelvic floor.

While some of the risk factors associated with prolapse are challenging to prevent, do not be discouraged! Steps you can take to decrease your risk of prolapse include:
- Managing your weight
- Avoiding vaping and tobacco use
- Eating a diet high in fiber (25 grams to 30 grams per day) to keep bowel movements soft and regular
- Managing constipation with appropriate use of stool softeners and laxatives (see Chapter 22)

HOW IS PELVIC ORGAN PROLAPSE TREATED?

If you have symptoms of pelvic organ prolapse, talk to your clinician. A physical examination will help your clinician determine your stage of prolapse, if any, and the best treatment for it. Pelvic organ prolapse is usually treated by doctors who specialize in women's health and conditions that affect the female reproductive system, such as gynecologists, urogynecologists and some urologists.

Nonsurgical options
There are several nonsurgical approaches to treating pelvic organ prolapse.

Monitoring Since pelvic organ prolapse is not life-threatening, it is an option to simply monitor the progression of your prolapse. There is no rush! It is possible that it may not advance beyond its current stages. This is an excellent option for women to do not have significant prolapse or bothersome symptoms.

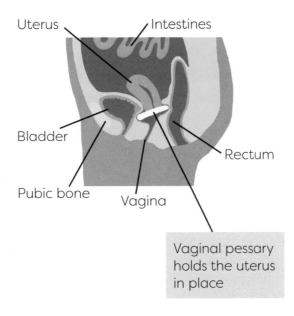

Uterus
Intestines
Bladder
Rectum
Pubic bone
Vagina

Vaginal pessary holds the uterus in place

Kegels and pelvic floor physical therapy These are exercises that help to strengthen the pelvic floor muscles. Working on these weakened muscles may help with the earlier stages of prolapse. Just as exercises at the gym require certain techniques, so do pelvic floor exercises. Ask your clinician for information on how to do them. There are also specialized physical therapists (pelvic floor physical therapists) who can assist you with advanced forms of these exercises.

Pessary A pessary is a silicone device that is inserted into the vagina. It comes in many different shapes and sizes. Pessaries work by pushing the prolapse back up into the vagina and by providing physical support.

During an office visit, your clinician can fit you for the correct size and shape. Some pessaries can be easily inserted and removed at home. Other pessaries used for advanced stages of prolapse can only be inserted and removed by your clinician. This is an ideal option for women who are not interested in having surgery or who are unlikely to undergo surgery because of another medical condition.

Surgical options
The overarching goal of surgery is to reconstruct the pelvic region, often by placing the organs back in their natural position. Different types of surgery can be performed through the vagina or the abdomen using a fiber-optic instrument called a laparoscope, or using a robot. Laparoscopic and robotic surgery allow for smaller incisions, faster recovery time and shorter hospital stays. However, keep in mind that not all medical centers or surgeons offer robotic surgery. For some women, surgery may involve a hysterectomy, or removal of the uterus. If a woman no longer has a uterus but is experiencing prolapse, surgical treatment involves repair of the vaginal vault only.

Apical suspension The purpose of this procedure is to restore the deepest or top part of the vagina (apex) to a more typical location. An apical suspension surgery may or may not include a hysterectomy. The surgery involves attaching the apex to strong ligaments in the pelvis to prevent further prolapse. The gold standard for apical suspension is a larger reconstructive surgery called a sacrocolpopexy. This procedure may not be the best option for older women, or those who are not and do not plan on being sexually active.

Anterior repair This procedure involves repairing the supportive tissue (fascia) that lies under the vaginal wall near the bladder. Essentially, anterior repair surgery creates a stable hammock for the bladder to rest on so that it no longer prolapses. An incision is made in the center portion of the vagina, under the bladder. The length of the incision depends on the severity of the prolapse. Repair of supportive fascia reestablishes support to the vaginal wall and bladder. No stitches (sutures) are placed in the bladder itself. Once the repair is made, the vaginal incision is closed.

Posterior repair This procedure is similar to an anterior repair but involves the part of the vagina that sits over the rectum. Repair of the fascia here creates a stable wall for the rectum to press against so that it no longer prolapses.

Obliterative procedure This procedure involves making incisions on the vaginal walls and sewing the segments of vaginal wall together so that the organs can no longer prolapse. It may be referred to as "closing" the vagina. The surgery has a high success rate but is not a good option for everyone. After this procedure is complete there is no option for vaginal intercourse.

To mesh or not to mesh? Some of the vaginal reconstructive procedures require the use of mesh. Currently, in the United States, mesh is approved by the Food and Drug Administration (FDA) for use in an abdominal sacrocolpopexy, a type of apical procedure. Mesh is not approved for use with anterior or posterior repairs. The use of mesh is a personal decision, so be sure to have a thorough discussion about it with your clinician.

If you still plan on having children, wait to have any reconstructive surgery to treat prolapse. In the meantime, using a pessary can be an effective treatment option.

WHY DOES PELVIC ORGAN PROLAPSE MATTER TO WOMEN?

Pelvic organ prolapse is unique to women. Men do not have a uterus or vagina so they are not affected by these conditions. For the most part, prolapse is not painful. Prolapse matters because it can affect a woman's quality of life, causing discomfort, painful sexual intercourse, vaginal infections, vaginal spotting and personal insecurity. At its worst, prolapse can affect kidney function by kinking or bending the ureters, the tubes that carry urine from the kidneys to the bladder.

QUESTIONS TO ASK YOUR HEALTH CARE TEAM ABOUT PELVIC ORGAN PROLAPSE

- What stage is my prolapse?
- Do you have experience doing prolapse surgeries?
- If I am interested in using a pessary, what type would be best and why?
- If I am interested in surgery, what are my options?
- Is it possible for a pessary to be placed to help relieve my symptoms until surgery is scheduled?
- Should I be worried about having issues with leaking urine after a reconstructive surgical repair?
- If mesh will be used, where will it be placed, what type of mesh is it, and what are the risks of using mesh?
  › What happens if I have issues with the mesh after surgery?
- What restrictions do I have after surgery?

PEARLS OF WISDOM

- There is no way to predict whether pelvic organ prolapse will progress or get better. Sometimes it can get worse, and sometimes it will remain the same for the rest of a woman's lifetime.
- Pelvic organ prolapse is not life-threatening, but it can drastically affect quality of life.
- It is not necessary to suffer in silence. There are many different treatment options, ranging from nonoperative management to complete surgical reconstruction.

"We empower our patients by educating them."

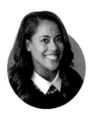

Nia Thompson Jenkins, M.D., M.P.H., FACOG - she/her
Dr. Thompson Jenkins is a female pelvic medicine specialist, reconstructive surgeon, and Assistant Professor of Obstetrics & Gynecology at University Health/ Truman Medical Center in Kansas City, Missouri. She specializes in prolapse repair, urinary incontinence, and minimally invasive gynecologic surgery.

"Women need to be heard in the decisions impacting their own lives, and health care is not an exception."

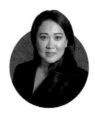

Stacey A. Scheib, M.D. - she/her
Dr. Scheib is the Division Director of Minimally Invasive Surgery for the Department of Obstetrics and Gynecology at Louisiana State University Health Sciences Center in New Orleans, Louisiana, and is the Director of Obstetric and Gynecologic Simulation. She specializes in chronic pelvic pain and minimally invasive gynecologic surgery.

54
Peripheral arterial disease

Camila Franco-Mesa, M.D., and Young Erben, M.D.

WHAT IS PERIPHERAL ARTERIAL DISEASE?

Peripheral arterial disease (PAD) is a condition that occurs when the arteries to your legs become clogged or narrowed with clumps of fatty, fibrous tissue (plaques). Arteries are tubes that carry blood from the heart to other organs and tissues in the body. Because arteries with PAD are not as wide as healthy arteries, there is less blood that can flow out to various parts of the body. Less blood flow means less oxygen to tissues, which can cause different symptoms. Leg pain is a common symptom of PAD, as tissues react to inadequate oxygen. People with PAD often experience pain in their calves when walking (claudication).

People with PAD have a high risk of heart attack and stroke. In all three of these diseases, narrowed arteries don't work as they should. The consequences depend on the location of the narrowed artery:
- A narrowed artery in the brain can cause a stroke.
- A narrowed artery in the heart can cause a heart attack.
- A narrowed artery in the legs can cause PAD.

CAN PERIPHERAL ARTERIAL DISEASE BE PREVENTED?

Yes, there are some important strategies you can use to help prevent PAD. This is true even when your risk of PAD is higher, such as with age or when diseases such as obesity, diabetes and hypertension run in your family.

Avoid cigarette smoking
This is probably the most important risk factor you can control. People who smoke tend to develop PAD more than twice as often as similar people who do not smoke. Also, smokers have more than double the risk of dying or developing severe complications from PAD when compared with nonsmokers.

Maintain blood sugar goals
Adequate nutrition and blood sugar management is extremely important in PAD. High blood sugar levels are associated with a worse outcome, especially because high blood sugar can accelerate PAD in the arteries below the knees, which correlates with a higher rate of amputation, surgical complications and death. It is estimated that for every increase of 1% in glycosylated hemoglobin (hemoglobin with sugar attached) the risk of PAD goes up by 26%.

How PAD affects leg arteries

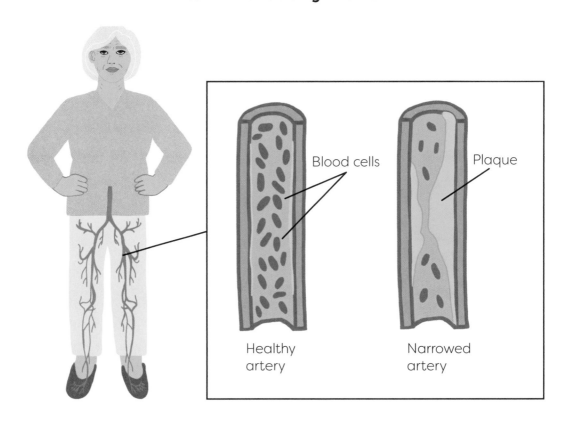

Blood cells

Plaque

Healthy artery

Narrowed artery

Maintain adequate blood pressure

High blood pressure levels damage the inside of the arteries and promote fatty tissue deposits. Each increase of 10 millimeters of mercury (mmHg) in systolic blood pressure, the top number in a blood pressure measurement, correlates with a 25% increased risk of PAD. Furthermore, the prevalence of PAD in people with high blood pressure is 6.9% compared with 2.2% in people who don't have high blood pressure.

Exercise

Regular exercise helps you maintain adequate blood sugar and blood pressure levels. It also helps improve the distance you can walk and decreases overall deaths related to cardiovascular health. It is esti-

mated that two or more exercise sessions a week improve walking distance by up to 200%.

Maintain a healthy weight

Being obese puts you at 1.5 times higher risk of developing PAD. A healthy weight is important for the health of your arteries.

HOW IS PERIPHERAL ARTERIAL DISEASE TREATED?

PAD requires a comprehensive treatment approach that typically combines lifestyle modifications, medications and, in some late-stage cases, surgery.

When you don't have symptoms or symptoms aren't worsening, lifestyle modifications and medications are key components of treating PAD.

Lifestyle modifications

Aerobic exercise, such as walking multiple times a week, is recommended. If you experience pain in your calves while walking, rest for a few minutes and then continue walking. Even if you do not have any symptoms of PAD, exercise programs are still effective in treating PAD. Eating a healthy, balanced diet reduces your risk of heart disease as well as PAD.

Not smoking is critical as well, since smoking is a known risk factor that speeds up the disease process. Additionally, cigarette smoking decreases the positive effects of exercise and medications.

Medications

Two types of medications are often used:
- Some medications are used to reduce the risk of PAD. These include medications to regulate blood pressure, blood sugar and cholesterol levels. Antiplatelet drugs such as aspirin or clopidogrel are also included in this category, as they can reduce the risk of developing a sudden and significant narrowing of an artery.
- Other medications are used to ease the symptoms of PAD, including cilostazol, pentoxifylline and prostaglandin E1. These medications aim to improve quality of life by decreasing pain while walking.

If you have diseases such as high blood pressure, elevated blood sugar or high cholesterol, be sure to take the medications for these conditions exactly as prescribed.

Surgery

If PAD symptoms are severe and do not improve with lifestyle measures and medication, surgery may be an option. Different procedures are available based on the severity of the disease. Such procedures can be as simple as going inside the blood vessel and unclogging it (revascularization procedure) or as complex as creating a new alternative pathway for the blood to flow and reach its target (bypass surgery).

WHY DOES PERIPHERAL ARTERIAL DISEASE MATTER TO WOMEN?

Even though PAD appears to be as common in men as it is in women, the outcomes of the disease differ between sexes. Women with PAD have a higher risk of heart attack and stroke than men with PAD and the rate of death due to heart disease is higher for women with PAD than for men. Although there's no single explanation for this, there are several theories:
- Women have higher inflammatory markers in the blood, which correlates with a higher degree of damage to the arteries and greater impairment of blood circulation.
- The drop in estrogen during the post-menopausal period seems to aggravate artery damage.
- Women are proportionally smaller than men, with smaller blood vessels. Thus, women's arteries may be more easily blocked.

Unfortunately, women also are subject to medical treatment disparities and less representation in clinical trials. These factors may contribute to worse outcomes.

QUESTIONS TO ASK YOUR HEALTH CARE TEAM ABOUT PAD

For anyone with PAD, regardless of the severity of their disease
- What are some strategies to improve my lifestyle habits?
  - Can you guide me in my weight loss process?
  - How can I learn to choose which foods to avoid and which to prioritize?
  - Can I get a referral to a registered dietitian or nutritionist?
- Will you work with me to create an adequate exercise program?
  - Can we set goals and work on them together?
  - Do you think I should see a physical trainer?
- Is there anything I can do to prevent:
  - High blood pressure?
  - High blood sugar?
  - Cholesterol?
- If I smoke, can you help me stop?

For people with mild to moderate PAD
- What medications should I take to prevent progression of the disease? In case that treatment is not enough, what other options do I have?

For people with severe PAD
- What is the risk of performing a procedure to unblock clogged arteries (revascularization procedure)? Would I benefit from it?
- What is the risk of my disease becoming so severe that I need an amputation of my lower leg? What can I do to prevent it?

PEARLS OF WISDOM

PAD is common. Severe PAD can lead to heart attack and stroke. Besides these life-threatening consequences, PAD has a profound impact on quality of life and overall health. The best treatment is early prevention by exercising, not smoking and managing chronic conditions such as high blood pressure, high blood sugar and high cholesterol. Women with PAD tend to have worse outcomes when compared with men, so early identification and treatment in women is particularly important to long-term health.

"We stand stronger when we stand together."

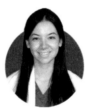

Camila Franco-Mesa, M.D. - she/her
Dr. Franco-Mesa is a General Surgery Resident at the University of Texas Medical Branch in Galveston, Texas. She is passionate about medical education and a strong advocate for women in medicine.

"I'm interested in women's health because I'm a woman. I'd be a darn fool not to be on my own side." – Maya Angelou

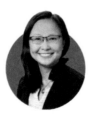

Young Erben, M.D. - she/her
Dr. Erben is Associate Professor of Surgery in the Division of Vascular and Endovascular Surgery at Mayo Clinic in Jacksonville, Florida. She has a special interest in the management of aortic, carotid and peripheral arterial disease in women.

55

Polycystic ovary syndrome

Iman Djarraya, M.P.H., M.B.Ch.B., B.Med.Sci.

WHAT IS POLYCYSTIC OVARY SYNDROME?

Polycystic ovary syndrome (PCOS) is the most common hormonal disorder in women of childbearing age, impacting 8% to 18% of women in this category.

PCOS impacts how our ovaries work. It causes the ovaries to produce higher levels of male hormones (androgens) than normal. This can lead to weight gain, abnormal hair growth on the face, chest or back, thinning of the hair on the head, male pattern baldness, oily skin, acne, and darkening of the skin in the back of the neck, the armpits, or the groin areas.

In some cases of PCOS, the body doesn't make enough of the hormones needed to release an egg (ovulate), which is part of a regular, healthy menstrual cycle. This can lead to irregular or absent menstrual cycles, heavy periods and difficulty getting pregnant.

The name PCOS refers to polycystic ovaries. Polycystic ovaries are enlarged ovaries that contain multiple fluid-filled sacs (cysts), which surround the eggs. However,

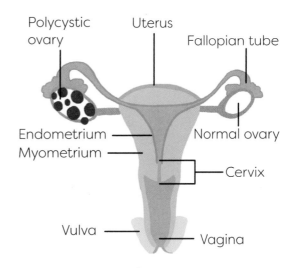

some women with PCOS do not have cysts, and some women without PCOS do have cysts.

Genetics, insulin resistance and inflammatory responses contribute to the development of PCOS. Insulin resistance occurs when the cells of the body do not respond normally to insulin, and blood sugar rises. Insulin resistance also increases your risk of developing gestational or type 2 diabetes. Additionally the pancreas, which is an organ in the abdomen, makes more insulin in order to lower blood sugar levels, which results in high levels of insulin that then trigger the ovaries to overproduce androgens.

Along with type 2 diabetes, women with PCOS also have a higher risk of developing:

- High cholesterol
- High blood pressure
- Metabolic syndrome and obesity
- Cardiovascular disease

In addition, women with PCOS can be at a higher risk of developing endometrial cancer. They are also more likely to experience anxiety and depression.

CAN POLYCYSTIC OVARY SYNDROME BE PREVENTED?

PCOS cannot be prevented entirely. However, if you have PCOS, you can employ several healthy lifestyle strategies to help you balance your hormone levels, improve your symptoms and prevent long-term complications.

Maintain a healthy weight
Weight gain in women with PCOS increases the body's resistance to insulin. Additional body fat increases the severity of the hormonal features of the syndrome. A weight loss of 5% to 10% of body weight improves many symptoms of PCOS.

Eat foods that reduce inflammation
Following an anti-inflammatory diet will help reduce the inflammation associated with PCOS, improving PCOS symptoms. For example, phytonutrients found in plants neutralize inflammation. Increase your intake of whole, plant-based foods,

including vegetables, fruits, whole grains, nuts and seeds. Try your best to avoid highly processed foods, added sugars, sweeteners, white flour and processed oils. Going dairy-free may also help improve PCOS symptoms, including acne. If you do avoid dairy, make sure you get your calcium and vitamin D from other sources.

Eat foods that have a low glycemic index and a low glycemic load
The glycemic index (GI) is a number between 0 and 100 given to a food item to represent how fast it can increase blood sugar levels in the body. Foods with a low glycemic index are more slowly digested, which helps reduce the speed at which your body absorbs sugar. The glycemic load is another important measure because it takes into account the serving size. It provides more accurate information about how the foods you eat affect your blood sugar levels.

Consuming a low glycemic index diet has been found to help with weight loss, improve insulin resistance and androgen levels, and reduce acne, abnormal hair growth and menstrual irregularities. Low glycemic index foods include green vegetables, mushrooms, beans, lentils, chickpeas, apples, strawberries, grapefruits and walnuts. If you are interested in learning more about the glycemic index and glycemic load values of different foods, consult a registered dietitian.

Eat more fiber
Most high-fiber foods are nourishing and help you stay fuller for longer. Fiber slows down digestion, which, in turn, slows down sugar absorption. High-fiber foods can help you maintain a healthy weight, healthy

blood sugar levels and healthy cholesterol levels.

Eat foods rich in omega-3 fats

Omega-3 fats, otherwise known as "good" fats, are found in avocados, nuts, olive oil, certain fish like salmon, and supplements made from fish. Omega-3 fats are associated with lower levels of triglyceride (a type of fat found in the blood), reducing the risk of high blood pressure.

Stay physically active

Physical activity plays an important role in managing PCOS symptoms and reducing complications. Regular exercise improves body weight, insulin resistance, cholesterol and triglyceride levels in the blood, and mental well-being. As a result of improvements like these, your risk of diabetes and heart disease will decrease. If you have other medical conditions, check with your doctor before you start physical activities.

Manage stress and your mental health

You may be experiencing stresses regarding weight loss, infertility, menstrual irregularities, excess hair growth, acne or the increased risk of diabetes, heart disease and endometrial cancer. In addition, women with PCOS are more likely to have anxiety, depression or both. You may also feel that you are not finding solutions to your PCOS symptoms from your clinician.

If you feel that the options offered to you aren't working, seek support from a gynecologist, a reproductive endocrinologist, an integrative medical doctor, a functional medicine doctor, a naturopathic doctor, a licensed nutritionist or a behavioral health therapist. At minimum, build yourself a health care team that consists of a medical doctor, a registered dietitian and a mental health professional.

Consider taking nutritional supplements

In addition to dietary and lifestyle changes, whole-food-based multivitamins can help ensure optimal health. In particular, the nutrients that can be particularly beneficial include:

- **Magnesium** This mineral plays a role in regulating blood sugar.
- **Vitamin D** Deficiencies of this vitamin have been associated with insulin resistance. Thus vitamin D supplementation may help with PCOS symptoms. Please discuss your vitamin D intake and correct dosage with your clinician. Also let your clinician know about any medications you're taking, as vitamin D supplements may interact negatively with certain medications.
- **Inositol** This substance is produced in the human body and is also found in fruits, beans, grains and nuts. Inositol improves insulin resistance and regulates hormones. Available clinical data show that Myo-inositol (MYO) and D-chiro-inositol (DCI) are two of nine forms of inositol that help with PCOS. MYO and DCI may cause low blood sugar, especially if taken with other medications or supplements that lower blood sugar. Always consult with your clinician before starting Inositol or other supplements.

If you're interested in taking supplements for PCOS, consult a specialist in functional medicine or a licensed naturopathic doctor. Ask them for names of trusted brands of supplements and the correct dosage. While supplements can be helpful, some should not be taken while you're trying to conceive or if you are pregnant, lactating, under the age of 18, taking certain medications or have other medical conditions. Consult your clinician before taking any supplements. If you experience negative side effects, discontinue use and let your clinician know.

HOW IS POLYCYSTIC OVARY SYNDROME TREATED?

As you've read, a healthy lifestyle can reduce PCOS symptoms and prevent complications. If those changes do not provide adequate relief, your clinician may recommend medical treatment. These recommendations will be customized for you depending on your symptoms.

Medications
Your clinician may recommend one or more of these medications to help treat PCOS. Be sure to ask your clinician about the risks of these treatment options.

Oral contraceptives (OCPs) Oral contraceptives can be used to treat PCOS if you're not trying to get pregnant. The combined oral contraceptive pill is a combination of estrogen and progestin. It is a common treatment for regulating the menstrual cycle in women with PCOS. This medication helps lower androgen levels and provides protection from endometrial cancer. Despite these benefits, oral contraceptives have been associated with negative effects, such as increases in the concentrations of low-density lipoproteins (LDLs), triglycerides and total cholesterol. The minipill (progestin-only birth control pill) is an alternative to the combined oral contraceptive pill. It contains progestin only and no estrogen.

Oral contraceptives are not recommended for women with certain health conditions, including but not limited to breast cancer, heart disease and stroke, because they increase the risk of complications from these conditions. Before taking any oral contraceptive, always discuss your current and past health conditions with your clinician, along with the benefits and risks of the medication.

Metformin is a medication commonly used to treat type 2 diabetes. It improves insulin sensitivity, androgen levels and ovulation in women with PCOS; however, it may cause gastrointestinal side effects.

Anti-androgens are medications used to reduce androgen levels or their effects on the body. These drugs can prevent excess hair growth and reduce acne. Because anti-androgens can cause birth defects, birth control (usually an oral contraceptive) is always recommended when taking this medication to prevent pregnancy.

Clomiphene citrate (Clomid) This medication is used to induce ovulation in some women with PCOS who are trying to become pregnant.

Laparoscopic ovarian drilling (LOD)
Laparoscopic ovarian drilling is a surgery done to trigger ovulation. The term laparoscopic refers to a surgical technique in which a thin tube attached to a tiny camera is inserted through a small incision in the abdomen. This allows the surgeon to view the organs and perform the procedure. LOD

is used to improve ovulation rates in women with an absence of ovulation (anovulation) who desire to get pregnant but did not respond to dietary changes, weight loss and fertility medicines such as clomiphene citrate. LOD has risks associated with it, such as infection, adhesions (internal scar tissue that can cause organs and tissues to stick together), ovarian scarring and premature ovarian failure.

WHY DOES POLYCYSTIC OVARY SYNDROME MATTER TO WOMEN?

PCOS is a common hormonal condition that affects women in different ways. The symptoms that women experience can have notable impacts on their mental health and emotional well-being. Women with this syndrome commonly face challenges in getting pregnant, which adds a lot of stress and uncertainty. Women may undergo fertility treatments that can take a physical, emotional and financial toll on them.

If left unmanaged, PCOS can cause serious health complications, including diabetes, heart disease and endometrial cancer. If you have PCOS it's important to take an active role in managing your symptoms by educating yourself, adopting a healthy lifestyle and seeking help from experienced clinicians.

QUESTIONS TO ASK YOUR HEALTH CARE TEAM ABOUT PCOS

- What can I do to better manage my PCOS?

- What are the side effects of medications for PCOS?
  › Is it safe to get pregnant or breastfeed while using them?
- Can you help me regularly monitor my blood pressure, fasting blood sugar and blood lipids (fats)?
  › How often should monitoring tests be done?

If you are overweight or experience obesity
- Can you help me lose weight?
- Can you refer me to a dietitian or
- nutritionist to help me understand what dietary changes will help me better manage my weight?

If you experience anxiety, low moods or depression
- Can you refer me to a mental health professional to help me with my mood?

If you have any other medical conditions
- Is it safe for me to exercise?
- What types of physical activities would you recommend for my situation?

Before trying to get pregnant
- Are the medications I currently take safe for pregnancy?
  › If not, when should I stop them?
  › At what point after stopping the medication is it safe to get pregnant?
- How can I increase my chances for a safe and healthy pregnancy?

If you are trying to get pregnant
- Do you recommend I take any medications to improve my chances of getting pregnant and having a safe pregnancy?

> › If yes, what are the best medication choices for my situation?
- How long should I try getting pregnant before consulting a fertility specialist?

PEARLS OF WISDOM

Women need to be informed about the hormonal disturbances and increased risks of certain medical conditions that accompany PCOS. It's especially important to get any insulin resistance under control, because it is often the root cause of PCOS hormonal imbalances.

Lifestyle modifications, such as proper nutrition, exercise and mental health therapy, can have significant positive impacts for women with PCOS. These strategies can also increase the chances of pregnancy.

When a woman takes an active role in managing her health and surrounds herself with experienced clinicians who listen, support and monitor her progress, she will feel more empowered. Taking care of your body, mind, and soul promotes total wellness!

"Empowering women to take care of their health and practice self-care is the key to women's wellness and results in healthier families and communities."

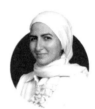

Iman Djarraya, M.P.H., M.B.Ch.B., B.Med.Sci. - she/her
Dr. Djarraya is a public health professional who has conducted research on PCOS. In her most recent position, she helped with the COVID-19 pandemic at the Tewksbury Public School District in Massachusetts. Her areas of focus are community health, disease prevention, nutrition, and wellness.

56
Rheumatoid arthritis

Courtney A. Arment, M.D.

WHAT IS RHEUMATOID ARTHRITIS?

Rheumatoid arthritis is an autoimmune disease, meaning the body incorrectly attacks itself. In the case of rheumatoid arthritis, the immune system starts attacking the joints. This is different from the most common type of arthritis, which is called osteoarthritis. With osteoarthritis, your joints wear down with time. With rheumatoid arthritis, joint damage is accelerated due to ongoing inflammation being driven by your immune system.

Rheumatoid arthritis affects 1 in every 100 people. The most common joints affected by rheumatoid arthritis are the small joints of the hands and feet. However, the condition also commonly affects large joints, such as knees, shoulders and hips. Compared to osteoarthritis, rheumatoid arthritis can cause more joint swelling as well as morning stiffness lasting for an hour or longer. Rheumatoid arthritis pain tends to improve with activities and worsen with rest (osteoarthritis pain typically does the opposite).

Rheumatoid arthritis can affect more than joints. The disease can impact the eyes, skin, nerves, glands, lungs and other organ systems. However, advancements in treatment options have led to better disease control, and it's now less common to have other organs affected beyond the joints.

CAN RHEUMATOID ARTHRITIS BE PREVENTED?

Unfortunately, there is no known way to prevent rheumatoid arthritis. A lot remains to be known about how rheumatoid arthritis develops in an individual. Current research suggests that certain genetic factors, environmental triggers and other risk factors (such as obesity and smoking) play a role.

The aim of treatment of rheumatoid arthritis is remission. This term is often used in cancer treatment to mean that there is no detectable cancer. In the case of rheumatoid arthritis, remission refers to a lack of ongoing symptoms in joints and no signs that the condition is affecting other organs. One of the many benefits of achieving remission in rheumatoid arthritis is preventing the involvement of additional joints and further joint damage. Thus, prevention of disease progression is possible if remission is achieved and sustained.

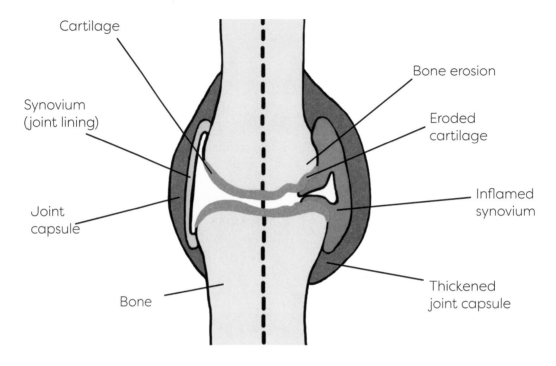

Healthy joint   **Joint with rheumatoid arthritis**

Cartilage

Synovium
(joint lining)

Joint
capsule

Bone

Bone erosion

Eroded
cartilage

Inflamed
synovium

Thickened
joint capsule

HOW IS RHEUMATOID ARTHRITIS TREATED?

In rheumatology, we use a "treat to target" approach. This involves a stepwise approach to treatment that targets the disease while ensuring that the treatment is based on your preferences and the severity of your symptoms and joint damage.

The ultimate goal of treatment is remission. Sometimes it can be challenging to know when remission is achieved. This can be due to other conditions, such as osteoarthritis and fibromyalgia, that can also be present in someone with rheumatoid arthritis. These conditions can cause pain in and of themselves and may not necessarily respond to treatments aimed at rheumatoid arthritis. People with rheumatoid arthritis require frequent monitoring with their rheumatolo-gist to adequately assess the severity of their disease. This may include additional imaging (X-ray studies), laboratory testing and physical examination.

If you're diagnosed with rheumatoid arthritis, your treatment plan may include one or more of several measures.

Medications

Medication is the first line of defense against rheumatoid arthritis, and thankfully we have many options available for treatment. While there are exceptions, most people with rheumatoid arthritis initially benefit from the use of both oral steroids and a second medication targeting the rheumatoid arthritis more specifically. This combination approach allows people to experience more rapid symptom relief.

Steroids Steroids such as prednisone can be a very effective way of controlling inflammation and reducing joint symptoms. They often begin providing relief within hours to days of treatment. However, steroids have many long-term side effects. Ideally, steroid treatment is tapered during the initial weeks to months of treatment as a second, more directed medication has time to take full effect.

Conventional synthetic disease-modifying agents (csDMARDs) These medications reduce symptoms by targeting the inflammation of rheumatoid arthritis in a more specific manner. They work more slowly than steroids, within weeks to months. Types of csDMARDs include oral medications such as hydroxychloroquine, methotrexate, leflunomide and sulfasalazine.

Targeted synthetic DMARDs (tsDMARDs) These drugs are a class of medication known as biologics. They can be taken by mouth, injection or infusion through an IV (vein). Examples of these medications include adalimumab, etanercept, abatacept, infliximab, tocilizumab, tofacitinib, updadacitinib and rituximab.

Nonprescription pain medications Nonprescription pain medications can also be used to help manage your symptoms, but they typically aren't designed to control the disease nor prevent it from causing further damage to your joints.

Your doctor may recommend taking several different csDMARDs together. Or you may be prescribed a combination of a conventional synthetic agent and a targeted synthetic one. However, research has not yet shown the safety and effectiveness of combining two or more targeted synthetic agents.

Because most disease-modifying medications tend to suppress the immune system, it's important to be up to date with infection screens and preventive measures before beginning treatment. This includes being tested for chronic hepatitis and tuberculosis. If possible and appropriate, it's also a good idea to update vaccines, including influenza, pneumonia, shingles and COVID-19 vaccinations, prior to starting treatment.

If you require long-term steroid treatment to control your rheumatoid arthritis, your doctor may prescribe additional medications to reduce the side effects of the treatment. For example, taking the equivalent of prednisone at a daily dose of 20 mg or more for longer than four weeks may increase your risk of developing pneumonia. To prevent that from happening, your doctor may suggest an antibiotic. Furthermore, even a low daily dose of prednisone taken for three months or longer can weaken your bones. In that situation, additional screens and measures for bone health may also be recommended.

Steroid injections
If one or a few of your joints are persistently bothersome, despite taking oral medications, your doctor may suggest an injection of a steroid medication into the joint or joints. Because there is a risk of infections in the joints, your doctor may first take fluid out of the joint through a needle to make sure no infection is present prior to proceeding with the injection. This procedure is typically done in the rheumatology office.

Therapy and massage

Another important part of treatment is physical and occupational therapy. Therapy may include exercises that maintain flexibility and promote strength to preserve healthy motion of the joints. Other pain management strategies can also be beneficial, such as applying heat and ice to sore joints. Massage can be helpful as well.

Support devices and tools

Some people benefit from use of devices to support joints and provide further pain relief. These include splints, braces and shoe inserts. There are also modified household tools that can make daily activities less painful. For example, enlarged handles on writing and eating utensils make grasping these objects easier and less painful.

An effective use of medication and other pain management measures can help relieve your symptoms. If you experience sustained remission for a year or longer, you may be able to successfully lower the amount of your medication(s). This option will need to be assessed and guided by your rheumatologist. Most people with rheumatoid arthritis require a medication long-term to manage their rheumatoid arthritis.

Ultimately, the goal of treatment is to use the least amount of medication possible to control rheumatoid arthritis activity. Currently, there is no way to predict the best regimen for each individual. Hopefully, in time, findings from additional research will assist in these efforts. Until then, the optimal treatment plan is determined by using different medications alone or in combination. Your rheumatologist will take many considerations into account to determine the most suitable approach for you. These include the severity of your rheumatoid arthritis and other personal factors.

WHY DOES RHEUMATOID ARTHRITIS MATTER TO WOMEN?

Rheumatoid arthritis matters to women because first and foremost, it is a disease that affects more women than men. This disease also can impact bone strength, leading to a higher risk of fracture. Women in general are more prone to weakened bones, namely osteoporosis, compared to men. Steroid medications often used to treat rheumatoid arthritis can further weaken bones. Fortunately, medications and other measures can be used to reduce the risk of fractures. If you have rheumatoid arthritis, discuss your bone health with your clinician.

Rheumatoid arthritis also increases the risk of heart disease. This is even more relevant for women, as the symptoms of heart disease may be less typical in women and therefore less recognizable. It's recommended that individuals with rheumatoid arthritis ensure that they are up to date with their cardiovascular health screens, particularly women. These screens are usually done through your primary care clinician and may include the use of another medication and/or lifestyle modifications to help lower cholesterol and maintain a healthy weight.

Medication safety during childbearing years, pregnancy and breastfeeding is another consideration. It's important to review rheumatoid arthritis medications in relation to family planning, because certain medications are not safe to use during conception and pregnancy. Unfortunately, rheumatoid arthritis symptoms can get worse with pregnancy and after delivery. To ensure that you receive appropriate care for your disease during these years, work closely with your rheumatologist.

As mothers, daughters, sisters, aunts, wives and grandmothers, we can have a tendency to become caretakers and neglect our own health. This can be detrimental in rheumatoid arthritis. Delayed treatment can lead to disease that is more difficult to control. It's important to seek help if you're experiencing symptoms of persistent joint pain. When in doubt, have it checked out.

QUESTIONS TO ASK YOUR HEALTH CARE TEAM ABOUT RHEUMATOID ARTHRITIS

- How severe is my rheumatoid arthritis?
  - › How does this impact the current treatment recommendations?
- Do I need additional health screening for cardiovascular risk given my diagnosis of rheumatoid arthritis?
- Do I have additional contributors to my pain, such as fibromyalgia and/or osteoarthritis?
- Are there lifestyle factors (diet and/or exercise) that I should implement to help my rheumatoid arthritis?
- What are my options for medications?
- For any given medications, what side effects and time to improvement should I expect?
- Do I need an additional medication to help reduce the side effects of steroid treatment, namely osteoporosis prevention?
- How long will I be on each medication?

- What medications can I add to my regimen for additional pain control if needed?
- How will we know when my rheumatoid arthritis is in remission?
- How often do I need lab monitoring for my medications?

PEARLS OF WISDOM

While less common than osteoarthritis ("wear and tear" arthritis), rheumatoid arthritis is the most common autoimmune cause of joint pain. People with this disease experience persistent joint pain and swelling, and prolonged stiffness upon waking up.

If you're experiencing persistent joint pain for six weeks or longer and joint stiffness in the morning lasting 60 minutes or longer with or without joint swelling, seek initial care with your primary care clinician. If necessary your clinician can refer you to a rheumatologist, who can help determine the cause of your symptoms and guide your treatment. Prompt treatment creates better outcomes, so it's important to not delay evaluation if you have ongoing symptoms.

"Self care is not selfish."

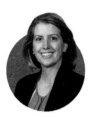

Courtney A. Arment, M.D. - she/her
Dr. Arment is an Assistant Professor of Medicine in the Rheumatology Department at Mayo Clinic, Rochester, Minnesota. She specializes in inflammatory arthritis and has a particular focus on both sarcoidosis and autoimmune hearing loss.

57
Shoulder pain

Vani J. Sabesan, M.D., and Laila H. Khoury, B.S., MS3

WHAT IS SHOULDER PAIN?

Shoulder pain is a common concern that can be caused by age-related tendon degeneration, arthritis, trauma (such as from a fall or a sport- or work-related injury), or other problems such as tumors and autoimmune conditions. It can also simply be due to overuse.

Different factors can trigger shoulder pain. Clinicians usually classify shoulder pain into one of two types.

Nonspecific shoulder pain

This is shoulder pain caused by conditions affecting other areas of your body but causing pain in the shoulder, such as a pinched nerve in your neck, or conditions that impact your whole body, including your shoulder, such as rheumatoid arthritis, diabetes-related complications or fibromyalgia. X-rays or other imaging tests of the shoulder are normal.

Specific shoulder pain

This is shoulder pain coming from a problem in the shoulder itself that can be confirmed by a physical exam or identified on an X-ray or other imaging tests of the shoulder. There are several common reasons for specific shoulder pain.

Osteoarthritis This condition occurs when the protective cartilage, which is the natural cushion between your joints, wears down over time and your bones begin to rub together, causing pain and swelling.

Rotator cuff tendon tear The rotator cuff is a group of four muscles that start on the shoulder blade and whose tendons insert into the upper arm bone. The rotator cuff keeps the shoulder joint in place and moves the arm in different directions. The most common of the tendons to tear is the supraspinatus tendon.

Frozen shoulder Your shoulder bones, ligaments and tendons are encased in a capsule of connective tissue. When that capsule of connective tissue thickens and tightens around the shoulder joint, it restricts movement of your shoulder, causing stiffness and pain. This is referred to as frozen shoulder, also called adhesive capsulitis.

Rotator cuff tendon tear

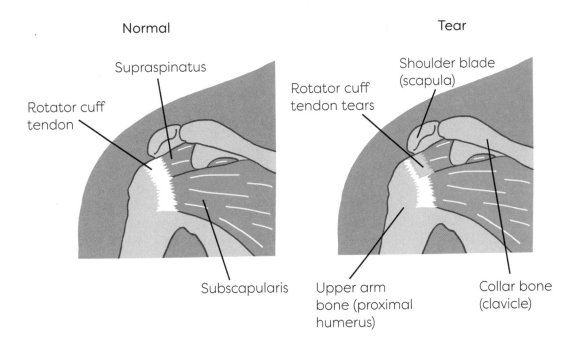

Normal

Rotator cuff tendon

Supraspinatus

Subscapularis

Tear

Shoulder blade (scapula)

Rotator cuff tendon tears

Upper arm bone (proximal humerus)

Collar bone (clavicle)

Frozen shoulder (adhesive capsulitis)

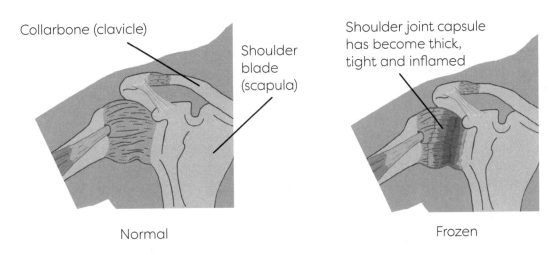

Collarbone (clavicle)

Shoulder blade (scapula)

Shoulder joint capsule has become thick, tight and inflamed

Normal

Frozen

CAN SHOULDER PAIN BE PREVENTED?

Yes, for many women. If you already have shoulder pain, incorporating exercises and other self-care steps into your routine can usually prevent progression of your shoulder pain or decrease the intensity of discomfort you feel.

Strengthen muscles

When doing the same task, women on average tend to use more muscles than men, meaning that women work harder and closer to their maximum capacity. By strengthening your muscles — especially the muscles in your arms, shoulder, neck and back — you build your muscle fibers and will fatigue less quickly. We recommend weight training with proper technique two or three times a week. This will allow your body to work smarter, not harder, and help prevent shoulder pain.

Stop smoking

Smoking is a risk factor for developing chronic pain because nicotine activates your immune system to cause inflammation. By quitting or at least reducing the amount you smoke, you can reduce inflammation and shoulder pain. The first step is to ask yourself if you want to stop smoking. Once you know that you do, you can assess whether you think you can stop and what motivations you have to stop. For example, you could say "I want to stop smoking, and I think I can stop smoking. My motivations to stop include my shoulder pain and the health of my family who live with me." You can join a smoking cessation group, call the national Tobacco Cessation Quitline (1-800-QUIT-NOW) or ask your doctor to help you create a plan to stop smoking.

Get annual blood tests

Annual blood tests are important to check your blood for signs of anemia, infection and overall health. They can also be used to identify diseases such as diabetes and hypothyroidism, which can be related to early development of rotator cuff disease in women. Knowing your blood test results can help you prevent or receive early treatment for conditions that can lead to different types of shoulder pain.

Vary your daily movements

Shoulder pain is one of the most common problems in female workers, especially when repetitive tasks and actions are part of the job. By repeating the same movements, you are placing a burden on certain muscles but not others. This underuse of some muscles weakens your total shoulder girdle, which is made up of many muscles. This creates a muscle imbalance and weakens your neck and other shoulder muscles. When you work, consider changing your hand, elbow and shoulder positions throughout the day, along with stretching your neck and shoulders.

At home, make sure your household cleaning tools fit you to prevent injuries.

Take quick breaks

Uninterrupted neck activity for more than four minutes at a time — for example, keeping your head in the same position for a prolonged period — is associated with shoulder pain. Along with changing up your movements throughout the day, take quick breaks from your current position every 5 to 10 minutes. Doing so releases the tension in your neck and shoulders, which can reduce the risk of shoulder pain.

Support your body

The body has natural curves in the neck, upper back and lower back. When these curves are not maintained, pain may develop in the shoulders, hips and even feet. Unfortunately, chairs, tables and beds are often made to provide support for the average man, making these items less supportive for the average woman. When choosing furniture or other supportive equipment, be sure to consider whether it will provide proper support for your height and natural curvature.

Adjust your work chair for your height and build, so that you can sit up straight against the back of your chair — sometime this requires putting a pillow or towel behind the small of your back — while making sure your feet are completely flat on the floor or on a footrest and your forearms can rest comfortably on your desk.

Also, use a small cylindrical pillow or rolled-up towel underneath the curve in your neck while sleeping face-up to relieve pressure in both your neck and shoulders.

HOW IS SHOULDER PAIN TREATED?

A lot of shoulder pain can be improved without surgery. However, surgery may be the best treatment for some women, depending on the cause of the pain.

Lifestyle modifications
The strategies mentioned in the preventive section are frequently recommended as first-line treatments as well, especially if the shoulder pain is the nonspecific type.

Physical therapy
Physical therapy is important to treat any type of muscle or joint pain. Physical therapy teaches you practical maneuvers to better use your shoulder, reduce pain and prevent further injury. If you cannot afford to see a physical therapist or do not have the time to go see one, look for videos online (such as on YouTube) demonstrating physical therapy for shoulder pain. If you do not know which one to pick, ask your doctor for recommendations.

Medications
The most common medications for shoulder pain include nonprescription painkillers such as acetaminophen (Tylenol), ibuprofen (Advil, Motrin, others) or naproxen (Aleve). However, if your shoulder pain is chronic, using these daily over many months can have side effects that affect your kidneys, stomach or liver. To minimize these other complications, follow the recommended dosing on the bottle, try not to use them every day and seek medical evaluation from a clinician if the pain continues for more than a few months.

Injections
Different types of injections may be given for shoulder pain, including corticosteroids and platelet-rich plasma (PRP). Corticosteroids and PRP can be injected into a space in your shoulder called the subacromial space or into your shoulder joint to provide pain relief and decrease inflammation. Pain relief from injection therapy varies from person to person and may be only temporary, so be sure to discuss your options with your clinician.

Acupuncture
Acupuncture has become more popular as a way to treat all kinds of muscle and joint pain. Although there is not very much research on its effects, this may be a consideration for you if other treatments are not available or not effective.

Surgery
If your shoulder pain is due to a rotator cuff tear or severe osteoarthritis, treatment may involve a rotator cuff tendon repair or shoulder joint replacement surgery. Most rotator cuff repairs involve arthroscopic

surgery, in which your surgeon uses small incisions to insert surgical instruments and a small camera to find the tear and reattach it to the bone. For severe arthritis, joint replacement may be appropriate. Less common reasons for surgery include the shoulder joint repeatedly coming out of the socket (dislocating) or being frozen (very stiff).

The prospect of shoulder surgery may make you feel anxious or worried about pain after surgery. The good news is that pain management after surgery has greatly improved with nerve blocks, inflammatory medications, nerve agents and nonaddictive pain medications. Be sure to discuss the recovery period, potential absence from work, and limitations on the use of your arm after surgery with your doctor. Last, to get maximum results from the surgery, you'll likely be asked to do certain exercises after surgery, which often can successfully be done at home or with a physical therapist.

WHY DOES SHOULDER PAIN MATTER TO WOMEN?

Shoulder pain can impact your mental and physical quality of life, as well as your finances. Shoulder pain can limit your activities, whether it be typing on the computer, housework, manual labor, working out, playing sports, or lifting heavy objects or groceries. Not being able to work at your job usually means less income.

Rotator cuff problems and work-related shoulder pain are more common in women than in men. This can be due to differences in daily activities (brushing longer hair or doing household chores such as dishwashing, vacuuming or laundry), job types (women often work at jobs that involve computer work, repetitive tasks and awkward postures), furniture design (chairs, tables and desks not designed for women) and body types (women on average are smaller and have less muscle mass than men).

Women are less likely to be referred for or receive shoulder surgeries. This delay in surgical treatment, either because women are not referred until later or because women delay their treatment, means that women often present to the surgeon with worse shoulder damage than men have. Greater damage to your shoulder can make surgeons more hesitant to treat you with an operation that may help you because the greater the damage, the greater the risk of complications. Seeking help early on can possibly reduce your symptoms and get you the proper treatment you need and deserve.

Despite women having more shoulder problems than men, there is little research on the difference between shoulder pain in men and women, let alone on the difference between white women and women of color. So, as women in medicine, we also want you to be educated on what we do know about shoulder pain, be aware of the disparities and the little research that has been done on them, and know that we are doing what we can to address this gap. Most important, we want you to know that your shoulder pain is valid and deserves proper and equal attention from your clinicians.

QUESTIONS TO ASK YOUR HEALTH CARE TEAM

Risk-reduction questions

- How do my occupation and daily activities affect my shoulder pain?
- I want to quit smoking, but I have tried and it never works. Can you help me figure out another way to stop?

Recommendation questions

- Can you recommend a weight-training regimen or other resources, such as a personal trainer, to help me strengthen my upper body and shoulders?
- Can you recommend any YouTube videos that I can follow for shoulder pain exercises?
- Do you recommend any injections for my shoulder pain?
  - › What are the risks and benefits of such an injection?

Diagnostic questions

- Can you run routine blood tests to check me for disorders that might increase my chances of getting shoulder pain?
- Do I need an X-ray or MRI of my shoulder? If not, why not?
- Can you explain my X-Ray or MRI results and what they mean to me?

Surgery questions

- Can you tell me the risks and benefits of getting surgery, both in general and specifically for my case?
  - › What kind of surgery do you recommend?
  - › What are the risks if I do not have surgery?
- If I undergo surgery, how long will my expected recovery time be?
  - › Will surgery affect my quality of life after the procedure?
- If I want to avoid opioid medications after shoulder surgery, can you provide me with an alternative pain management plan after surgery?

PEARLS OF WISDOM

Advocate for yourself! You should know that when women speak, doctors are supposed to listen. It is important that you know that a doctor's job description includes first and foremost listening carefully to you to understand your goals and figure out why you have shoulder pain. Further, your clinician is supposed to do a physical exam, run diagnostic and imaging tests when appropriate, and most important, provide you with quality care and treatment options specific to you (while also making sure you know the risks and benefits of each option). Your shoulder pain matters, so do not be afraid to question your clinician about the care or treatment options you are given.

"The success of every woman should be the inspiration to another. We should raise each other up. Make sure you're very courageous: be strong, be extremely kind, and above all be humble." – Serena Williams

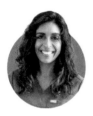

Vani J. Sabesan, M.D. - she/her
Dr. Sabesan is former Lang Family Endowed Chair at Cleveland Clinic Florida and currently Shoulder and Elbow/Sports Medicine Specialist at Palm Beach Shoulder Service in Atlantis Ortho-paedics. She is Associate Professor at FIU, FAU, Nova Southeastern University, and University of Miami. She specializes her clinical practice, education, and research in complex shoulder and elbow surgery, diversity, and bone health.

"Keep going and keep speaking up, even if your voice shakes." – Allyson Felix

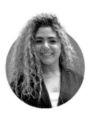

Laila H. Khoury, B.S., MS3 - she/her
Laila Khoury is a third-year medical student at Charles E. Schmidt College of Medicine in Boca Raton, Florida. She participates in orthopedic research at Palm Beach Shoulder Services, Atlantis Orthope-dics, with research interests in opioid usage in different orthopedic populations.

58
Stroke

Cynthia L. Kenmuir, M.D., Ph.D., FSVIN

WHAT IS A STROKE?

A stroke occurs when the blood supply to your brain is suddenly disrupted, preventing brain tissue from getting oxygen and resulting in brain cells dying. This injury to the brain causes a neurologic deficit (impaired functioning, such as an inability to speak or walk normally).

There are two forms of stroke:
- **Ischemic stroke** This type of stroke is caused by a blockage in one of the blood vessels to the brain. The blockage starves the brain of needed oxygen and nutrients, causing brain cells to die. Approximately 85% of strokes are ischemic.
- **Hemorrhagic stroke** This less common type of stroke occurs when there is bleeding into the brain caused by a broken blood vessel. Only 15% of strokes are hemorrhagic.

Stroke is a medical emergency. Both types of stroke can cause permanent disability or even death if left untreated. Brain cells die quickly — approximately 2 million brain cells are lost each minute during a stroke. However, it's very important to know that

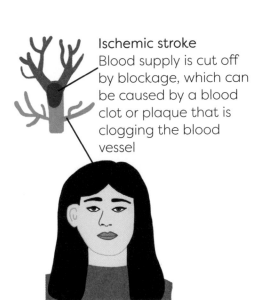

Ischemic stroke
Blood supply is cut off by blockage, which can be caused by a blood clot or plaque that is clogging the blood vessel

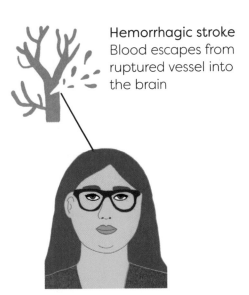

Hemorrhagic stroke
Blood escapes from ruptured vessel into the brain

Stroke signs and symptoms

Men

- Severe headaches
- Vision problems
- Face droop
- Difficulty speaking
- Weak arms
- Difficulty walking

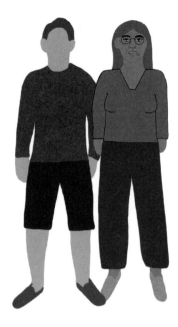

Women

- Confusion
- Fatigue
- Severe headaches
- Vision problems
- Face droop
- Difficulty speaking
- Nausea or vomiting
- Weak arms
- Difficulty walking
- General weakness

in many cases brain cells can recover (and stroke symptoms can improve) if blood flow is quickly restored by removing the blockage causing the stroke. When recognized early, strokes can be treated and result in good outcomes.

Common symptoms of stroke include:
- Weakness or numbness on one side of the face, arm or leg
- Trouble speaking or understanding
- Loss of vision
- Dizziness

Sometimes a blood vessel is blocked only briefly and symptoms are temporary. This is referred to as a transient ischemic attack. A transient ischemic attack still requires medical attention because it may be a warning that you could have a more serious stroke in the future.

CAN STROKE BE PREVENTED?

Yes — but not always. There are many things that you can do to keep your heart and blood vessels healthy to help prevent a stroke. Studies show that 90% of strokes are due to risk factors you can change or control.

Practice healthy habits
The following lifestyle modifications are very important for stroke prevention.

Eat healthy foods A Mediterranean-style diet that focuses on plant-based foods (vegetables, fruits, nuts, whole grains) and fish and limits sugars, saturated fats and cholesterol is protective against stroke. Diets high in fats, processed meats and sugar-sweetened beverages have been associated with nearly a 40% increase in strokes.

Maintain a healthy weight Obesity is associated with increased stroke risk. A weight loss of only 5%-10% of your body weight can reduce your risk of stroke and heart disease.

Be physically active You don't need to run a marathon. Studies show that even a little exercise each day can reduce your risk of stroke. Always talk to your clinician before starting an exercise regimen. A good goal for most people is to gradually build up to a 30-minute daily walk or swim.

Do not smoke or use tobacco products Smoking doubles the risk of a first stroke and increases the chance of a brain bleed from an aneurysm rupture (when a weak spot on a blood vessel bursts).

Do not drink alcohol, or drink sparingly Women who drink more than seven alcoholic drinks per week have a higher risk of stroke.

Assess your family history

Genetics may also play a role in stroke. If you have family members who had strokes at a young age or who died from a brain bleed, you may be at a higher risk of having a stroke. If you yourself have had a stroke, you have an increased chance of having another stroke, currently estimated as a 12% chance over the next five years. People with certain conditions, such as migraine with aura, diabetes, atrial fibrillation and carotid stenosis, also have an increased risk of stroke. If you fall into any of these higher-risk categories, the following measures are recommended where applicable.

Take precautions if you experience migraine with aura

Migraine with aura is a specific type of headache that has warning signs, such as seeing sparkles, dots or zig zags. This type of headache doubles your risk of having a stroke. Notably, this risk increases seven-fold if you also use oral hormones (birth control pills). If you have migraine with aura and you also smoke, the risk increases ten times. Women with migraine with aura should not smoke and only rarely use hormone-based treatments.

Maintain healthy blood pressure and cholesterol levels

Aim to maintain a blood pressure of less than 130/80 mmHg, using medications if needed. It's recommended to have your fasting cholesterol levels checked at least annually and maintain LDL ("bad") cholesterol levels of less than 70. If you have high cholesterol, your clinician may suggest using a statin medication. If you have trouble taking statins, an injectable medication may be an option.

Manage blood sugar if you have diabetes

Because diabetes increases the risk of stroke, it's important to carefully manage your blood sugar levels. A target HbA1c (average blood glucose level) of less than 7% can reduce stroke risk.

Take precautions if you have atrial fibrillation

Atrial fibrillation (irregular or very rapid heartbeat) is associated with twice the risk of stroke in women compared to men with the condition, and women are less likely to receive oral blood thinners than are men. Oral blood thinners (apixaban, dabigatran, edoxaban, rivaroxaban, warfarin) are recommended to help prevent first or recurrent stroke if you have been diagnosed with atrial fibrillation and are at low risk of bleeding complications. If you have high bleeding risk, your doctor may recommend alternative procedures to treat your condition.

Manage obstructive sleep apnea

Sleep apnea is a sleep-related breathing disorder. If you have sleep apnea and have had a stroke, treatment with a CPAP (continuous positive airway pressure) device is recommended to reduce risk of another stroke. Anyone who has been told that they stop breathing at times overnight or who snores heavily should have a sleep study to screen for sleep apnea.

Explore treatment for carotid artery stenosis

Carotid artery stenosis is a narrowing of the large arteries on either side of the neck that carry blood to the brain. The narrowing occurs when plaque (fatty, waxy deposits) builds up in the artery over time. If you've had a stroke and have severe narrowing of the carotid on the side where your stroke occurred, your clinician may recommend a procedure to reverse the narrowing. A stent (small mesh tube) may be placed to widen the artery, or the plaque buildup may be removed from the artery (endarterectomy). If your artery stenosis is mild to moderate, experts recommend that it be monitored while other stroke risk factors are treated, especially cholesterol, blood sugar and blood pressure.

Ask about blood thinners

For most people who have had a stroke, a daily dose of baby aspirin (81 mg) is recommended for prevention of recurrent stroke. Exceptions include people who are at increased risk of bleeding or who are allergic to aspirin. A second blood thinner, such as clopidogrel (Plavix) is usually recommended for a few weeks after a stroke to reduce the risk of another stroke. Stronger blood thinners, such as warfarin (Coumadin), apixaban (Eliquis), dabigatran (Pradaxa), rivaroxaban (Xarelto) and edoxaban (Lixiana), are not routinely recommended due to bleeding risk, unless another condition like atrial fibrillation has been identified.

HOW IS STROKE TREATED?

If you are having a stroke it is critical to seek emergency medical care, because the outcomes of many strokes can be improved with medicine or procedures received close to the time of the stroke.

Ischemic strokes can be treated with an intravenous (IV) medication called a thrombolytic (Tenecteplase, Alteplase, others), which breaks up blood clots. However, currently this medication can only be given safely up to 4.5 hours from when stroke symptoms begin, and they work best the earliest they can be given.

Some strokes can also be treated with an emergency procedure called a thrombectomy. During the procedure, a doctor places a catheter (small tube) into an artery in the groin or wrist. The doctor then moves the catheter inside the blood vessels and up through the body to the brain to remove the blockage causing the stroke. In some people, a thrombectomy can be done up to 24 hours after symptoms begin but, again, it works best the earliest it can be performed. Sometimes the damage from a stroke is too severe to safely perform the procedure.

Treatment for a hemorrhagic stroke focuses on minimizing the bleeding and reducing pressure in your brain. If you take blood thinners, you may receive medications to counteract their blood-thinning effects. Your health care team will also monitor your blood pressure.

WHY DOES STROKE MATTER TO WOMEN?

There are several reasons why stroke matters to women.

Women are more likely than men to have a stroke

One in five women will have a stroke in her lifetime. Among women, Black women have the highest chance of having a stroke. Women tend to be older than men are at the time of stroke and are 20% more likely to have significant disability from a stroke. Stroke kills more women than men and is the number four cause of death in women, killing over 80,000 women each year.

Women may present with nontraditional stroke symptoms

Compared with men, women more often report less-specific symptoms of stroke, including headache, lightheadedness or passing out, fatigue or generalized weakness, a "funny" feeling that's difficult to describe, chest pain, racing heart or shortness of breath, sudden behavior change, such as confusion, agitation or hallucinations, and nausea or vomiting. These less-specific symptoms can often be missed or misdiagnosed by both women and clinicians, resulting in treatment delays and worse outcomes.

Risk factors specific to women

Pregnancy changes can thicken the blood, increasing the risk of a blood clot forming and causing a stroke. Stroke risk is highest around the time of childbirth and normalizes by six weeks after giving birth. Women who develop pregnancy-specific high blood pressure (including preeclampsia and eclampsia) have two to five times the stroke risk later in life compared with women who don't have high blood pressure during pregnancy.

Hormones, including oral birth control pills and non-oral hormones such as Nuvaring, can increase the risk of blood clots that can cause stroke. These medications should be used with caution prior to age 35, and only after a discussion with your clinician that includes your individual stroke risk. Similarly, taking hormones later in life (more than 10 years from menopause) increases stroke risk. The age of menopause may also be a risk factor, with some studies suggesting that the earlier a woman reaches menopause, the greater her risk of stroke may be. However, not all experts agree and more research is needed.

Women are also less likely to be treated for stroke

After a stroke, women are less likely to be prescribed appropriate blood thinners and medications intended to lower blood sugar and cholesterol. They are less likely to be treated with emergency IV thrombolytic medication for their stroke, possibly related to delayed recognition of less typical symptoms by clinicians. Studies have shown that women are more prone to depression after a stroke and report a poorer quality of life after a stroke.

QUESTIONS TO ASK YOUR HEALTH CARE TEAM ABOUT STROKE

If you have a family history of stroke
- What is my risk of stroke and how do I lower it?

If you have had a stroke
- What caused this stroke?
  - › What tests can show the cause?
  - › Can I see a picture of my stroke and will you explain it to me?
- What degree of recovery should I expect?
  - › Over what time period should I expect recovery?
  - › When can I expect to go home?
- When can I safely begin to exercise or drive?
  - › Do I have any restrictions?
- What are the risks and benefits of any new medications and how will they interact with my other medications?
- What are the risks and benefits of any proposed treatment?
- What can I do to decrease my chance of having another stroke?
- When should I follow up and with whom?
  - › How do I reach my health care team with questions?

Always feel free to ask your doctor about her degree of experience or ask for a second opinion if you would like one. A good doctor will never be offended to have more input from colleagues.

PEARLS OF WISDOM

Listen to your body. If something doesn't feel right, it probably isn't. As you've read, women can have more subtle symptoms of a stroke, especially in the early phases, when the stroke is often treatable with a good possible outcome. Women are less likely to have their stroke symptoms recognized as a stroke, less likely to be seen by a stroke specialist and less likely to have the standard medical evaluation after a stroke.

Time is brain! If you're concerned that you or someone else is having a stroke, please call 911 immediately. Please do not call your neighbor, child or friend for a second opinion or try to drive yourself to the hospital. Strokes can worsen quickly, and you could miss your opportunity to get help, leaving you with permanent disability. Strokes can be treated, sometimes with complete recovery, if you get medical help quickly.

"Women have unique health care challenges ranging from having different risk factors for stroke, to having different symptoms of stroke, to responding differently to treatments for stroke, and sometimes being treated differently by health care providers. Women need to listen to their bodies and be open with their health care providers."

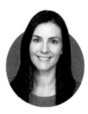

Cynthia L. Kenmuir, M.D., Ph.D., FSVIN - she/her
Dr. Kenmuir is the Director of the University of Pittsburgh Medical Center (UPMC) Altoona Stroke Program and the Director of the UPMC Altoona Neurointerventional Program and Assistant Professor of Neurology at the University of Pittsburgh. She specializes in diagnosing and treating stroke and head and neck blood vessel diseases.

59
Thyroid disease

Laura E. Ryan, M.D., and Rebecca D. Jackson, M.D.

WHAT IS THYROID DISEASE?

Thyroid disease is common in women. To understand the disease, it helps to first understand the basics of how the thyroid works. The thyroid is a small, butterfly-shaped endocrine (hormone-producing) gland located at the base of the throat. As an endocrine gland, the thyroid makes and releases thyroid hormones, which travel in the blood. Thyroid hormones impact almost every tissue in the body, affecting important chemical processes that allow the body to function normally. These processes include the conversion of nutrients from our food and drink into energy (metabolism) and processes that build, repair and support body systems.

The thyroid gland produces two related hormones: thyroxine (often called T4) and triiodothyronine (also known as T3). Most of the thyroid hormone made by the thyroid gland is T4. However, T4 is not the active form and doesn't affect metabolism — that's the role of T3. When needed, the body can elegantly transform T4 into T3.

One of the most useful methods for determining whole-body balance of thyroid hormone levels is to test for another hormone, called the thyroid stimulating hormone (TSH). TSH comes from the pituitary gland, located in the brain. It helps to regulate the release of T3 and T4 by telling the thyroid to increase or decrease hormone production. When there is adequate thyroid hormone in the body, the TSH levels will be in the normal range. High levels of TSH may indicate a thyroid hormone deficiency (hypothyroidism), whereas a low TSH level often indicates that thyroid hormone levels are too high (hyperthyroidism).

Thyroid conditions
Thyroid disease falls into several categories, depending on the cause.

Hypothyroidism (not enough!) Hypothyroidism is the most common thyroid condition and is found in approximately 4% to 10% of adults living in the United States. Hypothyroidism is anywhere from five to eight times more common in women than in men.

The most common cause of hypothyroidism in women is an autoimmune disease called Hashimoto's thyroiditis. In Hashimoto's thyroiditis, the body makes antibodies that attack and slowly break down normal thyroid tissue, reducing the thyroid gland's ability to make thyroid hormones. For this

Hyperthyroidism

- Unintentional weight loss
- Rapid heart rate or feeling like the heart is racing, pounding or skipping beats
- Anxiety/nervousness
- Irritability
- Shaking/trembling of the hands
- Sweating, and sensitivity to heat
- Fatigue
- Insomnia
- More frequent bowel movements
- Changes in the menstrual cycle (lighter, shorter periods)
- Brittle hair and nails; hair loss
- Muscle weakness

Hypothyroidism

- Fatigue
- Muscle weakness or muscle aches
- Constipation
- Weight gain and/or difficulty losing weight
- Frequently feeling cold/ greater sensitivity to cold
- Dry skin and hair; hair loss
- Worsening depression
- Forgetfulness
- Hoarse voice
- Changes in the menstrual cycle (usually longer, heavier periods)

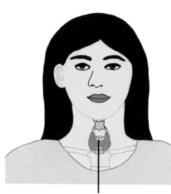

Thyroid gland

reason, doctors may test for these antibodies to predict a person's risk of developing a thyroid hormone deficiency or to help diagnose hypothyroidism. This test can be tricky to interpret, since many people who test positive for antibodies will never develop hypothyroidism. Thus, if you have an abnormal antibody result but have normal thyroid hormone levels, you don't need to be treated for thyroid disease.

Symptoms of hypothyroidism can include fatigue, muscle pain, constipation, weight gain and feeling cold. Other symptoms include hair loss, brittle hair and brittle or ridged fingernails. Hypothyroidism can worsen depression, create "brain fog" or sluggish thinking, result in heavy or irregular menstrual cycles and make it more

difficult to get pregnant. This condition can also contribute to the development of heart disease, abnormal cholesterol levels and anemia. When hypothyroidism is discovered and treated, most of the symptoms, including difficulty in getting pregnant, will go away.

Hyperthyroidism (too much!) Hyperthyroidism is much less common than hypothyroidism, occurring in about 0.2% to 1% of the population. But, like hypothyroidism, this condition is more common in women. Hyperthyroidism is most often caused by an autoimmune disease called Graves' disease. Graves' disease can cause the body to make antibodies directed against the thyroid. However, rather than destroying the thyroid tissue (as in Hashimoto's disease), these antibodies stimulate the thyroid gland to produce and release too much thyroid hormone. These antibodies can occasionally cause other effects on the body, such as swelling and expanding of the tissues around the eyeballs, which creates a bulging appearance of the eyes, so-called thyroid eye disease.

Hyperthyroidism can also occur when the thyroid gland becomes inflamed (thyroiditis), such as during a viral infection, and releases large quantities of stored thyroid hormone. This form of hyperthyroidism is short-lived hyperthyroidism, usually lasting 8 to 12 weeks and often requiring no treatment.

Differentiating amongst the various causes of hyperthyroidism (such as Graves' disease vs. thyroiditis) can be tricky, but your clinician can recommend tests to help unravel the cause and guide the best treatment. Tests used in the evaluation of hyperthyroidism include thyroid function studies, antibody measurements and sometimes imaging techniques such as ultrasound or a thyroid uptake scan.

The symptoms of hyperthyroidism can be dramatic and include feeling shaky or having tremors, feeling as though the heart is racing or skipping beats (palpitations), feeling very hot, having increased perspiration, having an increased number of bowel movements and experiencing insomnia. Weight loss, despite an increase in appetite, may also occur. Menstrual cycles can become irregular and sometimes light. In women after menopause, hot flashes can recur or worsen. Hyperthyroidism can also contribute to difficulty in conceiving or lead to miscarriages. Excessive thyroid hormone may cause worsening anxiety, irritability or mood swings. Not surprisingly, it is important to recognize, diagnose and treat hyperthyroidism quickly.

Thyroid goiter and nodules Goiter is a term used to describe a generalized enlargement of the thyroid gland. Sometimes this condition can cause a sense of fullness in the neck, trouble swallowing or discomfort when lying flat in bed. However, a goiter (even a very large one) usually does not cause symptoms. When a goiter is discovered, further evaluation is necessary to make sure the gland enlargement is not due to one or more lumps within the thyroid (thyroid nodules) and that the condition is not contributing to hyperthyroidism.

Thyroid nodules are relatively common. Although 94% of thyroid nodules are noncancerous (benign); up to 6% are cancerous. For those nodules that do contain a cancer, the vast majority of cases are readily treatable and curable. Thyroid nodules are often found during routine physical exams or tests for other conditions, such as during unrelated CT scans of the chest or neck. Thyroid nodules usually cause no symptoms, but they can sometimes lead to a feeling of fullness in the throat when at rest or when swallowing.

CAN THYROID DISEASE BE PREVENTED?

In most cases, no.

There is no evidence that a change in diet or nutritional supplements can prevent the development of thyroid disease and dysfunction. While celiac disease (an immune reaction to eating gluten) and hypothyroidism are both autoimmune diseases and can occur in the same person, adopting a gluten-free diet will not prevent thyroid disease, regardless of whether you have celiac disease. Similarly, while the mineral selenium is important in the creation of thyroid hormones, selenium naturally is found in most diets, and taking selenium does not reduce the risk of thyroid disease.

The mineral iodine is also an essential element for the synthesis of thyroid hormones. However, most diets in the United States contain plenty of iodine: It's found in salt, dairy products, some vegetables, and breads purchased in a grocery store. Iodine is also found in pretty much any pre-made foods, including fast foods. In fact, eating just one fast food meal a month provides most people with more than enough iodine. While adequate dietary iodine is important to thyroid synthesis, excessive iodine intake can cause thyroid function to cease, or cause inappropriately high thyroid hormone levels.

HOW IS THYROID DISEASE TREATED?

If you develop thyroid disease, your treatment will depend on your specific condition and symptoms. There are several common treatments for the different types of thyroid disease.

Treating hypothyroidism
Treatment of hypothyroidism is focused on thyroid hormone replacement medications, including:
- **Levothyroxine (T4)** This form of thyroid hormone is most often used to treat hypothyroidism and is recommended by the American Thyroid Association. The medication is well-tolerated and inexpensive. Usually generic levothyroxine works just as well as brand-name forms of the thyroid supplement. Once a person is started on thyroid hormone, it often takes a few months to adjust the dose and find just the right fit.
- **Liothyronine (T3)** For most people, being on levothyroxine can get them back to their healthy, productive selves. Occasionally, combination therapy with both levothyroxine and liothyronine may be used to treat hypothyroidism. Combination therapy can be more expensive and more complex, and occasionally requires taking the medications multiple times a day. Recent research has shown that long-acting T3 therapy could be a promising new treatment for hypothyroidism.

Most current thyroid hormone medications are synthetic, meaning they are entirely human-made. However, some T3 hormones are derived from pig hormone glands. This form of hormone is called desiccated thyroid hormone (Armour Thyroid). It can cause symptoms not common with synthetic levothyroxine, such as palpitations or insomnia. However, some studies have shown that desiccated thyroid hormone may lead to a slightly higher improvement in a person's quality of life.

Taking thyroid hormone every day is vital if you have hypothyroidism. It's important to take the medication by itself, 60 minutes before the intake of any other medications, food or beverages, such as coffee. Your clinician may need to adjust your dose to help your body maintain healthy levels of thyroid hormones. It often takes five to six weeks for thyroid hormone levels to stabilize after a dose adjustment, and often this is the timing for your clinician to retest your thyroid levels. If you're pregnant, your thyroid levels will likely be tested every four weeks. Once your thyroid levels have stabilized, your clinician may test your levels less frequently.

Many people wonder if being on a little extra thyroid hormone than needed might help them feel even better. The answer is no. The number one symptom of being on excessively high doses of thyroid hormone is fatigue. Too much thyroid hormone can also cause abnormal heart rhythms, irregular or rapid heartbeat (atrial fibrillation) and bone fractures.

Treating hyperthyroidism

The treatment of hyperthyroidism depends upon its cause. In some cases, your clinician may recommend a beta-blocker to treat your symptoms while closely monitoring your thyroid hormone levels with regular blood tests. Your clinician may also prescribe medications such as methimazole to reduce the amount of thyroid hormone your thyroid gland produces. Occasionally radioactive iodine or surgery may be necessary to treat hyperthyroidism. If you have Graves' disease and develop thyroid eye disease, your clinician may recommend a recent FDA-approved medication, teprotumumab, to treat the condition.

Treating thyroid goiter and nodules

If a large goiter is causing discomfort or difficulty with swallowing or breathing, or if it's contributing to hyperthyroidism, surgery can be performed to remove all or part of the thyroid gland. If a thyroid nodule is cancerous, treatment depends on the extent of the cancer and may include surgery, radioactive iodine, hormone replacement, radiation and, rarely, chemotherapy. Thyroid cancer is best treated by a team of health care specialists at a cancer center.

WHY IS THYROID DISEASE IMPORTANT TO WOMEN?

Thyroid diseases of all types are eight times more common in women than in men. White women are more likely to suffer from thyroid disease than Hispanic or Black women are. Thyroid nodules are also more common in women, and anywhere from 25% to 75% of women over the age of 50 will develop a nodule.

Thyroid hormone release and function is very sensitive to estrogen. Changes in estrogen levels can change the thyroid hormone levels in the blood, potentially contributing to the development of autoimmune thyroid disease. For women who are in their childbearing years, maintaining healthy thyroid hormone levels is important to reduce the risk of infertility. For women who are pregnant, maintaining healthy thyroid hormone levels is critical to ensure healthy fetal development.

If you have thyroid disease, estrogen plays a huge role not only in your thyroid hormone levels but also in determining the right dose of thyroid hormone medication. With any change in your estrogen levels, it's recommended that your thyroid hormone levels be checked, typically after six weeks. In particular, menopause is notoriously a time when thyroid hormone levels go up and down. Sometimes you just have to ride it out and have your blood checked often.

QUESTIONS TO ASK YOUR HEALTH CARE TEAM ABOUT THYROID DISEASE

- If I have a first-degree family member (parent, sibling or child) with thyroid disease, should I be screened for the disease?
- If I have hypothyroidism, how can I maximize my thyroid hormone therapy and dosing?
- How should I take my medication?
  - › *Be sure to tell your clinician if you are taking vitamins or supplements – especially biotin, which can interfere with thyroid lab tests.*
- Treatment for my thyroid disease has brought my thyroid hormones to a healthy level, but I still have some nagging symptoms. Should we consider another type of therapy or combination therapy?
- Do I just need to add some exercise into my weekly routine?
  - › *Two large studies have shown that increasing exercise frequency can improve the symptoms of hypothyroidism as effectively as taking liothyronine.*
- What impact will changes in my estrogen levels have on my thyroid treatment, such as if I add (or eliminate) birth control, become pregnant or go through menopause?
- I see (or feel) a new lump in my neck. Should I have an ultrasound?

PEARLS OF WISDOM

Thyroid disease is definitely more common in women than in men, and it can be tricky to diagnose because the symptoms can be vague and nonspecific. If you have a family history of thyroid disease (hypothyroidism, hyperthyroidism or thyroid nodules), then you are also more likely to develop those issues. Talk to your clinician, who may recommend screening you for thyroid disease more frequently.

If you do have thyroid disease, there is nothing more valuable than working in close partnership with your clinician. This kind of partnership can make all the difference. You should feel comfortable asking your clinician questions about your treatment and the right dose of medication for you, but also know that sometimes finding that sweet spot with your dosage can take time.

"When women and their clinicians work together, as a team, the best possible health can be achieved."

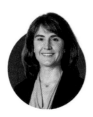

Laura E. Ryan, M.D. - she/her

Dr. Ryan is an Associate Professor of Clinical Medicine at the Center for Women's Health at The Ohio State's Wexner Medical Center, Division of Endocrinology, Diabetes and Metabolism. She holds the position of Director of Special Events, and plans and directs many educational events at the medical center. She is a clinical endocrinologist with a specialty in metabolic bone disease, benign thyroid disease, and ultrasound-guided thyroid biopsy.

"Research that includes the unique perspectives of women and clinicians has the greatest impact on improving health for both women and our communities."

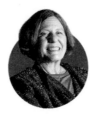

Rebecca D. Jackson, M.D. - she/her

Dr. Jackson is a Professor of Medicine in the Division of Endocrinology, Diabetes and Metabolism, The Ohio State University College of Medicine, and Principal Investigator of the Women's Health Initiative for the last 28 years — a landmark study of the factors impacting postmenopausal and older women's health. She is also Director and Principal Investigator of the Center for Clinical and Translational Science at The Ohio State University. Her clinical practice focuses on diagnosis and treatment of endocrine diseases that disproportionately affect women including metabolic bone disease, osteoporosis and thyroid disease. Dr. Jackson's research interests center on women's health, from identifying risk factors and genetic predictors of osteoporosis and osteoarthritis to addressing the opioid epidemic in Ohio, aiming to reduce overdose deaths.

60
Urinary incontinence

Angelish Kumar, M.D., and Alexandra R. Siegal, M.D.

WHAT IS URINARY INCONTINENCE?

Urinary incontinence is the involuntary leakage of urine which many women experience after childbirth, with aging or in association with other medical problems, such as diabetes mellitus or stroke. Incontinence can occur when exercising, laughing, coughing or sneezing, or when there is a strong urge to urinate and not enough time to make it to the bathroom.

While incontinence is not normal, it is extremely common in women. Studies show that at least 40% of women over 40 suffer from urinary incontinence. Yet most women are not receiving adequate medical attention or treatment for it. According to the National Poll on Healthy Aging, only 34% of women who experienced incontinence spoke to their doctor about it. This is because many women do not feel comfortable discussing this problem — they may feel it is something they are supposed to "just live with" — or they are not referred to urologists or urogynecologists, doctors who specialize in female incontinence and can offer effective treatment options.

To understand why women develop urinary incontinence, it helps to know how the urinary system works. The kidneys produce urine, which flows into the bladder through tubes called ureters. The bladder, which sits deep in the pelvis, stores the urine until you have decided it is an appropriate time to go to the bathroom. When you're ready to urinate, the pelvic floor muscles relax, the inner urethral sphincter muscle opens and the bladder muscle contracts. As the bladder contracts, urine flows out through a short tube called the urethra, which is just in front of the vagina.

The pelvic floor muscles and connective tissue on the outside of the urethra help to stabilize its position and maintain it in a closed state. Urinary leakage occurs when the urethra is unable to maintain adequate closure (stress incontinence) or the bladder muscle contracts inappropriately (urge incontinence).

Stress incontinence
This type of leakage occurs when a sudden increase in pressure is placed on the abdominal cavity, say when you sneeze, cough, run or jump. The pressure from the abdomen bears down on the bladder. Normally, the pelvic floor muscles and connective tissue are strong enough to keep the urethra closed even under pressure. But when there is

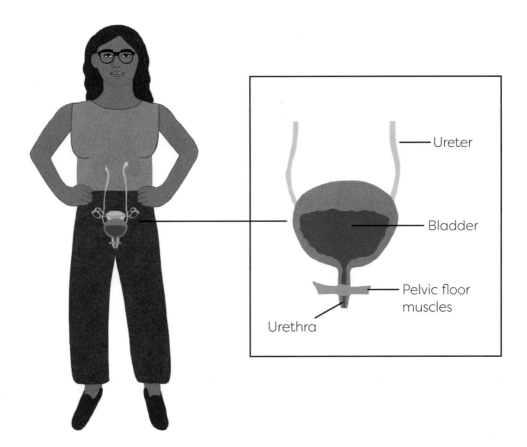

Ureter

Bladder

Pelvic floor muscles

Urethra

weakness in the pelvic floor or the internal urethral sphincter muscle, strong pressure on the bladder forces urine out.

Urge incontinence

The classic example of urge incontinence is that moment when you arrive home, and as you turn your key in the door, the urge to urinate is so strong that the urine starts to dribble out before you make it to the bathroom. Urge incontinence happens when the bladder muscle begins to contract and expel urine before you're actually sitting on the toilet. This occurs when the signals that normally prevent your bladder from contracting become weaker, which can happen with age, other illnesses or neurologic (nervous system) changes. Urge

incontinence can also result when the bladder is more sensitive due to urinary infections, medications or menopause. Women who have urinary urgency (the sudden need to urinate) and urge incontinence (leakage) may also feel they need to urinate frequently. Together, urinary urgency and frequency are referred to as "overactive bladder."

Many women have a combination of both stress and urge incontinence. While there are some common strategies that help with both of these problems, the treatments for each type of incontinence are different. To be offered comprehensive and effective treatment, it's important to have a thorough evaluation by a urologist or urogynecologist.

In addition to discussing your medical history with your doctor, you should have a physical exam and a urine sample checked to make sure you don't have an infection or blood in your urine. You should also be assessed for any other symptoms that could be related to incontinence, such as a neurologic problem.

CAN URINARY INCONTINENCE BE PREVENTED?

There are several ways to prevent urinary leakage.

Pelvic floor physical therapy

The pelvic floor muscles are integral to preventing leakage. They can become weak during pregnancy or childbirth, or from activities that cause significant bearing down (applying pressure to the abdomen), such as sports or chronic coughing. A common way to strengthen the pelvic floor and prevent urinary incontinence is to perform Kegel exercises, which involve tightening and releasing pelvic floor muscles. Many women try to do Kegel exercises on their own, but studies show that a more effective approach is to do pelvic floor physical therapy with a dedicated physical therapist. Ask your doctor or clinician for a recommended pelvic floor physical therapist.

Other types of exercise, such as Pilates, are also beneficial for core and pelvic floor strength. Pilates and pelvic floor physical therapy are both great forms of exercise that can be done during and after pregnancy.

Weight loss

Multiple studies have shown that in women who are overweight, weight loss helps with both stress and urge incontinence. Weight loss can improve quality of life by decreasing incontinence episodes and overactive bladder symptoms, and it can also decrease the risk of type 2 diabetes, hypertension and hyperlipidemia and improve mood. Weight is a complex issue that involves social, emotional, and genetic factors and deserves the same type of medical attention paid to other health issues like high blood pressure or high cholesterol. If you struggle with weight, you can find help from doctors who specialize in weight loss medicine and functional medicine and from cognitive behavioral therapists. Both can make a big difference in your ability to lose weight.

Quitting smoking

Smokers are twice as likely to develop incontinence compared to nonsmokers. Smoking leads to degradation of collagen, which is necessary in maintaining pelvic floor strength and healthy supportive tissue around the urethra. Longtime smokers also tend to have chronic cough and chronic obstructive pulmonary disease. The constant coughing and bearing down puts significant pressure on the already weak pelvic floor. Additionally, smoking is a major risk factor for bladder cancer, among many other types of cancers.

Managing constipation

Many women notice that their bladder symptoms are worse when they're constipated, or that they are not emptying their bladder fully when they also have constipation. Maintaining regular bowel movements is helpful not only for gastrointestinal health but for bladder health as well. Fiber supplements and stool softeners are good options to promote soft, well-formed and regular bowel movements. Taking a magnesium supplement can also help with constipation. Fiber-rich foods that can be added to your daily diet include prunes, chia seeds, and green leafy vegetables like spinach and kale. (See Chapter 22.)

HOW IS URINARY INCONTINENCE TREATED?

If you develop urinary incontinence, your clinician will likely suggest conservative treatments at first. Behavioral modification and pelvic floor physical therapy are considered the best treatments to start with for both urge and stress incontinence.

Behavioral modifications
It can be useful to keep a bladder diary, which is a record of how much liquid you consume throughout the day, how much liquid you urinate and when you urinate. A bladder diary can help you evaluate how much total fluid you're consuming and how much urine you're producing. It can also assist with identifying whether any type of caffeine, carbonated beverage, juice, alcohol, artificial sweeteners or diuretics (medications that cause the kidneys to make more urine) may be irritating your bladder or causing you to produce excess urine.

For some women, frequent urination is a habit that causes them to feel the need to urinate before the bladder is full. A bladder diary can also help your clinician assess your voiding habits to see whether a program of timed voiding (urinating on a fixed schedule) or bladder retraining (slowly stretching out the periods between timed urination) may help you. Bladder retraining techniques can help to rewire the signals so you can store urine for longer periods of time.

Pelvic floor physical therapy
While many women are told to do Kegel exercises on their own at home to strengthen their pelvic floor muscles, women who work with a pelvic floor physical therapist experience a greater improvement in their incontinence symptoms. Many women incorrectly contract their gluteal, abdominal or inner thigh muscles, and a dedicated therapist can make sure you are doing the exercises correctly. Pelvic floor physical therapists also use a technique called biofeedback that allows you to make sure you are contracting and relaxing the right muscles.

Strengthening the muscles so that they can protect you from leaking requires doing the exercises regularly and with greater intensity over time. This is more likely to be accomplished with a therapist than if you are trying to do it on your own. Once you have a good grasp of the correct muscles and what to do, there are good devices you can use at home for maintenance, such as Elvie and Leva.

If these measures don't relieve your symptoms, your doctor may recommend more aggressive or invasive treatments. These differ for urge incontinence and stress incontinence.

Treatment options for urge incontinence
Several options are available to treat urge incontinence.

Medications A number of FDA-approved medications can treat overactive bladder symptoms (urgency, frequency and urge incontinence). These medications help the bladder to store urine more comfortably. While these drugs can be effective, side effects can include dry mouth or constipation. Sometimes the first option you try may not be right for you, and you should ask to be switched to something else. If you have tried more than two medications and they are not effective, or if you're having unwanted side effects, speak to your urologist or urogynecologist about the non-medication options that follow in this section.

Nerve stimulation During this office procedure, a thin, acupuncture-size needle is inserted through the skin for gentle electrical stimulation of the posterior tibial nerve, which is located near the ankle. This nerve communicates with the sacral nerve, which regulates signals of urinary urgency and frequency coming from the bladder. Studies show that posterior tibial nerve stimulation is as effective as medication and is extremely simple and virtually pain free. However, it requires an office visit once a week for twelve weeks to do the full therapy. After that, people often need maintenance sessions about once every one to three months.

Bladder Botox In the same way that Botox works to reduce wrinkles by preventing contraction of facial muscles, this medicinal form of the toxin botulinum can also prevent inappropriate contraction of the bladder muscle. Bladder Botox is an office procedure that is very effective for overactive bladder and urge incontinence. It involves injecting Botox medication evenly in multiple places on the bladder wall.

Effects last about six to nine months before they begin to wear off. In some people, effects last longer. When they start to wear off, you can schedule a repeat injection. There is a small risk of urinary retention, meaning that you may have difficulty emptying your bladder. It is usually temporary but if it does happen, your urologist or urogynecologist can guide you on how to manage it.

Sacral nerve stimulation The bladder, rectum and pelvic floor communicate through a nerve called the sacral nerve. Sometimes, the signals traveling through this nerve create an inappropriate sense of needing to urinate or have a bowel movement. Sacral nerve stimulation delivers gentle electrical impulses directly to the nerve to improve the symptoms of urinary frequency, urge incontinence, fecal incontinence (inability to control bowel movements) and pelvic floor dysfunction.

This therapy involves surgically implanting a device that delivers electrical impulses to the sacral nerve. Just as a pacemaker controls a heartbeat, this device helps to control movements of the bladder, bowel and pelvic floor. Sacral nerve stimulation is one of the few therapies for incontinence that does not carry any risk of difficulty emptying the bladder, and in fact, it may help people who do not empty their bladder completely.

Treatment options for stress incontinence

There are several ways to treat stress incontinence.

Vaginal devices (pessaries) To support the urethra and bladder and prevent urinary leakage, your doctor may recommend using an insert inside your vagina. These inserts include medical-grade silicone pessaries, which are fitted for you by a clinician and which you insert yourself. There are also over-the-counter inserts, including the Poise Impressa, which looks and feels like a tampon but is designed to prop up the bladder and the urethra. In women who only leak when they exercise, this can be a nice option because it is disposable. You can wear it just for exercise and then remove it when you're done.

Urethral bulking injection This is a simple office procedure in which a sterile water-based gel is injected under the mucosal lining along the inner wall of the urethra.

This procedure gives the lining more volume, which helps create a tighter seal on the inside of the urethra so urine can't leak out. The injection is effective immediately.

Bulking injections work well in about 70% to 80% of women who suffer from stress incontinence, and women are very satisfied with not having to undergo a surgical procedure. There is a small risk of not being able to completely empty your bladder immediately after the procedure, but this is usually temporary.

Urethral sling surgery Sling surgery is an extremely effective and durable way to treat stress incontinence. A sling is a ribbon-shaped strip of mesh that prevents urinary leakage by restoring support around the urethra. The surgery involves placing the strip of mesh underneath the urethra through an incision in the vaginal wall. The mesh should not be seen or felt after the surgery. For women who wish to have the surgery but prefer to avoid mesh, a strip of your own

Urethral bulking injection

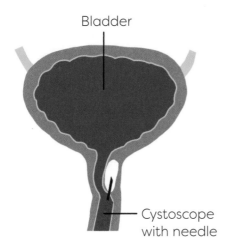

Bladder

Cystoscope with needle

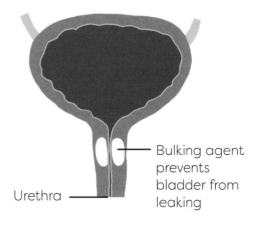

Urethra

Bulking agent prevents bladder from leaking

tissue can be harvested and used as the sling material, but this involves a separate incision and a longer recovery.

While sling surgery is an effective treatment for stress incontinence, it does carry small risks of injury to the bladder or urethra, pain from the mesh, exposure of the mesh or difficulty emptying the bladder. These concerns can usually be managed by a simple loosening of the mesh or removing the section that is causing the problem.

WHY DOES URINARY INCONTINENCE MATTER TO WOMEN?

Urinary incontinence is one of the most prevalent and bothersome health issues for women. It is especially common in women over 50, and it affects twice as many women as men. Several risk factors make women more prone to developing incontinence, such as number of pregnancies, vaginal deliveries, menopause and prior pelvic surgeries.

One-third of women experience stress incontinence after childbirth and notice that they no longer can exercise without wearing a pad or leakage garment. Stress incontinence is especially common after childbirth because pregnancy and vaginal delivery can cause the muscles and ligaments supporting the bladder and urethra to stretch and even tear. Many women are told that leaking after childbirth is "normal," and they should accept the need to wear a pad or avoid vigorous exercise. However, in the postpartum period, pelvic floor physical therapy

can be very effective in helping women to regain continence.

Women are also more prone to incontinence because the female urethra is very short (only four centimeters long). Even slight changes in the surrounding tissue and musculature can make it difficult for the urethra to stay closed while the bladder is filling with urine. The short urethra also makes women more prone to getting urinary tract infections from bacteria that reside in the genital area. Chronic bladder inflammation from urinary tract infections can lead to overactive bladder or urge incontinence symptoms. Some women notice they develop urge incontinence when they have a urinary tract infection because the bladder muscle spasms due to the inflamed lining.

As women age, hormonal changes lead to a loss of collagen and healthy blood supply around the urethra, which also results in a loss of support. A decrease in estrogen levels also affects the bladder, urethra and pelvic floor, increasing the risk of both stress incontinence and overactive bladder symptoms. The overall changes in genitourinary (vaginal and urinary) health, including urinary frequency, urgency, burning with urination, urinary incontinence, vaginal dryness, irritation, pain with intercourse and increased tendency to get urinary tract infections, are collectively known as the "genitourinary syndrome of menopause." Very often, these symptoms can be alleviated by using low-dose estrogen cream in the vagina, which is different from hormone replacement therapy in that it does not cause a systemic rise in the blood levels of estrogen.

While issues related to male aging have been treated by the medical community for decades, the genitourinary syndrome of menopause only received recognition as a medical condition in 2014. For years, women have been told to "just live with it," while men have been referred to specialists for erectile dysfunction and low testosterone. In the medical community we are finally addressing quality-of-life issues related to female aging!

QUESTIONS TO ASK YOUR HEALTH CARE TEAM ABOUT URINARY INCONTINENCE

If you are seeking care for urinary incontinence

- Can you provide me a referral for a pelvic floor physical therapist and for a urologist or urogynecologist?

If you have been prescribed medication for urinary incontinence

- What are the potential side effects?
- If the medication is not working in four to six weeks, can we try a different medication or therapy?

If you are about to undergo a procedure to treat urinary incontinence

- What realistic expectations should I have about the effectiveness of this procedure?
- What are all of the potential risks?
- What is the risk for infection, bleeding or injury to surrounding structures?
- How long will the recovery period be?
- Will I need to take time off work?
- Will I need to arrange for child care?

PEARLS OF WISDOM

See a urologist or a urogynecologist

If you have urinary problems that aren't improving under the care of your gynecologist or primary care clinician, ask for a referral to a doctor who is trained specifically to treat incontinence. Visiting this type of specialist can also help you learn more about your treatment options.

Ask for a referral for pelvic floor physical therapy

This is especially important for postpartum mamas. If an athlete injured a muscle or tendon, he or she would go through physical therapy and rehabilitation to regain strength and function. The same goes for your pelvic floor after childbirth.

Don't be afraid of getting a second opinion

Many clinicians have niches within their specialty or favor one treatment or procedure over another because of their own experience. If you're unsure about what you are being offered, ask who else you should see for a second opinion.

Speak up

If you have seen a good doctor, or you have received an effective treatment, tell your friends. Many women suffer in silence with incontinence because it is such a taboo topic in our society. Letting other women know they can access treatment is doing them a great service.

Give a thorough medical history

Let your clinician know when you've noticed new or worsening urinary symptoms, such as with childbirth, menopause, surgery, intercourse, weight gain, change in diet or hydration, or starting a new medication. Also mention any other symptoms you experience around the same time, such as muscle weakness or numbness in your extremities. These details are all important in the evaluation of urinary incontinence.

Trust your body

If you are experiencing any pain or see blood in your urine, or if your symptoms are not responding at all to conventional therapies, your incontinence could be the result of an underlying medical issue such as a urinary tract infection, kidney or bladder stone, interstitial cystitis or bladder cancer. Ruling out these causes may require one or more tests — such as a CT scan, ultrasound, MRI, or a cystoscopy — to evaluate the inner lining of the bladder.

"Women want to trust that their doctor understands their issues, and can offer them practical and effective treatments."

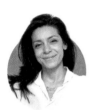

Angelish Kumar, M.D. - she/her
Dr. Kumar is the founder of Women's Urology New York and a Clinical Instructor of Urology at Mount Sinai School of Medicine in New York City. Dr. Kumar focuses her entire practice on women's genitourinary health and founded her practice to improve the urology experience for postpartum, middle-aged and post-menopausal women. She specializes in treating recurrent urinary tract infections, urinary incontinence, overactive bladder, bladder pain syndrome and genitourinary syndrome of menopause.

"It's important to create an environment where women's health care concerns are perceived as legitimate and approached with compassion."

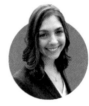

Alexandra R. Siegal, M.D. - she/her
Dr. Siegal is currently a urology resident at Mount Sinai Hospital in New York City. She is interested in pursuing a career in female pelvic medicine and reconstructive surgery.

61

Urinary tract infection

Imari C. Faceson, D.O., and Elodi Dielubanza, M.D.

WHAT IS A URINARY TRACT INFECTION (UTI)?

A urinary tract infection (UTI) occurs when bacteria enter the urinary tract — the system of organs that consists of the bladder, urethra, kidneys and ureters. The bowels and anus are the most common source of bacteria that cause UTI. Often, the friendly E. coli bacteria that live in the gut can cause problems when released during bowel movements. This leads to the bacteria spreading up the urinary tract and into the bladder. This series of events is responsible for about 80% to 95% of all confirmed UTIs.

UTIs are categorized based upon the location of the bacteria:
- **Urine (asymptomatic bacteriuria)** Asymptomatic bacteriuria occurs when bacteria are present in the urine but do not cause any symptoms.
- **Bladder (cystitis)** Cystitis occurs when bacteria attach to the bladder lining, which can cause inflammation, lower abdominal pain, pain with urination, increased urge to urinate, increased frequency of urination and blood in the urine.
- **Kidney (pyelonephritis)** Pyelonephritis occurs when bacteria from the bladder travel up the ureters to the kidney. This causes symptoms of cystitis along with fever and new back pain on the same side as the affected kidney.

To diagnose a UTI, your clinician will ask about your symptoms and will probably conduct certain urine tests:
- **Urinalysis** This is a rapid screening test for signs of infection in the urine, including inflammatory cells (such as leukocytes or white blood cells), blood and byproducts of bacteria.
- **Urine culture** This is the definitive test that identifies the type and number of bacteria present in the urine, as well as the appropriate antibiotics needed to treat the infection. It takes 24 to 48 hours to obtain the results of this test.

It is important to understand the results of your testing because urine culture testing can confirm the diagnosis of UTI, identify the bacteria causing the infection and identify any patterns of antibiotic resistance. Tests that are ultimately negative for infection may point to a different medical problem. Visible or microscopic blood in the urine that persists even when urine tests are negative, or between proven infections, can indicate a need for more detailed testing to look for causes other than infection.

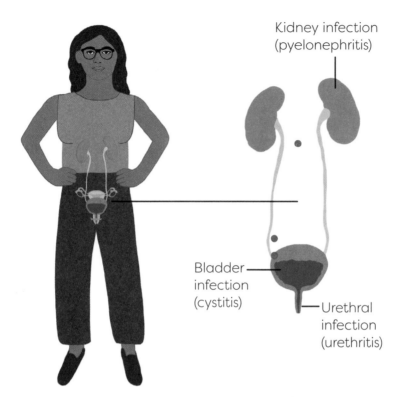

Kidney infection
(pyelonephritis)

Bladder
infection
(cystitis)

Urethral
infection
(urethritis)

Urinary tract infections that cause symptoms are classified as complicated or uncomplicated based on various factors.

- Uncomplicated UTIs occur in healthy women who do not have any medical risk factors that would impair the clearance of bacteria from the urinary tract.
- Complicated UTIs occur in women who have certain medical risk factors that either increase the risk of infection or decrease the chance of clearing bacteria. These risk factors include:
  › Use of immunosuppressant medications
  › Immune disorders
  › Spinal cord injury
  › Use of a urinary catheter
  › Anatomic abnormalities of the urinary tract (such as kidney stones)
  › Recent urinary tract surgery

Up to 20% of women experience recurrent UTI, defined as more than two infections in 6 months or more than three infections in 12 months. It is important to know that recurrent infections can still be uncomplicated and do not require longer antibiotic courses.

CAN UTIs BE PREVENTED?

The body's best defense against UTI is the strong, forward flow of urine to expel bacterial invaders from the urinary tract. Adequate hydration (drinking at least 48 ounces of fluids a day) and avoidance of holding in urine are important strategies to prevent infections.

It is important to wipe from front to back after a bowel movement to minimize transfer of bowel bacteria to the vagina and tissues surrounding the urethra. In addition, the population of healthy bacteria in the vagina (vaginal microbiome or flora) helps prevent colonization of infection-causing bacteria and UTI. Excessive vaginal cleaning practices can disturb these healthy bacteria and be counterproductive when it comes to UTI prevention. Avoid douching, using antibacterial or harsh soaps on the vagina, and cleansing the vagina very frequently.

These additional strategies can decrease the risk of UTI:

- **D-Mannose supplement** This daily supplement allows a simple carbohydrate to stick to E. coli bacteria, which keeps the bacteria from attaching to urinary tract tissue.
- **Cranberry supplement** Cranberries contain proanthocyanidins, a natural chemical in plants that can keep bacteria from attaching to the urinary tract.
- **Methenamine** This prescription medication produces ammonia and a weak formaldehyde in the urine, which can damage bacterial proteins and DNA and prevent infection. Methenamine works best when the urine has an acidic pH, so it is often taken with vitamin C.
- **Vaginal estrogen therapy** This treatment is useful for women who are near menopause (perimenopausal) or postmenopausal. Vaginal estrogen therapy helps support healthy vaginal tissue and restores healthy vaginal bacteria, thus decreasing the risk of UTI. It is available by prescription, after a consultation with your clinician. (It is important to note that oral estrogen does not have the same effect in decreasing the risk of UTI.)

- **Probiotics** These live microorganisms (such as bacteria or yeast) may help to fortify the populations of "good" bacteria in the gut and vagina. Probiotics are found in fermented foods (such as yogurt, kombucha or sauerkraut) and oral and topical supplements. Probiotics are generally safe, and there is evolving research that suggests that bacterial populations in the body are vital for immune function. However, if you have an immune disorder or you take immunosuppressant medications, talk to your clinician before using these supplements.
- **Antibiotic prevention** This approach may be considered for certain recurrent UTIs when non-antibiotic strategies have failed. Antibiotic prevention may also be used to prevent more serious problems, such as kidney infections. When sexual activity is a trigger for infections, a single low-dose antibiotic can be taken directly after sexual activity to prevent bacteria from growing in the urine. When there is not a clear trigger for infection, a daily low-dose antibiotic may be appropriate for several weeks.

The goal of antibiotic prevention is to reduce the frequency of UTIs and overall use of antibiotics (since more UTIs require more antibiotics). Because antibiotics can alter the balance of good bacteria in parts of the body outside of the urinary tract, it is important to limit the amount of time that antibiotic prevention strategies are used and have a plan in place to transition to non-antibiotic prevention.

A pelvic examination can reveal changes in the muscles and structures in the pelvis that support the bladder (such as bladder prolapse) as well as menopausal changes that might impact emptying of the bladder and increase the risk of UTI. If you continue to experience recurrent UTIs despite prevention measures, ask your clinician to check for these types of changes during a pelvic exam.

HOW ARE UTIs TREATED?

Before receiving treatment for UTI, be sure to discuss the details of your symptoms with your clinician to ensure that there are no other likely diagnoses. The goal of UTI treatment is to relieve symptoms and control the infection-causing bacteria while minimizing unwanted side effects of antibiotic treatment. An over-the-counter pain reliever that soothes bladder discomfort (phenazopyridine) and nonsteroidal anti-inflammatory drugs (NSAIDs), such as ibuprofen and naproxen, can help to alleviate symptoms. Antibiotics help eliminate bacteria and are best used at the lowest necessary dose and for the shortest duration. (Long courses of antibiotics can lead to development of drug-resistant bacteria and other infections, such as yeast infections and intestinal infections, as well as diarrhea.)

The type and duration of antibiotics is determined by a woman's health, whether an infection is complicated or uncomplicated, and sometimes by urine testing.
- For uncomplicated UTI, three to five days of first-line antibiotics such as nitrofurantoin, trimethoprim-sulfamethoxazole and fosfomycin are recommended, unless drug allergies or urine culture indicate use of different drugs.
- For complicated UTI, a course of 7 to 14 days of antibiotics may be needed. Urine

testing may help identify the best antibiotic to treat a complicated UTI.

Antibiotic drugs work in different ways, and some may take longer to produce relief than others. Don't hesitate to ask about medications to help relieve your symptoms. Ninety percent of UTIs get better when treated appropriately. If you have recurrent infections, strongly consider a prevention strategy or talk to your clinician about setting one up. Additionally, note that as you get older it's common to have bacteria in your urine without having symptoms, and antibiotic therapy isn't always necessary.

WHY DO UTIs MATTER TO WOMEN?

Almost half of all women will have at least one UTI in their lifetimes. UTI is one of the most common reasons that women visit a clinician or the emergency department.

Women are twice as likely as men to experience UTI because of their anatomy. The female urethra is short and close to the anus, where bacteria that cause UTI naturally reside. As a result, bacteria travel a shorter distance to enter the bladder in women compared to that for men.

Conditions that cause bacteria to come in closer proximity to the urethra can increase the risk of UTI. For example, sexual intercourse can be a trigger for infections. Additionally, using spermicide with barrier contraceptives (such as condoms, diaphragms or cervical caps) increases the risk of UTI. However, lifestyle practices such as using tampons, wearing tight clothes and wearing thong underwear have not been shown to increase the risk of UTI.

Other changes specific to women, such as hormone loss during menopause, can make women more susceptible to UTI. This is due to changes in vaginal tissue and disturbance of healthy vaginal bacteria, which can lead to harmful bacterial colonization of the vagina and result in a UTI.

QUESTIONS TO ASK YOUR HEALTH CARE TEAM ABOUT UTIs

- Do I have any anatomic factors that increase my risk of UTI? If you experience recurrent UTI, ask your clinician to check for structural or menopausal changes to your pelvic muscles and tissues during a pelvic exam.
- Do my symptoms or test results suggest something other than UTI?
- If I am being treated for a UTI, when should I start to feel better? How can I get relief from my symptoms?

PEARLS OF WISDOM

UTIs are common conditions and can range from having no symptoms to a recurrent serious infection. Keep these tips in mind:
- Maximize your body's natural protections by maintaining good hydration and urination habits. Consider non-antibiotic approaches to prevention
- Approach antibiotic use with an understanding of benefits and harms. More antibiotics are not always better. If appropriate antibiotic therapy fails to improve symptoms, it may be time to consider other explanations for your symptoms.
- Symptoms of vaginal itching or burning, increased vaginal discharge and persistent pelvic or vaginal pain are not typical symptoms of UTI and should heighten your suspicion of other causes, such as vaginal infections or menopausal changes in the vaginal tissue.
- If symptoms recur but urine cultures do not show that bacteria are present, talk to your clinician to explore other causes of bothersome symptoms, including overactive bladder syndrome.

"Women need to feel empowered when discussing their health with physicians."

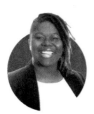

Imari C. Faceson, D.O. - she/her
Dr. Faceson graduated from the New York Institute of Technology College of Osteopathic Medicine at Arkansas State University in May 2022 and is currently in Urology residency.

"Education is the most important tool for women to navigate their health care."

Elodi Dielubanza, M.D. - she/her
Dr. Dielubanza is the Director of Female Pelvic Medicine and Reconstructive surgery in the Division of Urology at Brigham and Women's Hospital in Boston, Massachusetts. She specializes in the management of female pelvic disorders including incontinence and pelvic organ prolapse.

62

Uterine fibroids

Sarah C. Baumgarten, M.D., Ph.D., and Elizabeth (Ebbie) A. Stewart, M.D.

WHAT ARE UTERINE FIBROIDS?

Uterine fibroids, also called uterine leiomyomas or myomas, are noncancerous (benign) growths in the muscle layer of the uterus.

Fibroids can vary in size, ranging from the size of a pea to larger than a basketball. They can grow, shrink or even disappear during a woman's lifetime, but most uterine fibroids have steady growth until menopause. Women can have one fibroid or dozens. Fibroids are sensitive to estrogen and progesterone, the hormones that the ovaries make during a woman's reproductive years. This is why fibroids are typically diagnosed at this time in a woman's life. After menopause, the ovaries stop producing significant amounts of these hormones and the fibroids usually shrink.

Fibroids are very common and affect approximately 70% of reproductive-aged women. Among Black women, nearly 80% are affected by fibroids, and the fibroids are often more severe. Not all women have symptoms from fibroids, but for some women the symptoms can interfere with their everyday life, general health, work life and relationships.

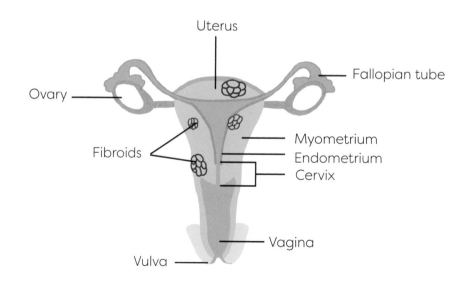

The most common symptom of fibroids is heavy or long menstrual periods, in which bleeding lasts seven or more days or there's a need to change pads or tampons every hour or two. This bleeding can result in anemia and fatigue, sometimes requiring blood transfusions. When fibroids are large, they can cause "bulk symptoms" that include abdominal pain or pressure and changes in bladder or bowel function, such as frequent urination, difficulty urinating or difficulty having a bowel movement. Fibroids can also cause painful menstrual periods and painful intercourse and can sometimes make women look like they are pregnant when they are not. Rarely, fibroids can cause problems with fertility, miscarriage or complications during pregnancy. Symptoms from fibroids differ depending on the number, size and location of the fibroids.

The initial evaluation for fibroids is typically a physical exam and an ultrasound of the uterus. The ultrasound can give information about the number, size and location of fibroids. Sometimes other imaging, such as an MRI, may be necessary. There are no lab tests needed for diagnosis; however, if a woman is experiencing heavy menstrual bleeding, a blood test to check for anemia or low blood count is important. Testing to rule out other common causes of heavy bleeding, such as thyroid disease, may also be done.

Fibroids are not cancerous or precancerous, but sometimes a cancer can look like a fibroid on routine testing. If you have new fibroids, fibroids that grow after menopause or fibroids with an unusual appearance on an MRI, there would be more worry about mistaking a cancer for a fibroid. Both fibroids and cancers can grow rapidly.

CAN UTERINE FIBROIDS BE PREVENTED?

Currently there are no measures known to prevent fibroids from forming. However, some studies suggest that certain lifestyle changes may reduce the risk of fibroids. For example, eating a diet rich in green vegetables and citrus fruits may decrease the risk of fibroids compared to a diet that is high in beef or red meats. Alcohol, particularly beer, may increase your risk of fibroids. Making these recommended dietary changes may help prevent fibroids while also helping you maintain a healthy weight and decrease your risk of heart disease and cancer.

There is evidence that low vitamin D levels may be a risk factor for the development of fibroids. Black women generally have lower levels of vitamin D, and this could be one reason why they are more likely to develop fibroids.

Reproductive factors also affect your risk of developing fibroids. Starting menstrual cycles at a young age, less than 10 years old, is associated with an increased risk of developing fibroids. Studies have shown that having pregnancies resulting in births strongly decreases the chance of fibroid formation. Also, certain hormonal contraceptives, such as birth control pills and depot medroxyprogesterone (a long-term injection for birth control), may be associated with a decreased risk of fibroids.

HOW ARE UTERINE FIBROIDS TREATED?

Fibroids can affect women in different ways, so your specific symptoms will help guide which treatment plan is right for you. The number, size and location of the fibroids and your plans for future pregnancy will then narrow treatment options. Generally, the least invasive approach to treating symptomatic fibroids should be considered first. However, new fibroids can form after most therapies, so the need for long-lasting treatment also has a role in decision making.

While fibroids sometimes are a problem for women actively trying to get pregnant, there are many women with fibroids who get pregnant without trouble. Therefore, completing a full fertility evaluation, including a sperm count if you have a male partner, is important for women with fibroids before doing any fibroid treatment.

Medical management options

Most medical treatments work best at decreasing heavy menstrual bleeding and pain.

Hormonal contraceptives Hormonal contraceptives in the form of birth control pills, vaginal rings or transdermal patches are often the preferred treatment for fibroids and heavy menstrual bleeding even if you don't need birth control. These medications have the benefit of being inexpensive and widely available. They also decrease iron deficiency anemia, uterine cancer, and ovarian cancer and provide contraception.

Hormone-releasing intrauterine device (IUD) For women who cannot or prefer not to use estrogen, hormone-releasing IUDs are an option. These IUDs release a progesterone-like hormone (levonorgestrel) that affects the uterus but doesn't change hormones in the rest of the body. The IUD, which is placed into the uterus by a clinician, can improve heavy menstrual bleeding and will last for three to six years before needing to be removed or replaced. However, women with certain fibroids that protrude into the uterine cavity may not be good candidates for an IUD.

Nonsteroidal anti-inflammatory drugs (NSAIDs) For women who cannot or do not want to take hormones, nonprescription or prescription NSAIDS such as ibuprofen or naproxen can help reduce heavy menstrual bleeding and relieve pain during periods. NSAIDS can also be used with the hormonal medications.

Tranexamic acid (TXA) Tranexamic acid is a pill that can be taken three times a day during the heavy days of menses to reduce heavy menstrual bleeding. TXA should not be combined with hormones.

Other medications For women with bleeding, bulk symptoms or both, medications that act on the brain to influence the reproductive system are effective medical therapy. Oral combination medications such as Oriahnn (twice daily) or Myfembree (once daily) are relatively new treatment options that decrease bleeding and bulk symptoms. This type of drug, which can be used for up to two years, contains medications that shut down the ovaries' production of hormones while giving back low levels of hormones to limit menopause-like side effects. Related medications available as injections, such as Lupron

Depot, are effective in reducing the size of fibroids. However, because they do not have the low dose of hormones added back, they have side effects such as hot flashes and bone loss. These injections are given monthly or every three months. They cause an initial increase in hormones, commonly called a flare, before hormone levels drop, which can lead to a heavy bleeding episode at the start of treatment. They are now typically only used to reduce the size of fibroids prior to surgical treatment.

Interventional management and surgical options

When medical management options are not appropriate or effective, surgery or other procedures can be considered to reduce heavy menstrual bleeding and bulk symptoms. Some of these treatments allow future pregnancy, and others don't. With most of these treatments, even if all the fibroids are removed or treated, new fibroids can form within a few years.

Myomectomy Myomectomy is a surgery that removes fibroids. For most women, this is the best option when you are actively trying for pregnancy. Myomectomies can be done using:

- An instrument called a hysteroscope, which can remove a small fibroid that is on the inside of the uterus without any skin incisions.
- An instrument called a laparoscope, which can remove a small number of fibroids by several small skin incisions through the belly button. A laparoscopic myomectomy may sometimes use an energy probe to destroy the fibroid (Accessa procedure).

- A larger abdominal incision, called an abdominal myomectomy, to remove very large or very many fibroids.
- Recovery is shortest for a hysteroscopic myomectomy and longest for an abdominal myomectomy.

Uterine artery embolization (UAE) Uterine artery embolization is a minimally invasive procedure that for most women is as effective as surgery for treating bleeding and bulk symptoms. In UAE, a small tube (catheter) is placed in a blood vessel in the groin (the femoral artery) and guided to the uterus, where the catheter delivers small particles to block blood vessels that feed the fibroids. This decrease in blood supply typically causes the fibroids to shrink and soften. Heavy menstrual bleeding can also improve after UAE. While early reports suggested UAE was not meant for women who wanted future pregnancy, newer efforts are encouraging and suggest that this may not be the case.

Rarely used techniques Several options are used less commonly. One technique, called ExAblate, treats some fibroids by sending powerful ultrasound waves through the belly while a woman lies in an MRI machine.

Another option, called endometrial ablation, destroys the lining of the uterus. In this procedure, the surgeon inserts an instrument into the vagina, through the cervix and into the uterus. The instrument destroys the lining of the uterus using heat, cold or a type of high-energy wave (radiofrequency ablation). This procedure reduces menstrual bleeding but does not treat the fibroids themselves.

Hysterectomy Hysterectomy is a commonly used surgery for fibroids that removes the whole uterus so new fibroids cannot form. While women get improvement in all their fibroid symptoms and enhanced quality of life, the procedure ends women's options for pregnancy. In addition, newer research suggests that other common medical problems, such as heart disease, depression and anxiety, may be increased in women many years after a hysterectomy. For most women having a hysterectomy for fibroids, preserving the ovaries helps maintain normal hormone production.

WHY DO UTERINE FIBROIDS MATTER TO WOMEN?

Fibroids are only found in women, and they can significantly affect a woman's day-to-day life. While some women have no symptoms, or mild symptoms that are easily manageable, others may have heavy menstrual bleeding, pain or other symptoms that can affect their quality of life. Their physical and emotional wellness, mental health and social function can be impacted. Fibroids are a disease of health disparities because they are more common, more severe and occur at an earlier age in Black women.

QUESTIONS TO ASK YOUR HEALTH CARE TEAM ABOUT FIBROIDS

- Which of my symptoms may be due to fibroids?
- Are there medications that would help with my symptoms?

- Are there surgical procedures that would help with my symptoms?
- What are my alternatives to hysterectomy?
- What treatment options are available at this institution?
- If I want to get pregnant now or in the future, how does this change my treatment options?

PEARLS OF WISDOM

Fibroids are common among reproductive-aged women and are often unrecognized by women and undiagnosed by clinicians. Eating a diet rich in fruits and vegetables, exercising, minimizing stress and maintaining a healthy weight is associated with decreased fibroid risk.

If you have heavy or long periods of menstrual bleeding, anemia, or symptoms of an enlarged uterus, be proactive and seek a clinician who is willing to investigate these symptoms and do an ultrasound to obtain a diagnosis. Likewise, before undergoing surgery or interventional therapy, consider a second opinion and seek out health care professionals who are knowledgeable in all fibroid treatment options and who will work with you to make a shared decision on therapy.

Finally, discussing your reproductive goals and minimizing surgical therapy before pregnancy will help optimize your outcomes. Nearly every woman has an alternative to hysterectomy for uterine fibroids.

"Women deserve to receive the most up-to-date and evidence-based care from their clinicians."

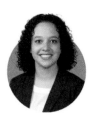

Sarah C. Baumgarten, M.D., Ph.D. - she/her
Dr. Baumgarten is a Clinical Fellow in the Division of Reproductive Endocrinology and Infertility at Mayo Clinic in Rochester, Minnesota. She provides clinical care to women with infertility and fibroids. She previously completed her PhD, and her research focused on the role of hormones and growth factors in ovarian follicle development.

"Research is urgently needed in many aspects of women's health to improve the quality of life women deserve in the 21st century."

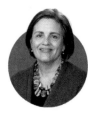

Elizabeth (Ebbie) A. Stewart, M.D. - she/her
Dr. Stewart is the past chair of the Division of Reproductive Endocrinology at Mayo Clinic in Rochester, Minnesota, and Professor of Obstetrics and Gynecology at Mayo Clinic Alix School of Medicine. She specializes in clinical care for uterine fibroids and infertility and clinical and translational research regarding uterine fibroids and adenomyosis.

63
Vaginal bleeding (abnormal)

Dana C. McKee, M.D., and Megan N. Wasson, D.O.

WHAT IS ABNORMAL VAGINAL BLEEDING?

Abnormal vaginal bleeding, simply put, is bleeding from the vagina that should not be occurring. This includes period (menstrual cycle) abnormalities, such as prolonged, heavy, or irregular periods. It may also refer to bleeding that occurs outside of the normal menstrual cycle.

A "normal" period — the time from the first day of one period to the first day of the next — can be anywhere from 24 to 38 days. Bleeding can last up to eight days, and "normal" flow is determined by each person. Heavy menstrual bleeding is medically defined as "excessive menstrual blood loss which interferes with a woman's physical, social, emotional and/or material quality of life." However, this definition can be challenging, since some women may not realize that the amount of bleeding they are experiencing is more than would be expected. Soaking through a heavy pad or tampon after less than two hours or passing blood clots greater than the size of a quarter is typically considered heavy flow.

It's important to note that any vaginal bleeding after menopause, defined as one year without a period, is considered abnormal and requires investigation with your clinician.

CAN ABNORMAL VAGINAL BLEEDING BE PREVENTED?

Many of the causes of abnormal vaginal bleeding cannot be prevented, but there are some things you can do to help decrease your risk of abnormal vaginal bleeding.

Maintain a healthy weight
Higher amounts of fatty tissue throughout the body can cause the lining inside your uterus to become thickened. This in turn can lead to abnormal bleeding episodes and can even develop into uterine cancer over time.

Conduct routine health care maintenance
Following screening guidelines for cervical cancer, including routine Pap smears, helps detect any precancerous or cancerous changes of the cervix, which may cause abnormal vaginal bleeding. Additionally, the human papillomavirus (HPV) vaccine is recommended for women up to age 45 to

protect against HPV, the leading cause of cervical cancer. Although a Pap smear is not required every year, it is still important to undergo an annual physical exam. If gynecologic symptoms or concerns are present, your clinician can assess for visual abnormalities of the vulva, vagina or cervix, as well as feel for any abnormalities of the uterus or ovaries.

Be aware of current hormonal treatments

Use of hormones (estrogen, progesterone or testosterone), such as those found in birth control or hormone replacement therapy, can lead to the development of abnormal vaginal bleeding. Talk to your clinician about the risks and benefits of discontinuing or changing these methods to help with abnormal bleeding.

HOW IS ABNORMAL VAGINAL BLEEDING TREATED?

Just like prevention, treatment depends on the underlying cause of bleeding.

Check for pregnancy

In a woman who is still having periods and therefore able to get pregnant, any new abnormal vaginal bleeding should prompt investigation to make sure that a pregnancy is not present. You can rule out pregnancy by taking a home pregnancy test or visiting your clinician or local health clinic.

Endometrial polyps

These are overgrowths of the lining of the uterus and are one of the most common causes of abnormal bleeding in women, both before and after menopause. Treatment

Tell your clinician if you experience vaginal bleeding

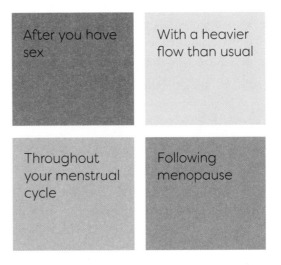

After you have sex

With a heavier flow than usual

Throughout your menstrual cycle

Following menopause

involves removal of the polyp from the inside of the uterus, which may be done in your gynecologist's office or during an outpatient surgical procedure. If a polyp is incidentally found in a woman who is still having monthly periods and is not having any issues with her bleeding, continued monitoring may be an option, as it's possible the polyp will be shed with the uterine lining during a subsequent period. It's recommended that polyps found in post-menopausal women be removed, as these will not shed on their own. The majority of polyps are noncancerous (benign), but on occasion cancerous (malignant) polyps are found in some women.

Uterine fibroids

Uterine fibroids (leiomyomas) are benign growths arising from the muscle of the uterus and are very common findings. These growths may not cause any symptoms in some women. However, in others they can lead to a variety of symptoms, including periods with heavy or prolonged bleeding.

Treatment options vary greatly, from conservative management with monitoring and medications, such as hormones as needed, to more aggressive options, including:

- Ultrasound-guided thermoablation, a procedure that uses high-intensity ultrasound energy or heat to destroy fibroids
- Uterine fibroid embolization, a procedure that injects small particles into the uterine arteries to block blood supply to the fibroids, causing them to shrink and die
- Surgical treatment with myomectomy (removal of only the fibroids)
- Hysterectomy (removal of the uterus)

If a woman wants to keep the option of pregnancy in the future, myomectomy is the best choice given that thermoablation and embolization are not advised prior to pregnancy. However, if there is no desire for future pregnancy, but a woman wants to keep her uterus, thermoablation or embolization are great options. If no symptoms are present and the fibroids are not causing any issues, no treatment is needed. (See Chapter 62.)

Adenomyosis

This is a benign condition in which the lining of the uterus grows into the muscle portion of the uterus, which can lead to heavy and painful periods. Adenomyosis is different from endometriosis, which is a condition in which cells similar to the lining of the uterus grow outside of the uterus (see Chapter 28). Imaging tests such as ultrasound or MRI may be used to help detect adenomyosis.

Less aggressive treatment includes the use of hormones, which may be in the form of pills or a progesterone intrauterine device (IUD). If hormones fail to improve symptoms, a hysterectomy may be the best option. A hysterectomy is also the only way to confirm the diagnosis of adenomyosis with certainty, as the tissues of the uterus can then be evaluated visually and a sample can be examined under the microscope.

Endometrial hyperplasia

Endometrial hyperplasia refers to thickening of the uterine lining (endometrium), which can cause abnormal vaginal bleeding. Hyperplasia can be benign or precancerous and may increase the risk of uterine cancer. Treatment for hyperplasia may involve close monitoring, progesterone-only therapies, birth control pills or hysterectomy.

Cancer

The first sign of uterine cancer is typically abnormal vaginal bleeding. If uterine cancer is diagnosed, treatment usually includes surgery to remove the uterus, fallopian tubes and ovaries. For women who desire pregnancy in the future, it is possible to treat uterine cancer with progesterone-only therapy and delay surgery until the option of becoming pregnant is no longer desired. Depending on the stage of cancer, further treatment with radiation or chemotherapy may be recommended (see Chapter 27).

Cervical cancer may also cause abnormal vaginal bleeding. Fortunately the Pap smear screening test allows most changes of the cervix to be identified when they are precancerous (a stage called cervical dysplasia) so that they can be treated before becoming a cancer (see Chapter 18).

Ovulatory dysfunction

Also referred to as anovulatory cycles, this condition occurs when a woman does not release an egg each month (ovulate). Without ovulation there is no menstrual period, but ovulatory dysfunction can lead to irregular and infrequent bleeding episodes. This condition is typically the cause of abnormal bleeding in women with polycystic ovary syndrome (see Chapter 55). Ovulatory dysfunction may also occur in relation to stress, intense exercise and body weight extremes, including underweight and obesity. Treatment for ovulatory dysfunction involves controlling the timing of periods with birth control pills or other hormonal treatments. Weight loss has also been shown to help regulate bleeding in women who are overweight or have obesity (see Chapter 48).

Infections

Genital tract infections of the vulva, vagina, cervix, uterus or fallopian tubes can lead to abnormal vaginal bleeding. Your clinician may recommend testing for sexually transmitted infections (STIs), such as gonorrhea, chlamydia or trichomonas, which are treated with antibiotics. Using condoms during sex can help prevent STIs.

Birth control or hormone use

Although birth control and hormones are often used in the treatment of abnormal vaginal bleeding, the most common side effect of all hormonal contraception also happens to be bleeding. When starting contraception, abnormal bleeding is experienced by almost everyone. Abnormal bleeding caused by birth control or hormones is not harmful but can certainly be bothersome. Treatment may involve changing the dose, frequency or type of birth control. However, it's also important for your clinician to evaluate for other potential causes of the bleeding, such as the ones listed in this section.

Other hormonal dysregulation

Examples of this include abnormalities of the thyroid hormone (see Chapter 59) or prolactin, a hormone the brain releases most commonly during pregnancy and during periods of breastfeeding. A hormone specialist (endocrinologist) can help with treatment of these disorders.

Bleeding disorders

Bleeding disorders are a rarer cause of abnormal vaginal bleeding. They include conditions such as a blood clotting disorder called von Willebrand disease and disorders of the platelets — blood cells that are essential for clotting, which is what stops bleeding — including low platelet levels (immune thrombocytopenia) or platelet function abnormalities. Your clinician might suspect a bleeding disorder if heavy or prolonged bleeding began with your first menstrual period, if you have a family history of a bleeding disorder, if you have a history of easy bruising or gum bleeding or if you're taking medications associated with an increased bleeding tendency. Diagnosis requires lab tests and consultation with a blood disorder specialist or hematologist. Treatment may involve use of hormones or other medications.

Abnormalities of the vulva, vagina or cervix

Most of the abnormal bleeding discussed so far comes from the uterus. However, the lower genital tract, including the vulva, vagina and cervix, may also be the source of bleeding. The best way to determine this is through a pelvic exam by your clinician. If lesions or growths are identified, they may be treated with surgical removal, burning or freezing the lesion (ablation), or heating the lesion (coagulation).

Postmenopausal bleeding

Bleeding after menopause should always be investigated to rule out cancer. Your clinician may recommend an ultrasound and a biopsy, if needed, from the uterus. A common benign cause of postmenopausal bleeding is genitourinary syndrome of menopause (previously known as vaginal atrophy), which occurs due to lack of estrogen. Treatment for this condition includes vaginal moisturizers, estrogen or both.

WHY DOES ABNORMAL VAGINAL BLEEDING MATTER TO WOMEN?

Abnormal vaginal bleeding is a condition unique to women and a common reason for a visit to a clinician's office. It may be a sign of an underlying medical condition, an abnormal growth of the genital tract or even cancer. In the teenage years, abnormal vaginal bleeding may be the first sign of an underlying bleeding disorder. Pregnancy is also an important cause of abnormal vaginal bleeding. If you're in your reproductive years, the first step is to check for pregnancy. If you're postmenopausal, any vaginal bleeding is a reason to make an appointment with your clinician.

QUESTIONS TO ASK YOUR HEALTH CARE TEAM ABOUT ABNORMAL VAGINAL BLEEDING

For all women to discuss with their primary care clinicians
- Am I up to date on my routine gynecologic screening (such as Pap smears)?
- Should I receive the HPV vaccine?
- Should I be tested for sexually transmitted infections?
- Am I at the weight I should be?
  › If overweight or with obesity: What resources are available to me for weight loss?

For women experiencing abnormal vaginal bleeding
- Is it possible I could be pregnant?
- Is the volume of bleeding I am experiencing normal?
- Is there an obvious cause of bleeding that you see on the pelvic exam today?
- Is there a reason to obtain labs or imaging for my bleeding?
  › Should a biopsy be performed?
- Is there concern that cancer is the cause of my bleeding?
- Could the bleeding be related to my birth control method?

For women who need treatment for abnormal vaginal bleeding
- For which hormonal treatments am I a candidate?
  › What are the side effects of each option?
- Are there any nonhormonal medication options for treatment of my condition?
- What surgical options are available for my condition?
- Is surgery a good option for me?

> What are the pros and cons of surgery for my condition?
- What options do I have other than surgery?
- If I delay surgery, could this condition go away on its own or could it get worse?
- What can I do to improve surgical outcomes and decrease my risk of complications?

PEARLS OF WISDOM

It's important for women to listen to their bodies and to know that abnormal vaginal bleeding may be an indication of a more serious medical condition. Keeping track of which days you are bleeding and the amount of bleeding you have may be a helpful tool for you and your clinician to better understand your bleeding patterns.

If a diagnosis has been made for your abnormal vaginal bleeding but your bleeding persists despite treatment, be sure to let your clinician know. You may require further evaluation or treatments. Most important, maintaining a healthy weight and staying up to date with routine health care maintenance, including yearly gynecologic exams, is vital for prevention of gynecologic conditions.

"I hope to educate and empower my patients so they can make health care decisions that align with their personal values and goals."

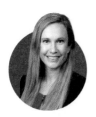

Dana C. McKee, M.D. - she/her
Dr. McKee is a fellow in Minimally Invasive Gynecologic Surgery at Mayo Clinic in Phoenix, Arizona. Her clinical and research interests focus on the medical and surgical management of complex benign gynecologic pathology including pelvic pain, endometriosis, abnormal uterine bleeding, fibroids, and adnexal masses.

"Women should be empowered to be advocates in their health journeys."

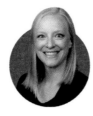

Megan N. Wasson, D.O. - she/her
Dr. Wasson is the Chair of the Department of Medical and Surgical Gynecology and Associate Professor of Obstetrics and Gynecology at Mayo Clinic in Phoenix, Arizona. She is a subspecialist in minimally invasive gynecologic surgery with a special focus on endometriosis and pelvic pain.

64
Vaginal infections

Faiza Yasin, M.D., M.H.S., and Chi-Fong Wang, M.D.

WHAT IS A VAGINAL INFECTION?

A vaginal infection occurs when there is an invasion of microorganisms that are not normally present within the vagina. These microorganisms disrupt the environment of the vagina or the external genitalia (vulva) — your labia, clitoris, and the area just beyond the vaginal opening.

Signs and symptoms
There are several signs and symptoms that may indicate a vaginal infection.

General discomfort, irritation or itching The words vaginitis or vulvovaginitis are general terms for inflammation of the vagina, or vulva and vagina, respectively. The term vulvar dermatitis describes the irritation of the vulvar skin (the term dermatitis specifically refers to irritation of skin). Symptoms such as irritation and itching of the skin often become worse at night or after physical activity, especially with heat and sweating. Chronic scratching can lead to redness of the skin, skin breaks and thickening of the skin.

Since the vulvar skin is sensitive, vulvar dermatitis can result from many different types of irritants and allergens including ingredients in lotions, toilet paper and detergents, especially fragrance or softeners. Vulvar dermatitis can also occur because of atopy — having an immune system that is predisposed to respond in an exaggerated way to common allergens. If you have eczema, asthma, or seasonal allergies, you may be more likely to develop vulvar dermatitis.

Changes in vaginal discharge Changes in the volume, color, or smell of vaginal discharge do not necessarily mean an infection is present. Normal vaginal discharge varies by person and the timing of discharge within the menstrual cycle. Discharge can be affected by many things, including but not limited to diet, pregnancy, menopause, stress, clothing, soaps and medications. To diagnose a vaginal infection, your clinician may examine the discharge by looking under a microscope during an office visit or ordering lab tests for a more detailed assessment.

Burning sensation It can be difficult to precisely locate where a burning sensation is coming from. Symptoms often overlap between different infections. Typically, burning that occurs primarily with urination is suggestive of a urinary tract infection, whereas burning that is unrelated to

Common vaginal infections

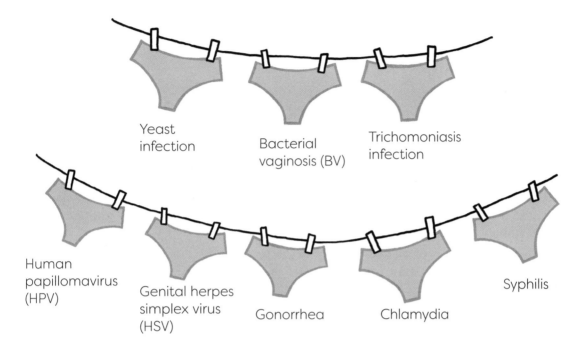

Yeast infection

Bacterial vaginosis (BV)

Trichomoniasis infection

Human papillomavirus (HPV)

Genital herpes simplex virus (HSV)

Gonorrhea

Chlamydia

Syphilis

urination or is located around the vulva instead of the urethra is more suggestive of vulvovaginitis.

Causes

Vaginal infections can be due to a variety of causes. Some vaginal infections are sexually transmitted; others are not. If you are experiencing any of the signs or symptoms listed in the preceding section, or if you have been with a new sexual partner, see your clinician to get tested for vaginal infections.

Yeast infection (Candida vulvovaginitis) Yeast infections are caused by an overgrowth of Candida (a type of yeast) in the vagina. This is one of the most common causes of vulvovaginal itching, redness of the vulvar skin and changes in vaginal discharge. Discharge is usually odorless, thick and white, with a

cottage-cheese-like consistency. Yeast can be a normal part of the vaginal ecosystem, and the presence of Candida without symptoms can be completely normal. A yeast infection can develop when an imbalance occurs in the ecosystem. Some women find they get yeast infections after taking antibiotics to treat an unrelated infection.

Bacterial vaginosis Bacterial vaginosis (BV) may occur when a change in the vaginal environment causes an imbalance or overgrowth of bacteria normally present in your vagina, most commonly a species called Gardnerella vaginalis. Bacterial vaginosis affects many women, and symptoms can range from very mild to severe. Symptoms include vaginal discharge that is thin and clear to white to gray, with a change in smell, often described as "fish-like," or an unpleasant smell. Symptoms may be more noticeable during or immediately after your period or unprotected intercourse, as these events may change the pH (acid-base balance) of your vagina.

Trichomoniasis is a sexually transmitted infection (STI) caused by Trichomonas vaginalis. Symptoms can vary from very mild to severe and include a thin vaginal discharge that is yellow-green in color and is unpleasant-smelling. Many women also experience urinary symptoms, similar to those they might have with a urinary tract infection, and pain with sexual activity. In addition, some women experience spotting after sexual activity. Although trichomoniasis is sexually transmitted, it gets categorized as a kind of vaginitis more often than other STIs because it causes more vaginal symptoms than the STIs described next.

Human papillomavirus (HPV) This is the most common STI, affecting most sexually active adults in the United States in their lifetimes. There are many different strains of HPV, most of which are cleared by the body without long-term effects. Some strains can cause disease — most notably precancerous and cancerous changes in the cells of the cervix. There are other strains that do not cause cancer but may cause genital warts, which can be bothersome.

Gonorrhea and chlamydia These are common sexually transmitted bacterial infections that typically do not cause symptoms in people with a vagina, in contrast to people with a penis, who usually do have symptoms. When symptoms occur in the vagina and are not treated in a timely manner, these

STIs can have long-lasting consequences, such as pelvic inflammatory disease (PID), pregnancy outside the uterus (ectopic pregnancy), typically in the Fallopian tubes, and infertility.

Mycoplasma genitalium (M. genitalium) This sexually transmitted bacterial infection can occur with no symptoms or with nonspecific symptoms such as pelvic pain, abnormal vaginal discharge or vaginal itching. The infection is associated with PID and may be linked to infertility, although additional studies are needed in this area.

Genital herpes simplex virus (HSV) This is a common sexually transmitted viral infection that can never be cured once contracted. However, suppressive antiviral treatments can effectively relieve symptoms and minimize outbreaks in healthy people.

Syphilis This sexually transmitted bacterial infection can have a variety of serious consequences affecting various areas in the body (such as the genital area, skin, brain and central nervous system) depending on how long it has been untreated.

CAN VAGINAL INFECTIONS BE PREVENTED?

Yes, sometimes vaginal infections can be prevented, depending on the cause. There are a number of steps you can take to minimize your risk of vaginal infections.

Vulvar hygiene
- Remove wet or moist clothing after swimming or after a strenuous workout to help limit excessive moisture on the

vulvar area. Moisture can create an environment conducive to certain conditions, such as yeast infections and vulvar dermatitis.

- Consider sleeping without underwear and avoiding tight-fitting pants to allow the vulva to breathe and to maintain a healthy vaginal environment.
- Avoid soaps, detergents and toilet papers that have a lot of potentially irritating fragrances, softeners or dyes.
- Avoid douching and cleaning inside the vagina, as these practices tend to disrupt the normal acidic environment of the vagina and may predispose you to bacterial vaginosis (BV) or yeast infections.
- Ask your clinician about estrogen-containing birth control pills and probiotics. These may have a role in preventing BV, but additional studies are needed.

Barrier protection

- Using a condom with sexual partners, for all sexual activity, is the most effective way to prevent sexually transmitted infections. The alkaline or basic pH of semen also can cause BV symptoms by disrupting the normal acidic environment of the vagina.

Vaccinations

- The HPV vaccine is a two- to three-part vaccine series that can protect you from some of the HPV strains that are more likely to cause cervical cancer. While it does not protect you from all HPV strains, it is very effective at protecting you from the strains that cause persistent infection and high-risk disease, especially if the vaccine is given before a person's first sexual encounter.

HOW ARE VAGINAL INFECTIONS TREATED?

Your clinician may treat the most likely cause of the infection based on your symptoms but will likely do a few tests in the office to make a definitive diagnosis. For example, sometimes removing a small sample of vulvar skin (vulvar biopsy) may be needed. The treatment choices may need to be adjusted depending on your allergies and interactions with other medications you are taking.

You can reduce general vaginal discomfort by limiting time in moist clothing and avoiding triggers (lotions and detergents, for example). If you continue to experience symptoms, do not use over-the-counter anti-itch creams without first speaking to your clinician. Many of these products contain ingredients that aren't treating but rather masking the symptoms. Your clinician may instead prescribe topical steroids, which can be applied to the vulvar skin to treat inflammation and irritation of the skin.

Treatment options depend on the type of infection.

Yeast infection (Candida vulvovaginitis)

Intravaginal antifungal medications (clotrimazole, miconazole) are inserted into the vagina for three to seven days. This is the preferred method for treating pregnant individuals. Another treatment option is an oral antifungal medication (fluconazole). It is taken as a pill once and can be taken again in 72 hours if you still have symptoms. Most people respond to treatment within a few days. Sexual partners do not need to be treated.

Bacterial vaginosis (BV)

Intravaginal metronidazole gel or oral metronidazole can be used for treatment. Both are antibiotics and have similar effectiveness. Choice of therapy depends on your preference and either can be used in pregnancy. It is important to avoid drinking alcohol if you are taking oral metronidazole due to side effects such as nausea, vomiting and abdominal pain, which can range in severity. This reaction to alcohol and metronidazole being taken together is known as a disulfiram-like reaction.

Trichomoniasis infection

Oral antibiotics (metronidazole or tinidazole) are used to treat trichomoniasis. Pregnant people are typically treated with metronidazole.

Human papillomavirus (HPV)

There is no complete cure for HPV infection, but there are treatment options to remove HPV-related genital warts and precancerous or cancerous lesions on the cervix related to HPV. It is very important to get routine Pap smears to detect early changes that might develop into cervical cancer if left untreated.

Gonorrhea and chlamydia

Gonorrhea is treated with an injectable antibiotic called ceftriaxone. Sometimes clinicians will offer empiric treatment — treatment before you have a laboratory-proven diagnosis. Chlamydia can be treated with a one-week course of an antibiotic called doxycycline, or a one-time dose of azithromycin if you are pregnant or allergic to doxycycline.

Mycoplasma genitalium (M. genitalium)

This infection is treated with a one-week course of an oral antibiotic (doxycycline) and is sometimes followed by an additional three to seven days of a second antibiotic.

Genital herpes simplex virus (HSV)

There is no cure for genital HSV. Some antiviral medications (most commonly acyclovir or valacyclovir) can be used to treat and prevent outbreaks and minimize spread to sexual partners. It is important to suppress symptoms of genital HSV during pregnancy around the time of a vaginal delivery.

Syphilis

The mainstay of treatment for syphilis is injectable penicillin, an antibiotic. The number of doses depends on when you developed symptoms and the stage of syphilis at the time of your diagnosis.

Other precautions

If you are diagnosed with and treated for gonorrhea, chlamydia, trichomoniasis, M. genitalium or syphilis, all of your sexual partners should also be treated. Expedited partner therapy (EPT) is often an option. It involves treating the sexual partner without that person first being examined by a clinician, although it's important that all partners also see a clinician for testing, if possible.

Avoid any sexual activity while undergoing treatment and for at least seven days after completing treatment to prevent reinfection. All sexual partners should do the same. For women who have had an STI, a repeat test, often called test of cure, is usually recommended in pregnancy but is not always necessary in nonpregnant people. You may also consider testing for other STIs, such as HIV and hepatitis B or C.

WHY DO VAGINAL INFECTIONS MATTER TO WOMEN?

Most women experience vaginal infections at some point in their lives. The symptoms of vaginal infections range from being bothersome to indicating more serious problems, including infertility and cancer. Some causes of vaginitis, such as bacterial vaginosis (BV), can increase the risk of contracting other infections, including HIV, gonorrhea, chlamydia and herpes viruses.

QUESTIONS TO ASK YOUR HEALTH CARE TEAM ABOUT VAGINAL INFECTIONS

- What do you think is causing these vaginal symptoms?
- How can we determine the cause of my vaginal symptoms?
  - › What testing is necessary, and what are the tests looking for?
- Can I get treatment before the test results come back?
  - › What are the harms and benefits of doing this?
  - › Does treatment need to change if I am pregnant or breast-feeding?
- What are the risks and benefits of treatment?
  - › Is there anything I should avoid doing while on treatment?
- Based on the symptoms or test results, could this infection be contagious to sexual partners or close contacts?
- If I get these symptoms very frequently, what can I do to prevent them in the future?

PEARLS OF WISDOM

Most causes of bothersome vaginal symptoms are treatable and can be quickly diagnosed by your clinician. The treatment will depend on the diagnosis. The diagnosis can be difficult to know without a physical exam or testing, so it is important to speak with a clinician if there has been a change in your vaginal health or if you are experiencing new symptoms.

Some symptoms may seem minimal or not too bothersome but can lead to a more serious condition. If you are experiencing a change in vaginal discharge, pain or discomfort with urination, or pain or discomfort with sex, it may be a sign of infection or inflammation and should be evaluated by a clinician.

"Women belong in all places where decisions are being made. It shouldn't be that women are the exception." – Ruth Bader Ginsburg

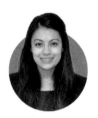

Faiza Yasin, M.D., M.H.S. - she/her
Dr. Yasin completed her residency training in Internal Medicine at Yale in New Haven, Connecticut. She is currently working as an adult internist in primary care at One Medical in San Francisco, California.

"A good laugh and a long sleep are the best cures in the doctor's book." – Irish Proverb

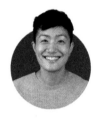

Chi-Fong Wang, M.D. - she/her
Dr. Wang completed her residency training at Women and Infants' Hospital/ Brown University in Providence, Rhode Island. She is now an attending physician and instructor in Obstetrics, Gynecology, and Reproductive Biology at Beth Israel Deaconess Medical Center and Harvard Medical School in Boston, Massachusetts.

65

When your illness is a mystery

Denise Millstine, M.D.

WHAT IS MY CONDITION?

Many women who pick up this book will have signs or symptoms of one or more of the conditions named in it, but a subset will have symptoms — often nonspecific and prolonged — that are not. In fact, millions of Americans live with what has been termed "undiagnosed illness" and "medically unexplained symptoms." The Diagnostic and Statistical Manual of Mental Disorders 5 (DSM-5) categorizes these conditions as "somatic symptom disorders."

Common symptoms include fatigue, dizziness, weakness, racing or pounding heart (palpitations), pain, and abdominal and pelvic discomfort. Most women with this constellation of symptoms will have started their health care journey in the emergency department or with their primary care clinician. Many will have been referred on to specialists. These women will have had labs, tests, maybe imaging and even diagnostic procedures — all of which likely failed to reveal an explanation for the symptoms. Medications

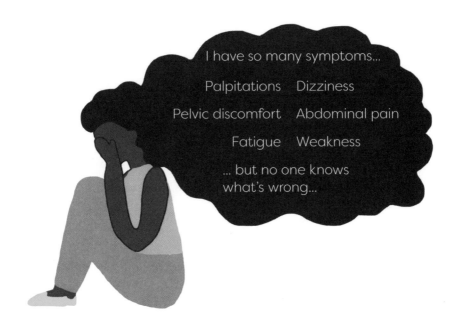

I have so many symptoms...

Palpitations   Dizziness

Pelvic discomfort   Abdominal pain

Fatigue   Weakness

... but no one knows
what's wrong...

and therapies were likely tried. Some treatments may have eased symptoms but others had no effect or made these women feel worse. While pieces and components may be revealed, most medical interactions will not converge on an "aha moment" in which the symptoms are explained.

Unfortunately, many women in this group will have had traumatic experiences in the context of their health care. They will have been dismissed or labeled "difficult." They might have been told the symptoms are "all in your head." It's likely they were referred to psychiatry or psychology to manage their anxiety disorder. While many women will indeed be anxious at that point, this will not explain their illness and its impetus.

How could this happen? With all of the research and resources funneled into our modern health care system, how is it possible that your illness is not understood and that your symptoms are unexplainable? It may be that you have a rare disease unfamiliar to the clinicians you've seen, and therefore they cannot recognize it. More likely, you have uncommon signs and symptoms of a common illness or you have a condition that is currently unknown. The good news is that you can still seek to improve your health even if what's disrupting it remains a mystery.

CAN MY CONDITION BE PREVENTED?

Probably not.

As these undiagnosed conditions are poorly understood, it's not possible to know how to prevent them. Yet some women are at higher risk of developing unexplained symptoms. Addressing the modifiable risk factors and living a healthy lifestyle may make symptoms less likely and less burdensome.

Manage stress

A higher stress burden will worsen almost all the common symptoms in undiagnosed illnesses. While a stress-free existence is not possible, recognizing and devising intentional plans for managing stress is beneficial. Common stress management approaches include relaxation, mindfulness and guided imagery. There are many platforms, programs and books addressing stress, and one option is *The Mayo Clinic Guide to Stress Free Living* by Amit Sood, M.D.

Recognize and address trauma

A history of trauma, even going back to childhood, increases the risk of developing medically undiagnosed symptoms. Strong associations exist with histories of sexual trauma and victimization. Trauma cannot be undone, but trained psychologists and other mental health professionals can assist with recognizing, facing and releasing trauma. Often this is accomplished through cognitive behavioral therapy (CBT). Having a history of difficult or challenging childhood events, including a parent who was ill, will also increase your risk of developing a somatic disorder. In a somatic disorder you think about your symptoms to a much greater extent than the seriousness of your symptoms would suggest is reasonable and you have a high level of anxiety about your symptoms and health.

Build a support system

Your health care team is crucial in determining whether you will get healthier or less healthy over time. Your social support network, including family and friends, is equally important. Having an undiagnosed illness can impact your relationships, especially when others don't understand how you're feeling or why you need to cancel plans when you're feeling worse. Do your best to communicate with people who are important in your life so they can understand and empathize with what you are going through.

Mind your diet, movement and sleep

While nearly every condition improves with a healthy lifestyle, how you live is particularly important when you have medically unexplained symptoms. A diet full of highly processed foods can be inflammatory, potentially worsening any type of pain and causing fatigue. Movement in proportion to what you are capable of doing — without worsening symptoms or requiring a prolonged recovery period — is imperative for all chronic fatiguing illnesses. High-quality sleep also allows the body and brain to heal.

Treat diagnosed conditions

Many people with diagnosed conditions still have symptoms that are unrelated to their known diagnoses and remain unexplained. People with a history of heart attack can have subsequent noncardiac chest pain. Those with a history of migraine headaches may have unrelated, episodic dizziness. Staying on track with recommended management for your known diagnoses is important when you are also managing undiagnosed symptoms.

HOW CAN MY CONDITION BE TREATED?

The broad range of symptoms in the undiagnosed illness makes generalized treatment recommendations difficult. Ideally, you'll receive treatment from a multidisciplinary team, which often includes your primary care clinician and a psychologist or other mental health therapist. Your team may also include medical subspecialists, a dietitian, exercise experts or physical therapists and a wellness coach.

If your health care team conducts any tests, be aware that medical laboratories determine ranges of normal for all of their results. The clinician ordering your tests will review the results and may not consider some numbers labeled as "out of range" to be significant. However, all results need to be considered in the context of your symptoms and within the known limits of each test to provide usable information.

Symptomatic management has been tried through the following methods.

Cognitive behavioral therapy (CBT)

A form of psychotherapy focused on thought patterns and specific behaviors, CBT shows the best evidence for treating medically unexplained symptoms. This approach looks at the patterns and habits that trigger symptoms or cause them to persist. Along with a trained therapist, you rewire your brain's response to certain triggers.

Antidepressants

It's common for people with undiagnosed illness to also have mood disorders, such as generalized anxiety, panic disorder and major depression. Treating these disorders can help with other unexplained symptoms. In addition, medications that treat mood disorders, such as antidepressants, also are effective in reducing pain symptoms in people with fibromyalgia and chronic pain syndromes.

Reassessment of pain medications

A common approach to treating pain is to start narcotic or opioid medications. These powerful substances can lead to misuse, dependence and addiction. Counterintuitively, using them for long periods of time can worsen pain and make the pain more difficult to treat. If you find yourself in the trap of requiring these medications, consider working with a trained professional who can help you reduce your dose or eliminate the medications from your treatment plan. Comprehensive, multidimensional pain management programs, such as the Mayo Clinic Pain Rehabilitation Centers, are an effective way to approach this.

Exercise and physical therapy

When you don't feel well, you probably move less. When you move less, you feel even worse. On and on the cycle continues. It's important to incorporate a regular movement practice that is matched in intensity, duration and frequency to your overall health status and goals — in other words, move however you can. A type of physical therapy called graded exercise therapy, and low-impact activities, such as walking and water movement, are good places to start.

Relaxation practices

These low-risk, low-cost and easily incorpo-rated activities are effective and often practiced in the context of a multidisciplinary approach to managing symptoms.

An active, trusting relationship with your clinician

The lack of diagnosis and limitations in treatment options are likely to place a strain on your relationship with your clinician. The best approach is to find someone with whom you can build a trusting relationship. Decide together how often you will have visits, and set boundaries around time spent and number of concerns addressed per session.

Additional support

While seeking treatment, it's a good idea to also seek quality information about your unexplained symptoms. Many academic medical centers have publicly available, high-quality health information, including **www.mayoclinic.org**. Another site focused on functional neurologic disorders is **www. neurosymptoms.org**. Finally, you can find regularly updated information through the National Institutes of Health (NIH) Genetic and Rare Diseases Information Center at **rarediseases.info.nih.gov**.

Online and virtual support groups exist on many social media platforms. While this is a great way to feel less alone with your experience, these commonly are not moderated by a health care professional and may include incorrect information. Additionally, stories shared on these platforms and in blogs or personal channels represent an individual's experience and should be considered anecdotal. While you might glean helpful information from these sites, be on the alert for advice that seems counterintuitive or has the potential for harm.

For truly unusual cases, a network of medical experts has formed the Undiagnosed Disease Network (UDN) (undiagnosed.hms.harvard.edu) in partnership with the NIH to assess and catalog possible genetic patterns associated with disorders that have remained undiagnosed after traditional medical evaluation. To be considered by the UDN, a clinician must submit a letter of application summarizing your condition, your evaluation and attempts at treatment.

WHY WOULD A MYSTERY ILLNESS MATTER TO WOMEN?

Women are more likely to experience medically unexplained symptoms compared to men. Traditionally, women have struggled to feel heard and understood in medical interactions. In addition, women are more likely to visit their clinicians with a higher number of symptoms. Other risk factors for an undiagnosed illness include being in a lower socioeconomic bracket and having a history of trauma, especially childhood trauma. Girls are slightly more likely than boys to have had childhood sexual trauma.

Fluctuations in hormone status, which affect women more than men, may also worsen or alleviate symptoms throughout menstrual cycles and during pregnancy, when breastfeeding, or through the postpartum state. This type of ebb and flow may make symptoms more difficult to understand, even for the women experiencing them, and more challenging to describe to others. Women are also traditionally and culturally caregivers for others, so they may delay or not pursue self-care for their vague or difficult-to-describe symptoms.

QUESTIONS TO ASK YOUR HEALTH CARE TEAM

- Who is on the health care team?
- Are my abnormal labs significant?
- Where can I seek quality information about my condition?
- Should I be referred to the Undiagnosed Disease Network (UDN)?

PEARLS OF WISDOM

While having an undiagnosed condition or medically unexplained symptoms can be frustrating and disheartening, it is possible to find and pursue health even without a diagnosis. Many psychological approaches, particularly CBT, have been shown to be effective in managing symptoms. Quality information is available. The enormous amount of information available on digital platforms and via social media should be considered carefully.

Many clinicians will want to help you. Recognize who you can trust and be wary of those who promise too much. Use the emergency department only for emergencies and not to seek answers to ongoing problems. Keep in mind that the lack of diagnosis and uncertain approach is often hard for your clinician to accept as well.

With medically undiagnosed symptoms, the clinician must switch from a "cure" to a "care" mentality.

Remember, you are your own best advocate. Develop healthy habits and approaches to cope with unexplained symptoms. Be intentional about choosing your health care team and support system. As someone with an undiagnosed illness, your health is very much in your own hands, even more so than for those with diagnosed illnesses.

"Health rarely comes from a pill bottle."

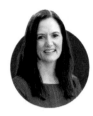

Denise Millstine, M.D. - she/her
Dr. Millstine is the Director of Integrative Medicine and Health and a consultant in Women's Health Internal Medicine at Mayo Clinic Arizona. She is an Assistant Professor of Medicine and a medical editor for Mayo Clinic Press. She specializes in natural approaches to health regardless of burden of disease and focuses on women and cancer care.

Part 3

Taking care of you

66

What contributes to your health?

Mary I. O'Connor, M.D., and Kanwal L. Haq, M.S.

Health is what we want for ourselves, our families and our communities. The World Health Organization (WHO) has a wonderful definition of health: a state of "complete physical, mental and social well-being and not merely the absence of disease or infirmity."

The factors that influence health are important to understand as you navigate the challenges of life. This chapter is devoted to broadening your understanding of the many factors that influence your health.

Many of us think that health is related to access to medical care. And it is. However, medical care contributes a surprisingly small amount to overall well-being — only 11%. Of course, this 11% is critical if you need medical care for a broken bone, for example, or if you have chest pain. And having great doctors and other clinicians who listen to you and care about you is crucial. But there are other vital factors outside of the medical care system that also have a strong influence on whether you get sick and on your potential for recovery.

GENETICS

We are who our parents made us to be from a genetic standpoint. Genetics contributes a significant 22% to our health and well-being. Some conditions — such as sickle cell disease, hemophilia and muscular dystrophy — are directly determined by your genes. If you carry the genes for these diseases, you will develop the disease. However, the connection isn't always so straightforward.

Oftentimes our genes may predispose us to developing certain medical conditions and diseases, but they don't automatically cause those conditions and diseases. Even within a family in which everyone has the same genetic predisposition, some may get the condition or disease and others may not.

Obviously, genetics cannot be controlled. However, you can try to learn the medical history of your family and share this with your clinicians. Your health care team can use this information to determine what screening tests, if any, are appropriate. Early detection usually allows for better treatment.

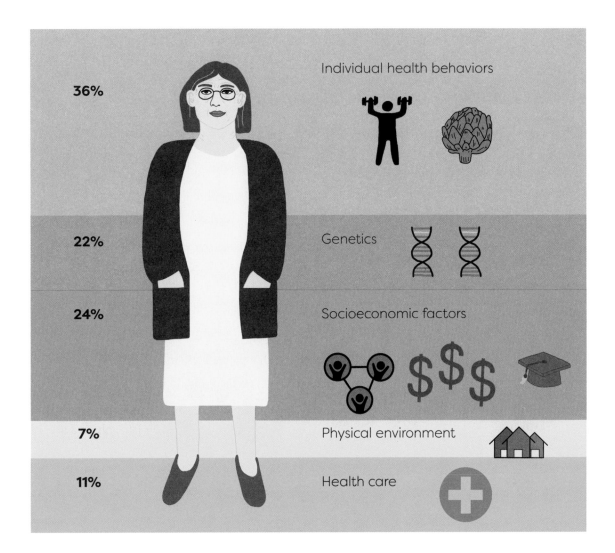

36%

Individual health behaviors

22%

Genetics

24%

Socioeconomic factors

7%

Physical environment

11%

Health care

PHYSICAL ENVIRONMENT

It's estimated that the physical environment in which we live influences our health and well-being by 7%. Air pollution can cause breathing illnesses. Living in a food desert — a neighborhood that lacks access to affordable fresh and nutritious foods — can lead to obesity, which promotes high blood pressure, arthritis, heart disease and diabetes. Safe drinking water is essential but not present in every community. In 2019 the administrator for the U.S. Environmental Protection Agency (EPA), Andrew Wheeler, stated that "92% of the water everyday meets all the EPA requirements for safe drinking water." There are neighborhoods where gun violence is far too common, creating the risk of direct and bystander injury. In our opinion, 7% is too low of an estimate of the importance of physical environment for women and their families who are in unsafe neighborhoods or homes.

SOCIAL CIRCUMSTANCES

Social circumstances contribute 24% to our health and well-being. Women of lower socioeconomic status tend to have less education, which is correlated with lower health literacy. Limited income often means purchasing less expensive foods. A study from 2013 shows that a healthy diet costs about $1.50 more per person per day compared to less healthy diets, or about $2,200 more in a year for a family of four. Discrimination and bias are frequently a part of a woman's social circumstances, particularly impacting women of color and those who are part of the LGBTQ community. Social connectedness also contributes to health and refers to the quality of support we receive from our various relationships including family, friends and community.

INDIVIDUAL HEALTH BEHAVIORS

The biggest factor in a woman's health and well-being, however, is her own behavior, contributing 36%. *This* is the biggest opportunity for women to take control of their health. The epidemics of obesity and sedentary lifestyles are dramatically impacting the length and quality of women's lives. Sleep is often sacrificed as women are overburdened with responsibilities both inside and outside of the home. Smoking is terrible for health, and more women than men die each year of lung cancer, mostly related to smoking.

PEARLS OF WISDOM

Medical care is essential to health but only contributes 11% to our overall health and well-being. Social circumstances and physical environment (social determinants of health) influence 31% of our health and well-being, but the strongest driver of our health and well-being is our individual behavior, at 36%. The following sections in this book aim to provide more context on how we can change our individual behaviors — such as nutrition, sleep, physical activity, hobbies, social relationships and more — to increase our health and well-being. We hope that each of you reading this book will make positive health changes in your own lives and support these positive changes for those around you.

"Health begins at home and in our communities; women must both create and demand healthier communities for themselves, their families and their neighbors."

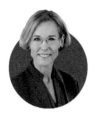

Mary I. O'Connor, M.D. - she/her
Dr. O'Connor is co-founder and Chief Medical Officer at Vori Health, an innovative health care enterprise with a mission to empower all people to lead their healthiest lives. She serves as Chair of Movement is Life, a national nonprofit coalition committed to health equity. Dr. O'Connor is a past chair of the Department of Orthopedic Surgery at Mayo Clinic in Jacksonville, Florida, and Emerita Professor of Orthopedics at Mayo Clinic. She specialized in bone and soft tissue tumor surgery and hip and knee replacement surgery.

"Being healthy is a revolutionary act."
– Unknown

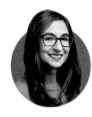

Kanwal L. Haq, M.S. - she/her
Kanwal is a medical anthropologist passionate about creating more connected, more informed, and more equitable systems of care. She specializes in community-based participatory research and builds accessible tools, resources, and programs for women around the globe. Kanwal currently leads the NYC women's health programs at the Arnhold Institute for Global Health at Mount Sinai's Icahn School of Medicine.

67
Nutrition

Jennifer Thomas, C.N.S., C.D.N.

WHAT IS NUTRITION?

Nutrition is the study of how our bodies function in response to what we eat and drink. The field of nutrition is food-based and food-focused — but nutrition professionals may also recommend supplements, botanicals, blood tests, genetics and lifestyle changes, such as those related to exercise and sleep. The goal of nutrition is to help your body and mind operate at their optimal levels.

HOW DOES NUTRITION CONTRIBUTE TO YOUR OVERALL HEALTH?

What you eat and drink is the raw material used to make every cell, organ, hormone, neurotransmitter and compound in your body. In this section, we'll use some common phrases about nutrition to delve into how your diet contributes to your overall health.

"You are what you eat."
While you won't literally turn into a burger after eating one, the very makeup of that burger — the proteins, fats, carbohydrates, vitamins, minerals and more — will become the building blocks of you. Because of this

unbreakable connection, your diet has a profound effect on your health and how you feel day to day. Do you have energy? Are you comfortable moving around? Do you suffer from pain or a preventable condition such as diabetes? How well are you aging? All of these factors are impacted by your nutrition.

"You can't outrun a poor diet."
Exercise, quality sleep and stress management benefit you greatly, but their benefits are all limited by a poor diet. Take weight training as an example: with poor nutrition you will not gain as much strength and definition, recover as quickly or feel as good before, during and after your workouts. Proper nutrition and refueling after exercise can dramatically improve your strength gains, body composition, recovery, energy production, metabolism and more.

"Let food be thy medicine."
Nutrition is a key part of avoiding many of the conditions that plague us today. It's also one of the best ways to improve these conditions if we do develop them. Many conditions are greatly improved and at times can be completely managed by diet and lifestyle, including diabetes, heart disease, some autoimmune conditions,

irritable bowel syndrome (IBS) or irritable bowel disease (IBD) and more.

WHY DOES NUTRITION MATTER TO WOMEN?

As our bodies change, our nutritional needs change with them. Over our lifespans we have different needs as adolescent girls, as women of reproductive age (nonpregnant, nonlactating), as pregnant and lactating women, as women who are perimenopausal and as postmenopausal women. At different stages in life, women require different amounts of nutrients to support proper body functioning.

From early childhood to early adulthood (up to age 35), it's vital for women to consume calcium-rich foods and take in adequate vitamin D3. This is when your body makes new bone at a faster rate than it breaks down old bone. Consuming calcium during these years helps your body build maximum bone mass, reducing your risk of developing osteoporosis, a condition that can lead to bone fractures (see Chapter 49).

During the reproductive years, consuming iron-rich foods is important because women lose 15 to 20 milligrams of iron every month due to menstruation. This can lead to iron deficiency anemia (see Chapter 11). Once women have reached menopause, iron generally increases because menstruation has ceased.

When it comes to caloric intake, the number of calories required varies from woman to woman based on several factors, including age and activity level. Generally speaking,

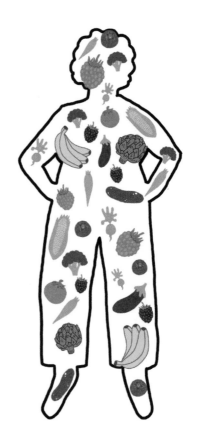

women aged 23 to 50 need between 1,700 and 2,200 calories per day to maintain their energy needs, while older women generally require fewer calories. However, consuming a diet too low in calories for your needs (even if you are trying to lose weight) can put you at risk of malnutrition and poor health. To learn more about calculating your nutritional needs, visit www.choosemy-plate.gov, which will provide a good starting point. A certified nutritionist or dietitian can guide you further.

HOW CAN A NUTRITION PROFESSIONAL GUIDE ME?

We all know that a well-balanced and diverse diet is best for our health, but often it's not crystal clear what such a diet looks like. Taking your individual lifestyle factors into consideration, a nutrition professional can help you answer these questions:

- What does a healthy diet look like, specifically for me?
- How could my energy, mood, weight or medical conditions improve with diet changes?
- What vitamins and minerals do I need?
  › Why are these important, specifically for me?
  › How much of each vitamin and mineral should my diet include?
  › What foods are good sources of these vitamins and minerals?
  › Are there any dietary supplements I should incorporate into my diet?
- How much fat and sugar is OK for me to consume on a daily basis?
  › What is a safe limit of saturated and trans fat in my diet?
  › What foods might be considered "empty calories"? How can I replace these foods with more nutrient-dense choices?
- How can I lose weight in a safe manner?

These are just some of the ways a certified nutrition professional can assist you. It's important to know that "nutritionist" is not a regulated title in many states. This means that people can call themselves nutritionists without actually having a background or education in nutrition. Always work with a certified nutrition professional who has either:

- A master's degree or a doctoral degree in nutrition as well as certified nutrition specialist (C.N.S.) credentialing from the Board for Certification of Nutrition Specialists (BCNS)

Or

- A bachelor's degree in nutrition as well as registered dietitian nutritionist (R.D. or R.D.N.) credentialing from the Academy of Nutrition and Dietetics' Commission on Dietetic Registration

To receive either of these credentials, a nutrition professional must pass a comprehensive exam, complete a supervised internship and continue receiving education credits to stay up to date with the most relevant nutritional information.

QUESTIONS TO ASK YOUR HEALTH CARE TEAM ABOUT NUTRITION

- Could I be low in any nutrients?
  › Are there tests to check if I am deficient in any nutrients?
- Do I need any supplements, such as calcium, magnesium, vitamin D3 or vitamin K?
  › If so, in what form should I take the supplement? How much should I take? How could it impact my risk of other diseases? Could the supplement interact with any other medications I'm taking?
- Is it possible for me to manage my medical conditions without medication?
  › Are there diet and lifestyle changes I could make instead of, or along with, medication?
  › What diet is best for me and why?
- Can you refer me to a credentialed nutritionist?
  › If I have a specific condition or concern, can you refer me to someone who specifically works with individuals who have my condition or concern?

PEARLS OF WISDOM

For overall health

The key to good health and longevity is eating a diverse, colorful diet that is high in vegetables. Aim for a diet that is visually around 50% vegetables. Every vegetable provides a different array of nutrients that nourishes your gut with helpful microbes. A diverse gut means better health. All the various types of healthful diets (Mediterranean, DASH, paleo, vegetarian, etc.) have one thing in common: high vegetable intake. This can be achieved by having a big salad every day, eating two to three vegetables with dinner and adding veggies to breakfast foods, such as eggs or smoothies.

Buy organic whenever you can — especially for thin-skinned produce like apples, strawberries and leafy greens, as well as for oats and oatmeal, meats and dairy. These foods, when not produced organically, have been shown to have the highest pesticide content.

Use healthy food preparation tips:
- Chop onions and garlic ahead of time and allow them to sit for 10 minutes before cooking. This allows the beneficial compounds to develop, maximizing their health benefits.
- Avoid or limit microwaving. Microwaving food rapidly destroys several nutrients, including B12, folate and vitamin C. When possible, use a stovetop pan, oven or toaster oven to reheat food.
- To drastically reduce the formation of carcinogens (cancer-causing substances) in grilled meat, soak the meat in a marinade at least 20 minutes before cooking. Include in the marinade something acidic like lemon juice or vinegar and, if possible, fresh herbs like rosemary and thyme.

As much as possible, avoid foods and ingredients that can only be made in a laboratory. Examples include food additives, preservatives, colorings, flavorings, artificial sweeteners and plant-based meats and cheeses. Stick to foods you can recognize in nature, such as vegetables, fruits, nuts, seed, legumes, meat, poultry, fish, eggs and whole grains. If it's not something you could make in your kitchen, then you're probably better off avoiding it. Avoid drinking calories or sweet beverages in general.

Practice overnight fasting. Aim for at least a 12-hour fast overnight. This practice may decrease your risk of certain cancers and help balance other important areas of the body. After about 8 hours of fasting (while you are asleep) a special part of your immune system kicks in, identifies precancerous or cancerous cells and eliminates them. These types of cells exist in every living body, at any given time, and are completely normal. However, if left unchecked by your immune system, they can continue to multiply themselves and eventually become something we would call cancer or a tumor.

For concerns with energy, mood or weight

Stabilize blood sugar levels by eating three balanced meals and up to one or two snacks a day. Aim to make your meals somewhat equal in calories. In general, a balanced meal would visually be around 50% vegetables, 25% proteins (about the size of your palm) and 25% healthy carbohydrates. A source of healthy fat, such as olive oil or avocado, is also part of a balanced meal. However, young women, pregnant women, lactating women or women who are very active may require a different balance of nutrients. Since everyone's nutrition needs are different, speaking with a credentialed nutritionist is the best way to identify what's right for you.

Stay hydrated throughout the day. Aim for 64 ounces to 80 ounces of fresh water daily. Prioritize proper sleep, time outdoors, physical activity and time spent doing something enjoyable.

Ensure adequate intake of B vitamins, vitamin C and minerals such as iron, magnesium and iodine by eating quality eggs, meat, fish, poultry, dark leafy greens, nuts, seeds, legumes and a variety of fresh vegetables. Work with a credentialed nutritionist to identify supplements that would best benefit you, such as D3, omega-3s and magnesium.

For supporting strong bones

Eat a diet rich in fresh vegetables and herbs. Aim for a daily diet that is visually around 50% vegetables. Avoid substances and activities that increase the withdrawal of calcium from the bones. These include sugar, alcohol, too much salt, highly processed foods and unmanaged chronic stress. Include quality food sources of calcium such as almonds, pinto beans, parsley, cooked, dark leafy greens, and dairy if tolerated.

Do strength-training exercises (such as pushups, lifting weights and using weight machines) and weight-bearing exercises (such as walking, dancing, and playing tennis) regularly. Work with a credentialed

nutritionist to identify which supplements, and how much of each, would best support your bones. Examples of supplements include D3, calcium, magnesium, vitamin K and more.

For prediabetes and type 2 diabetes

Stabilize blood sugar levels by eating two or three balanced meals and one or two snacks a day, focusing on low glycemic foods. Include a variety of vegetables, such as dark leafy greens, onions, garlic, broccoli, cauliflower, cabbage, Brussels sprouts, asparagus, bell peppers, mushrooms and more. Avoid sugar when possible. Also limit fruit sugars, such as those from tropical fruits such as banana, mango and pineapple and from dried fruits such as raisins and dates. Exercise regularly, including walking, cardio, and strength training.

Work with a credentialed nutritionist to assess what foods to include in your diet, how many carbohydrates to eat and what supplements might best support healthy blood sugar levels and long-term health. Supplements might include omega-3s, magnesium, chromium, cinnamon, a quality multivitamin and others.

For lowering risk of heart disease

Eat a diet that is visually around 50% vegetables and around 25% proteins and 25% healthy carbohydrates. Focus on foods found in nature that have been minimally processed. Exercise regularly, including activities such as walking, cardio and strength training. Ensure quality sleep and prioritize managing stress. Manage your risk factors, such as high blood pressure, diabetes or sleep apnea. Work with a credentialed nutritionist to identify supplements that would best support your heart health, such as omega-3s, magnesium and CoQ10.

For those fighting cancer

Eat a diet that is visually around 50% vegetables and contains adequate protein. Include a wide range of fresh, colorful produce, including broccoli, cauliflower, cabbage, kale, dark leafy greens, onions, garlic, mushrooms, berries, pomegranates and more. Choose organic and locally produced food items whenever you can. Drink green tea plain or with lemon. Adding milk or calcium to green tea negates much of the tea's health benefits.

Avoid or limit sugar, alcohol, highly processed foods, cured and charred meats, fried foods, smoke and excessive sun exposure. Exercise regularly, including activities such as walking, cardio and strength training. Ensure quality sleep and prioritize managing stress. Aim for at least 12 hours between the last time you eat before bed and the first time you eat the next day.

"Nutrition has a major impact on women's health and quality of life."

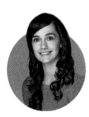

Jennifer Thomas, C.N.S., C.D.N. - she/her
Jennifer Thomas runs a private nutrition practice, Evolved Nutrition, in Cheshire, Connecticut. She specializes in individualized nutrition and lifestyle approaches to a variety of conditions including diabetes, hypothyroidism, and weight loss.

68
Sleep

Kanwal L. Haq, M.S., and Nishi Bhopal, M.D.

WHAT IS GOOD QUALITY SLEEP?

A good night's sleep can a make a world of difference on the following day. While you may think that your body is doing nothing during sleep, many parts of your brain are actually quite active, busily directing your body to repair itself while you rest. During sleep, your cells are building bone and muscle, regenerating tissue, and strengthening your immune system!

Sleep also allows your brain to flush out toxins that build up during the day via your glymphatic system. Thus, sleep is not something you can simply neglect — sleep is restorative. Getting good quality sleep is vital for good physical and mental health.

While there is not an exact definition of quality sleep, the National Sleep Foundation proposes four measures to help assess good quality sleep:
- Sleep latency: Being able to fall asleep within 30 minutes or less of getting into bed
- Sleep waking: Not waking up at all during the night, or only once after you fall asleep
- Wakefulness: If you wake up, being able to fall back asleep in 20 minutes or less

- Sleep efficiency: Overall, sleeping for at least 85% of the time you are in bed

The measures listed are primarily focused on sleeping without waking up too much. However, another way to gauge the quality of sleep is by how deeply we've slept. Deep sleep occurs when we are getting enough uninterrupted sleep. Adult women usually need about 7 to 9 hours of sleep per night (although this can vary slightly due to age). During these 7 to 9 hours of sleep, our bodies cycle between deep and non-deep sleep, completing a cycle every 100 to 110 minutes. The 4 stages of a sleep cycle include:
- Non-REM Stage 1:
  › This is when you are transitioning between being awake and being asleep.
- Non-REM Stage 2:
  › This is when your body starts preparing for deeper sleep, your body temperature drops and your heart rate slows down.
- Non-REM Stage 3:
  › This is the deepest level of sleep; it is very hard to wake up in this stage.
- REM Stage 4:
  › Your body is no longer in the deepest level of sleep, your brain becomes

more active, you have rapid eye movement (REM), and you may have intense dreams during this time; however, your muscles are temporarily paralyzed so that you do not move.

HOW CAN I TELL IF I AM EXPERIENCING QUALITY SLEEP?

The best way to know if you're getting quality sleep is to consider how you feel when you wake up.

We all tend to have our own personal markers that let us know we've experienced quality sleep. We may wake up feeling refreshed, having more energy or better concentration, being more alert or clear-headed, having better emotional regulation, or feeling calmer and less stressed out.

If you're having trouble sleeping or wake up feeling tired, it may be time to look at your sleep hygiene habits.

HOW CAN YOU PRACTICE GOOD SLEEP HYGIENE?

Good sleep hygiene empowers you to promote your body's own natural ability to sleep well. Good sleep hygiene actually starts way before bedtime. Here's what you can do during the day to have a restful night.

In the morning
Aim to wake up sometime between 6 a.m. and 7 a.m. so that you can wake up with bright light (although this time may alter slightly due to season and location).

Consistency is key. Aim to wake up at the same time every day. (Yes, even on weekends. It may be difficult at first, but try not to sleep in more than an hour on weekends. If we deviate too far from our weekday routines, we have trouble getting to sleep on time on Sunday nights, and Mondays become more difficult.)

Start your day with some light exercise — such as a stretching, yoga or meditation practice. Have some breakfast and caffeine (if you like) and make your day's to-do list. For the rest of the day, do not spend time in bed. Doing so trains your brain to associate being in bed with being awake.

At midday
Between 11 a.m. and 2 p.m., eat lunch, which should be your main (biggest) meal of the day. After lunch do some light movement — take a walk, or do yoga, tai chi or qi gong. These are all effective strategies for better sleep. By 2 p.m., stop your caffeine intake for the rest of the day. After 3 p.m., do not take naps.

In the early evening
Wrap up work, avoid vigorous exercise, and use the rest of the evening for relaxation. Enjoy a light dinner at least three hours before bedtime (avoid any food or drink after dinner, including alcohol, which is a sleep disruptor). Some people wake up at night from hunger. If you tend to get hungry at night, consider a high-fiber snack an hour before bedtime. A handful of nuts or some almond butter with fruit is a great option!

At bedtime
Try to incorporate habits like these in your bedtime routine:

- Aim for a bedtime somewhere between 10 p.m. and 11 p.m.
- Dim the lights about an hour before bed to promote melatonin production.
- Stop using digital screens 30 minutes prior to the time you intend to fall sleep.
- Build a relaxing routine that calms down your body and mind before bedtime (brushing teeth, doing a skincare routine, reading, journaling and so on).
- Consider showering or taking a bath before bed. It lowers your core body temperature, which is essential for sleep onset.
- Keep your bedroom dark and cool (60 to 67 degrees Fahrenheit).
- Sleep in natural fiber clothing (such as cotton, linen or silk) and use natural fiber bedsheets (cotton percale sheets can be helpful for those who get hot at night).
- If you can't fall asleep, don't try to "make yourself" sleep. Focus on relaxation techniques instead.

HOW DO SLEEP-RELATED FACTORS IMPACT WOMEN?

Compared to men, women are more likely to not get enough sleep. Not getting enough quality sleep can lead to multiple health concerns, impacting your immune system, metabolism (body weight, hunger, blood sugar), blood pressure, heart health and brain health.

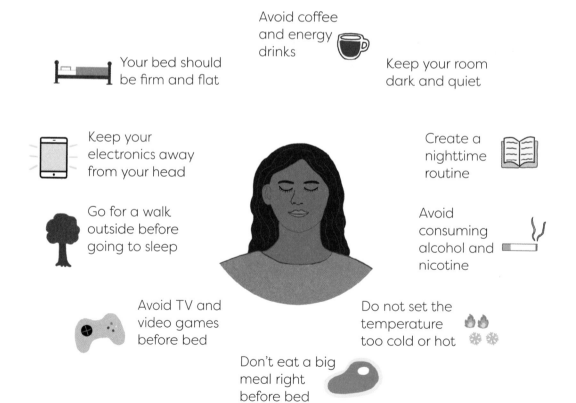

Avoid coffee and energy drinks

Keep your room dark and quiet

Your bed should be firm and flat

Keep your electronics away from your head

Create a nighttime routine

Go for a walk outside before going to sleep

Avoid consuming alcohol and nicotine

Avoid TV and video games before bed

Do not set the temperature too cold or hot

Don't eat a big meal right before bed

Studies show that women experience insomnia 40% more than men. Lack of sleep can affect how you think and how you feel. Anxiety and depression, conditions that impact women almost twice as much as men, are strongly correlated to insomnia. Often, true insomnia needs treatment with a kind of talk therapy called cognitive behavioral therapy for insomnia (CBT-I).

Other factors that impact sleep quality in women include the following.

Hormone shifts

During monthly menstruation, many women have trouble sleeping due to cramps, bloating, body aches and headaches. Many women also report higher levels of daytime sleepiness, tiredness and fatigue. We may feel like we need more sleep than usual during these times because we are not getting enough quality sleep. Additionally, our hormones shift during this time, which in turn impacts our body's internal clock (circadian rhythms). Keeping a consistent schedule — waking up, eating meals, exercising and going to bed at the same time every day — can help minimize the impact of hormone shifts.

Restless legs syndrome

Restless legs syndrome (RLS) is another condition that impacts women more than men. RLS causes an intense urge to move your legs, often in the evening and when lying down, which makes it difficult to fall asleep. RLS is associated with iron deficiency. Due to menstruation, women's iron stores are lower than men's, which may help explain why RLS is more common in women. RLS is also more common during pregnancy. One hypothesis suggests that

high levels of estrogen play a role in RLS, but the link is still unclear.

Pregnancy

During pregnancy, women face additional sleep challenges. Changing hormone levels, pain or discomfort, and the need to urinate frequently can disrupt sleep. These issues often continue after childbirth, compounded by the demands of taking care of a newborn with a developing sleep cycle. Obstructive sleep apnea also becomes more common during pregnancy. Sleep apnea is a serious disorder in which your breathing stops repeatedly, sometimes hundreds of times during the night, severely disrupting sleep even if you don't wake up.

Menopause

Menopause also can bring sleep challenges in the form of hot flashes. Approximately 85% of women going through menopause experience hot flashes during this time. Hot flashes can occur at night and disturb your sleep, waking you up in a sweat. Sleep apnea also becomes more common around menopause.

Underlying conditions

Sleep apnea, RLS, and insomnia are primary sleep conditions that can impact older women. Older women also may experience secondary sleep challenges due to other underlying medical conditions such as COPD, acid reflux (GERD), osteoarthritis, urinary incontinence, dementia, heart conditions and lung conditions. Medication side effects can affect sleep quality, as well.

Conditions contributing to lack of quality sleep can drastically impact your quality of life. Lack of sleep can also become a safety issue for those around you, increasing the risk of transportation-related accidents and workplace injuries. If you are consistently experiencing sleep-related challenges, it's important to speak to your clinician about what steps you can take to improve your sleep.

QUESTIONS TO ASK YOUR HEALTH CARE TEAM ABOUT SLEEP

- Do I need any blood tests?
  › For example, do my thyroid, iron, vitamin D and vitamin B12 levels need to be checked?
- Are there any vitamins or supplements that I should be taking?
- Are there any foods that I should be eating?
- Are there any foods that I should avoid?
- What is the best time to exercise for me?
- If I have sleep apnea, what are alternatives to CPAP?
- Could any of my medications (for other conditions) be causing my sleep issues?
- How can I minimize using medications for sleep?
  › *Mindfulness, meditation, yoga, tai chi, and qi gong are effective strategies for better sleep.*
- Should I see a sleep physician?
  › *Sleep medicine is an interdisciplinary field. Depending on your needs, you may be referred to a sleep specialist who is a psychiatrist, neurologist, pulmonologist, ENT doctor, internist, or pediatrician.*
- Should I see a sleep psychologist?
  › *CBT-I is often the first-line treatment for insomnia, and it can be more effective than medications because there are no side effects. Mindfulness practice has been shown to be a similarly effective alternative to CBT-I.*
- Do I need a sleep study?
  › *A home sleep test (HST) looks at breathing and oxygen levels, and sometimes leg movements. But it can miss mild sleep apnea, so if your HST is negative and you continue to have trouble sleeping, pursue a lab sleep study.*
  › *A lab sleep study, or polysomnogram, is a comprehensive study that looks at breathing and oxygen levels, limb movements and brain waves (to observe sleep stages). A lab sleep study can assess sleep apnea and other conditions such as periodic limb movements (sleep-related movement disorders).*
  › *If you have excessive daytime sleepiness, you may need a multiple sleep latency test (MSLT). MSLT is used to assess sleep disorders such as narcolepsy and idiopathic hypersomnia.*

PEARLS OF WISDOM

Good sleep starts during the day! You can start optimizing your sleep by being active during the day, which will increase your sleep drive. Adenosine, a naturally occurring molecule in our bodies, builds up the longer we are awake, and it makes us feel sleepy at night. Caffeine is a sleep disruptor and blocks adenosine, which is why limiting caffeine can be helpful. In addition to limiting your caffeine and alcohol intake, get better sleep by improving your sleep environment, developing a calming bedtime routine and keeping a consistent schedule. Getting eight hours of sleep at irregular times does not have the same effect as getting eight hours of consistent sleep, every day. Remember, better sleep leads to a better life with higher levels of happiness, well-being and overall life satisfaction. So get some rest!

"Health is not valued till sickness comes."
- Unknown

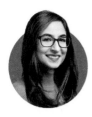

Kanwal L. Haq, M.S. - she/her
Kanwal is a medical anthropologist passionate about creating more connected, more informed, and more equitable systems of care. She specializes in community-based participatory research and builds accessible tools, resources, and programs for women around the globe. Kanwal currently leads the NYC women's health programs at the Arnhold Institute for Global Health at Mount Sinai's Icahn School of Medicine.

"Every woman deserves to experience deep, restful, restorative sleep."

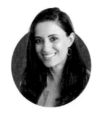

Nishi Bhopal, M.D. - she/her
Dr. Bhopal is the founder and CEO of Pacific Integrative Psychiatry in the San Francisco Bay Area and IntraBalance, an online platform educating patients and clinicians about the intersection of sleep and mental health. She specializes in integrative psychiatry and sleep medicine.

69
Physical activity

Mary I. O'Connor, M.D.

SITTING TO YOUR DEATH

Sitting is killing you. It is just that simple. And women sit more than men. The gender gap in physical activity is real, and it impacts your health and that of your mothers, sisters, daughters and female friends. There is also a racial and ethnic gap, with women of color having lower levels of physical activity than white women. I could share alarming statistics with you, but you are not a statistic. You are a woman with a life that is more likely to be long, healthy and happy if you are physically active.

As an orthopedic surgeon, I have cared for thousands of women over my career. Women come to see me for joint pain, especially in the knee, hip or back. On occasion the woman sitting in front of me is physically active, but often she is sedentary. As I spend time with these women, I share the importance of physical activity to their health, and especially to their bones and joints. However, the goal of becoming more physically active is daunting for many women.

WHY DO WOMEN EXERCISE LESS THAN MEN?

Is there something in our XX chromosomes that is anti-exercise? Of course not! Common reasons why women do not exercise include lack of time, family and household demands, financial pressures including the need to work, and lack of motivation. I totally get it. You are really busy and have a lot of responsibility. However, by being healthier — by exercising — you can feel more energized and better meet the demands of your life!

WHAT ARE THE BENEFITS OF REGULAR PHYSICAL ACTIVITY FOR WOMEN?

The benefits of physical activity, especially for women, are numerous. Here are some of the most important ones.

Living longer
People who are physically active for about 150 minutes a week — only 30 minutes a day for five days a week! — have a 33% lower risk of dying prematurely than those

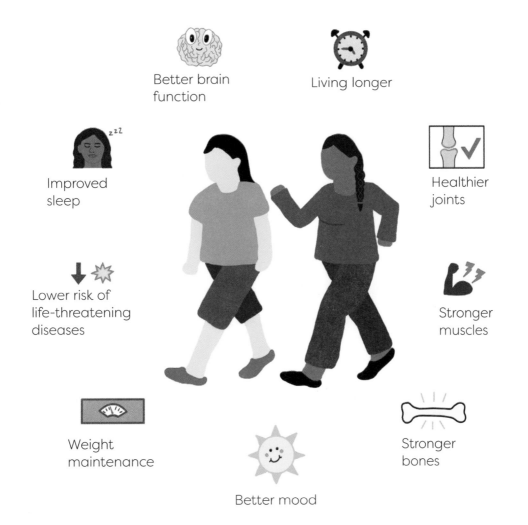

Better brain function

Living longer

Improved sleep

Healthier joints

Lower risk of life-threatening diseases

Stronger muscles

Weight maintenance

Stronger bones

Better mood

who are inactive. Of all the things you can do for your health, regular exercise is the most important.

Better brain function
Staying active keeps your thinking skills and memory sharp as you age. Exercise lowers your risk of dementia.

Improved sleep
You need good-quality sleep. I know you probably do not get enough sleep, just as

you probably don't get enough exercise, so improve the sleep you get with exercise.

Lower risk of life-threatening diseases
Exercise lowers your risk of all kinds of serious health conditions, such as heart disease, diabetes, stroke, high cholesterol and cancer, including breast cancer.

Weight maintenance
Exercise helps you maintain a healthy weight, which is so very important for your

health. This is especially important for women as we age and our metabolism slows down.

Better mood

Exercise promotes feelings of well-being and reduces symptoms of anxiety and depression. When you exercise you change the balance of hormones and chemicals in your brain, decreasing stress hormones and increasing natural pain killers and mood elevators (endorphins). Exercise gives you a "natural high."

Stronger bones

This benefit of physical activity deserves your full attention. With age, women develop osteoporosis much more frequently than men and experience fractures of the hip, back and wrist. I have treated hundreds of women with hip fractures, and it is a devastating event for the woman and her family. Over 20% of people who have a hip fracture are dead within a year of the fracture. Less than 50% are able to recover their pre-fracture level of function. Please remember that weight-bearing exercise, such as walking, jogging and playing tennis, is key to improving and maintaining strength in your bones!

Stronger muscles

As we age, we lose muscle strength and muscle mass more than men do. I wish this were not so, and if I had a magic wand, I would make all women have stronger muscles. But this is our reality. This weakness increases our risk of falling (and breaking bones) and puts more stress on our joints, contributing to arthritis. Thus, strength-training exercises, such as lifting weights, is a requirement.

Healthier joints

Strong muscles help protect your joints from arthritis by absorbing some of the stress to the joint. Strong muscles in your thighs, for example, will help prevent knee arthritis, which affects women more than men (see Chapter 39).

MOVING FOR YOUR LIFE

Creating a regular exercise program for yourself will help you live longer and healthier. National U.S. guidelines recommend that adults engage in at least 150 minutes a week of moderate-intensity aerobic physical activity or 75 to 150 minutes of vigorous or high-intensity aerobic physical activity (aerobic exercises are those that get your heart rate up). On two or more days a week, also do muscle-strengthening activities of moderate or greater intensity. If you're an older adult, include balance training in your exercise routines, too.

Does the thought of meeting these goals seem overwhelming? It might. But remember that any exercise is good for you. You can start increasing your level of physical activity at any age and gain benefit. It is never too late to start.

Here are my personal tips for getting started.

Start small

Find even 10 minutes to do something active five days of the week. You can build up your time! Don't paralyze yourself by thinking that if you can't do 150 minutes a week then it's better to do nothing. You are not a failure if you are doing something.

Make exercise part of your "must do's"

Too often women do not prioritize their own health. This is not fair to them and it is not fair to their loved ones. You are no good to your family if you are sick (or dead). Stop thinking of physical activity as optional, something that you squeeze in if you have the time. Think of it as an essential part of your self-care routine — like brushing your teeth.

Blend physical activity with other enjoyments

For myself, I like to do aerobic exercise on a machine while watching Netflix. I find a series or movie that I like, and this helps me come back to the machine. Maybe you enjoy exercising with music. Whatever your preference, try to make your exercise routine something you look forward to and it will be easier for you to be consistent.

Exercise with others

Women are social beings. Sometimes it is easier (it is for me) to exercise with others at the gym. Plan to meet a friend for an exercise class. Take your daughter, sister or mother with you to the gym. Make it a family and friends activity. What about dancing? Turn the music up and move!

Don't forget the benefit of walking

While walking is not as vigorous a form of exercise as other activities, it is still a wonderful way to get moving. You can have alone time while walking, or walk with friends or family. When you walk outdoors, you are away from the stressors of your home and work environment. You can appreciate the wonders of nature as you walk.

PEARLS OF WISDOM

Of all the things you can do for your health, exercise is one of the most important. There are many factors that influence our health, some of which we can control and some of which we cannot. We cannot control our genetics — certain diseases may be more likely in some women than others based on heredity factors. Similarly, we cannot always control our environments or how we respond to medical treatments. However, we can determine our level of physical activity.

Physical activity is a big part of self-love and care, and you deserve the best you can give yourself. So, move for your life! You are important and the world needs you.

"Movement is LIFE! Divine Mother gave us bodies that move. We honor her by using them."

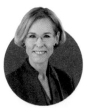

Mary I. O'Connor, M.D. - she/her
Dr. O'Connor is co-founder and Chief Medical Officer at Vori Health, an innovative health care enterprise with a mission to empower all people to lead their healthiest lives. She serves as Chair of Movement is Life, a national nonprofit coalition committed to health equity. Dr. O'Connor is a past chair of the Department of Orthopedic Surgery at Mayo Clinic in Jacksonville, Florida, and Emerita Professor of Orthopedics at Mayo Clinic. She specialized in bone and soft tissue tumor surgery and hip and knee replacement surgery.

70
Purposeful activity

Hena S. Ahmed Cheema, M.D., and Kanwal L. Haq, M.S.

WHAT IS PURPOSEFUL ACTIVITY?

It is widely known that physical activity improves our health. In much the same way, purposeful activity also betters our well-being. Purposeful activity is defined as a task or behavior that you intentionally engage in by taking on an active and voluntary role that is "effort-requiring." Effort in this context can be defined in a variety of ways but generally refers to any action involving the mind, body and soul and therefore engages the physical, mental, emotional and spiritual self.

Purposeful activity can be anything that requires an investment of your time, energy and resources. It is something that you personally enjoy and that holds a deeper meaning for you. The combination of activities that involve active participation and result in joy are beneficial to individual well-being. In a sense, a purposeful activity is a hobby that contributes to personal growth, development and enrichment. Hobbies can teach us new skills, sharpen our minds, provide supplemental income or lead to new social connections. Here are just a few examples of purposeful activity:

- Meditation and reflection
- Spending time outdoors with nature
- Cooking, baking and other culinary activities
- Individual and team recreational sports
- Individual or group dance
- Socializing with loved ones or people who share your interests
- Spiritual or religious endeavors
- Learning languages
- Listening to or creating music
- Traditional arts or crafting
- Traveling
- Taking care of pets

Regardless of the activity, the guiding principle is that purposeful activity brings you fulfillment.

Often, purposeful activity is influenced by our social support networks, cultures and environments. From an evolutionary perspective, purposeful activities may have originated as necessary for human survival, helping provide necessities such as food (from cooking and traveling), clothing (from crafting) and psychosocial support (from activities such as socializing, learning languages or playing sports). The fact that many purposeful activities require you to integrate into the social fabric of your community shows how these activities ultimately benefit both the individual and the collective unit.

WHAT DOES PURPOSEFUL ACTIVITY LOOK LIKE IN ACTION?

Every morning, a 53-year-old woman living in our neighborhood performs the ancient tradition of tai chi, arguably one of the earliest forms of purposeful activity. Tai chi is typified by slow or active movements using the hands, fists and body to channel the two characteristically opposing forces of yin and yang. The tradition is grounded in the idea of expressing internal power rooted in the tension of natural opposing forces and serves as a form of mental strengthening by way of meditation. There is simultaneous engagement of the frontal cortex with rhythmic body movements. The daily practice of this combination has been linked with improved stress levels, joint mobility, and mental and physiological balance. There is an added benefit of improving self-defense abilities.

Other purposeful activities may look a bit different. A woman in her 40s sitting in a coffee shop in London spent her days writing about a magical place, filling thousands of sheets of paper, only later to be rejected by over a dozen publishing houses. Those stories later became the famous Harry Potter franchise that we all know today. Creative writing is a purposeful activity that provides active mental engagement. Harnessing the power of the mind's executive functions with creativity and the physical motion of a pen on paper, or fingers on a keyboard, aligns the body and mind axis, resulting in a form of mental ease and comfort.

HOW DOES PURPOSEFUL ACTIVITY IMPACT HEALTH?

Recent research shows that purposeful activity can be especially helpful during stressful times and in post-stress recovery periods. Activities that require us to take a break from the hustle and bustle of everyday life and actively engage in something that is personally meaningful can serve a restorative function and reduce levels of the stress hormone cortisol.

The cost of stress
Cortisol is produced as a short-term fix for helping our bodies become more efficient in times of high demand. For example, cortisol can help us to be more alert while studying late into the night for an exam or become more focused while trying to score that final touchdown in the last few minutes of a football game.

However, chronic elevations of cortisol result in a kind of toxic stress load on the body and mind — like flooring the gas pedal in a car for too long, causing the engine to stall and overheat. Eventually, with chronic stress, our bodies "throw in the towel," which can result in medical conditions such as chronic fatigue, heart disease, diabetes mellitus, liver disease, vision problems, cognitive fatigue and memory loss, weight gain, muscle and hair loss, and autoimmune conditions. To mitigate the risk of developing such conditions, it is vital to reduce the role of stress in our lives.

Benefits of stress reduction
A large body of research shows us that we need to find active ways to reduce or manage stress — ways that are

"effort-requiring." Initially, it may seem easier to engage in inactive stress-reduction methods, such as binge-watching TV, surfing social media or playing video games, but these behaviors do not result in long-term benefits. Think about stress reduction as your body and cells trying to clean house — it's an active process. Similarly, self-renewal is an active process that engages your physical, mental, emotional and spiritual self.

Research shows that purposeful activities improve physiological function and clinical health outcomes and increase longevity. Research on purposeful activity also shows improved restorative functions, specifically thinking and memory outcomes. This is in line with the notion that health requires a two-fold investment:

1. Physical activities, which strengthen the unconscious physiologic functions of the body.
2. Mental activities, which strengthen the conscious activities of the mind and body.

Different purposeful activities can strengthen either or both health investments. Most of us are familiar with the first investment, physical activities, but what about the second investment?

Many mental activities are regulated by a part of our brain called the frontal cortex. The frontal cortex is like the brain's "executive suite." It is the area of the brain that is responsible for executive functions such as attention, memory, comprehension, problem solving, reasoning and judgment, decision making, emotional responses and impulse control, to name just a few.

Developing strong executive functions, through intentional use and practice, improves life outcomes in a cyclical way. For example, learning how to drive a car leads to better focused attention, hand-eye coordination and rapid decision-making skills, safer behavioral patterns such as sober and defensive driving, and caring about the larger driving population, which results in care for the community and belief in the greater common good. You get all of these benefits from learning to drive a car — imagine the benefits from other recreational activities! (We note — and agree — that driving with the windows down on a beautiful weekend afternoon would count toward purposeful activity!)

Strengthening executive functions

While engaging in purposeful activities, we can strengthen our executive functions by engaging in several complementary practices.

Gratitude and joy The more grateful thoughts we have, the better we feel. Some ways we can practice gratitude are writing or saying what we feel grateful for, listening to or saying positive affirmations, thinking of someone who helps or has helped us, and extending gratitude to those around us.

Even when it may feel very difficult to be grateful, you may want to start by expressing gratitude for something you might take for granted, such as the sun rising. Doing so shows us what we have overlooked and how much we have to be grateful for. Cultivating gratitude can broaden our minds and create a healthier, more positive cycle of thinking and behaving.

Strengthen your executive suite!

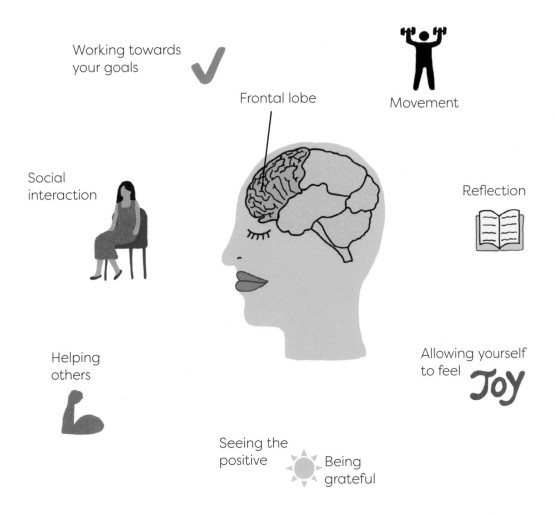

Working towards your goals

Frontal lobe

Movement

Social interaction

Reflection

Helping others

Allowing yourself to feel JOY

Seeing the positive

Being grateful

Practicing gratitude allows us to feel and express joy, and joy can help reduce negative emotions and stress. Optimistic thoughts are a quick way for us to boost serotonin levels and release dopamine!

Movement Moving our bodies requires attention, memory, and mental discipline to coordinate our actions, enhancing our neural activity.

Reflective practices Engaging in reflective and mindful practices, such as meditation, requires awareness, concentration and decision making, which can help us better understand what we are feeling and how we may (or may not) respond to those feelings.

Goal setting Setting goals requires our brains to evaluate how important a goal is to us. Our frontal lobes then break down the details of what the goal entails. Different parts of our brain work together to keep us focused and moving toward achieving our goals, literally contributing to the reshaping of our brain (neuroplasticity). The more challenging our goals, the quicker our brains will change to help us achieve our goals!

Social interaction We are social creatures, and when we are around others, we want to present ourselves in a positive light. This alone can help us engage in purposeful activities. Having one or two strong companions with whom we interact regularly requires us to continue strengthening our social brain functions. When it is not possible to have individuals nearby, pets can serve as strong social companions too!

Helping others Volunteering is a great way to keep our brains engaged and healthy. One study showed a win-win situation in which older adults delayed or reversed declining brain function by tutoring children!

WHY DOES PURPOSEFUL ACTIVITY MATTER TO WOMEN?

The most important aspect of purposeful activity is its relationship to our sense of self as portrayed through intentional, effortful behavior. For many women, this is paramount, as a sense of self-expression often arises from our daily activities, and we tend to experience the highest sense of satisfaction through meaningful engagement. Meaningful engagement requires maximum sustained attention for a prolonged period, typically ranging from 30 minutes to several hours, and results in a form of cognitive ease that positive psychology refers to as a state of "flow."

Flow state can be described as being "in the zone" — a state of mind in which you are so focused that your mind has moved past all distractions. You feel that time has slowed down and that you are "at one with" the task you are engaged in, that your mind and body are in sync allowing you to be completely immersed in what you are doing. Anyone can achieve flow state, whether it is through a creative pursuit, physical or mental activity, or even a simple everyday task. Flow states have been widely studied, with researchers investigating how we can enter a flow state as well as what activities help us achieve flow states. Flow states can be achieved whether we are climbing mountains, creating art, baking a cake or playing chess. Anything that requires full engagement of the self into a single goal can result in flow.

You might be asking, well, what about multitasking? How does the common assumption that women multitask as part of family and communal duties play a role? Does it result in a detriment to their well-being? If a flow state is the mark of ultimate happiness, then yes. Constant multitasking — including disruptions from electronic devices, loved ones or work partners — keeps us away from achieving flow. In fact, these disruptions are proven to lead to chronic fatigue and elevated stress levels. Perhaps collective efforts to reevaluate societal expectations that women "do it all" would benefit all of us. It would reduce the amount of "required" burdens we carry in our professional and personal lives, and it would bring about more opportunities to increase our engagement in purposeful activities that can bring about real meaning, happiness and health!

QUESTIONS TO ASK YOUR HEALTH CARE TEAM

- Which activities would best help me meet my physical and psychosocial needs and goals?
  - › What type of evaluation would help determine the best activity for me?
  - › Are there recommended ways to combine activities?
- What is considered an active versus inactive activity?
- If I have a medical condition, what activities might help me?
- What am I fundamentally able to do based on my current physical abilities?
  - › What activities might be detrimental?
- Are there professionals I could meet with for short-term and long-term consultation on lifestyle activity modifications?
- How will my lifestyle changes impact my family?

PEARLS OF WISDOM

Start small
The point of a purposeful activity is not to add to your "to do list" but rather to help you recharge and conquer such a list. Go for a daily five-minute walk. Play with your pet. Talk to your plants while watering them. Give an old friend a call during your walk to the parking garage. Start with anything that will brighten both your and someone else's day!

Put on blinders
Everyone will have their own version of purposeful activity. And yes, they may very well be posting about it every day on Instagram, Facebook, Twitter, TikTok, and so on. Stop the comparisons. Although some parts of our brains know that the filtered photo worlds are not real, other parts may take in all of the visual cues and process them as facts, making us believe the unreal is real. If seeing such posts is having a negative effect on you, delete your social media accounts. Learn to disengage for the sake of your mental well-being. Live in the physical world instead of the photo world. You will quickly discover that calling up a dear friend is worth so much more than seeing what a high school acquaintance ate for lunch that weekend.

Be courageous
Courage means the act of going beyond what is familiar to you. No, you do not need to take up bungee jumping. However, you should try out that new restaurant or museum you have been meaning to check out. Or grab dinner with a new student in class, or a new colleague at work (who knows, you may end up writing a book together). Expand your horizons in whatever sense that means to you. Novel experiences have been shown to not only improve our well-being but to also strengthen the bonds we have with our intimate partners, family members and friends.

Dream big
There is such a vast array of purposeful activities! Never feel pressured to take on something that you truly don't enjoy. If you don't enjoy the outdoors, then don't try to make camping happen. If you enjoy singing '90s hits with your friends instead, karaoke can certainly be your go-to purposeful activity!

Have fun!

The bottom line is to have fun with your chosen purposeful activity. And although it's easier said than done, don't criticize yourself for what you enjoy. Holding back criticisms of your own choices is the first step to true mental freedom. Embrace your chance to do something truly for yourself.

Load up on the fun! As women, we do so much for others that we often neglect ourselves as a result. Make yourself a priority because when you benefit, everyone around you will benefit, too.

"It's time for women's health to be health care's highest priority."

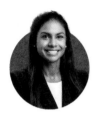

Hena S. Ahmed Cheema, M.D. - she/her
Dr. Ahmed is currently a PGY-4 Diagnostic Radiology resident at the Hospital of University of Pennsylvania and is serving as Chief Resident. She plans to subspecialize in breast imaging and interventions with a dual certification in nuclear medicine and therapeutics.

"Don't get so busy making a living that you forget to make a life." – Dolly Parton

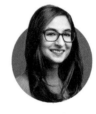

Kanwal L. Haq, M.S. - she/her
Kanwal is a medical anthropologist passionate about creating more connected, more informed, and more equitable systems of care. She specializes in community-based participatory research and builds accessible tools, resources, and programs for women around the globe. Kanwal currently leads the NYC women's health programs at the Arnhold Institute for Global Health at Mount Sinai's Icahn School of Medicine.

71
Social relationships

Teresa M. Cooney, Ph.D., and Kanwal L. Haq, M.S.

WHAT ARE SOCIAL RELATIONSHIPS?

Humans are social creatures and our social relationships (or lack thereof) noticeably impact our mental and physical health. Social relationships are connections between two or more people that have purpose and meaning for all involved. Some examples of social relationships include romantic partners, family members, friends, and colleagues. In many cases, social relationships are a resource to the people involved, providing benefits such as intimacy, companionship, and/or economic, practical and emotional support.

However, social relationships can have a downside, too, such as when our loved ones criticize us or place demands upon us, causing stress. We may also feel distressed or worry about situations happening in the lives of those with whom we are connected. Finally, when close relationships (of any kind) dissolve, we may often encounter feelings of loss and grief. These varied relationship dynamics and situations can all impact our health.

HOW CAN SOCIAL RELATIONSHIPS BENEFIT HEALTH?

There are many ways that our social interactions and ties can promote better health. Some very practical ways include the ability to utilize a partner's or parent's employer-provided health insurance or receiving help from family or friends when we are ill.

In more nuanced ways, our social relationships can influence and impact our health-related behaviors. For example, those close to us may discourage unhealthy habits such as drinking and smoking, and instead encourage us to exercise and schedule regular medical checkups. Our social relationships can also impact how our bodies function. Caring behaviors trigger the release of stress-reducing hormones, mitigating the negative effects of stress on our coronary arteries, gut function, insulin regulation and immune system. For example, individuals with high levels of social support are less likely to become ill when exposed to a virus than those with more limited support are. Individuals with a variety of satisfying relationships with friends and family also have the lowest risk for dementia.

Let's further explore a few types of social relationships, along with different types of positive effects these relationships can have on our health.

Family
- Among teens who experience depression, parental (but not friend) support reduces the impact of depression on the body's ability to function properly.
- Teens who feel they can count on their parents' support consume fewer unhealthy foods and are less sedentary. Black teens, in particular, report greater support and more suggestions for healthy behavior from parents than from siblings and friends. They view parents as role models and managers of home eating and diet.
- LGBTQ young adults who perceive greater parental acceptance report less depression and substance abuse, fewer suicidal thoughts and attempts, and better overall health.
- Adults with strong family support have lower stress hormone (cortisol) levels along with faster recoveries and fewer post-surgical complications when undergoing surgery.
- Adults with greater family and social support report less pain following a musculoskeletal (bone, muscle, ligament, tendon) injury.
- Having cohesiveness and closeness with family members is linked to fewer health problems overall in adulthood.

Friends
- Among young teens, peer support appears to have a greater impact on physical activity than parental encouragement does. In particular, engaging with friends can lead teens to exercise more and play sports.
- Having more "real-world" friends and feeling close to them is linked to better mental health and lower body mass index (BMI) for adults.
- Having supportive relationships with friends and community members is linked to longevity.

Workplace relationships
- Adults reporting greater social support at work experience fewer major depressive symptoms.
- Women who experience greater understanding and trust with co-workers and managers report less stress and fewer risky health behaviors (such as smoking or poor diet).

Marriage
Across cultures, races, ages and socioeconomic groups, marriage is associated with better health. Compared with unmarried people, those who are married have lower rates of illness, chronic conditions, functional limitations and premature death from all causes. Other examples include:
- Married and cohabiting adults report fewer depressive symptoms and thoughts of suicide than people who are single.
- Married individuals have a reduced risk of cardiovascular disease and chronic heart failure, and higher heart attack survival rates, compared with unmarried people.

- Adult smokers are more likely to stop smoking if a spouse stops than if a friend or sibling gives up the habit.

HOW CAN SOCIAL RELATIONS HARM HEALTH?

While supportive relationships can have a positive impact on health, as noted thus far, strained relationships and loss of relationships often contribute to poorer health.

Although our health may benefit from supportive social relationships, as described in the previous section, those close to us may also encourage unhealthy habits such as drinking, smoking, and eating in unhealthy ways. For example, your risk of obesity is influenced by others. Having a friend (especially a same-sex friend) become obese increases your own risk of obesity by 57%. Similarly, if a sibling becomes obese, your own risk increases by 40%, and if your spouse becomes obese, your risk increases by 37%.

In ways separate from health behaviors, emotions that result from strained social interactions, such as anger and anxiety, may increase the risk of certain health conditions and premature death. This is because emotions impact our body's functioning, contributing to factors such as elevating the risk of diabetes, cardiovascular disease, cancer and other serious conditions.

Some specific social relationships and their negative effects on health include those described in the following:

Strained family and friend relationships
- Conflict in relationships is associated with a disrupted immune response, negatively impacting the body's ability to heal from injuries and fight off infection. For example, women reporting more social strain (such as demands from others, or people getting on their nerves) have a significantly greater risk of coronary heart disease.

Strain in the workplace
- Women who feel they've received unfair treatment at work and have low levels of co-worker support experience higher blood pressure.
- Being the recipient of workplace bullying increases the risk of long-term work absences due to sickness.

Strain in marriage
- Women who experience high levels of criticism and long-term aggression from a spouse produce higher levels of the stress hormone cortisol, which is linked to poor health outcomes.
- Adults with low spousal support experience heightened inflammation in the body and poorer health outcomes.
- Marital conflict, especially for low-income adults, can impact a person's ability to function well in daily life.
- Compared with married men who experience illness, married women (both heterosexual and same sex) who experience illness say their illnesses cause greater stress in their marriages.

Divorce
A risk faced with any relationship is its potential loss. Research done primarily on

divorce and spousal death finds mostly negative consequences of this loss. Though divorce may bring positive changes for someone in a distressed marriage, unfavorable health consequences can still result, likely due to the loss of financial and personal resources, the emotions related to ending a marriage and the possible judgment of others. Here are some specific health-related outcomes of divorce:

- Compared with continuously married women, divorced women report reduced vegetable intake after a marriage has ended, a greater tendency to skip mammograms and, if they were former smokers, higher rates of returning to smoking.
- Divorced women report greater short-term psychological distress than married women. They also report heightened physical illness, often a decade after divorce.
- Rates of illness-related work absences increase in the months prior to divorce and peak during the year of divorce. Although the rates of absences due to illness decline after a divorce, they never drop back to pre-divorce levels.

Social isolation and loneliness

A lack of social ties, referred to as social isolation, has overwhelmingly negative effects on health. In fact, people who lack strong social relationships have a 50% higher risk of premature death from all causes compared to people with strong social bonds. This risk effect is similar to smoking up to 15 cigarettes a day! Social isolation often leads to feelings of loneliness, which impacts health. In the United States, many adults report feeling lonely, often. Loneliness isn't limited to those who are isolated. It can affect people who have social ties as well. One example is that adults who spend more time on social media report poorer self-rated health and higher BMI. Loneliness further raises the risk of conditions such as depression, coronary heart disease and stroke.

WHY DO SOCIAL RELATIONSHIPS MATTER FOR WOMEN'S HEALTH?

Women are socialized to be nurturing and caring, and they tend to engage in social relationships differently than many males do, often forming deeper social bonds. For example, men often engage in group interactions, but women appear to be more drawn to one-on-one interactions. Women are more likely to turn to others when in need, and also more likely to offer assistance to others. Women tend to be the caregivers and nurturers for their families and loved ones.

Compared to men, women are also more likely to experience more stress and the associated psychological distress and physical symptoms. This difference is largely due to women's greater concern about people in their social networks and events occurring in others' lives. It is important for women to recognize the ways in which they interact with others and how these social relationships impact their well-being.

PEARLS OF WISDOM

Our social relationships with others can both help and hurt our health behaviors and outcomes. If strains exist, be proactive to address the challenges rather than letting them magnify and create more stress for you. At the same time, it's also important to nurture the social relationships that provide reciprocity and benefits to you. It is good for your health and the health of others to receive and accept assistance when you need it. Finally, remember that by encouraging your friends to engage in healthy habits with you, you are positively enhancing your own health too!

"Communities and countries and ultimately the world are only as strong as the health of their women." –Michelle Obama

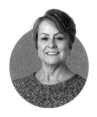

Teresa M. Cooney, Ph.D. - she/her
Dr. Cooney is a professor of sociology and Sociology Department Chair at the University of Colorado Denver. She also is a fellow of the Gerontological Society of America. Her research focuses on aging and families; she has written extensively about the roles adults play in caregiving and support to their family members, up and down the generational lines.

"Each time a woman stands up for herself, without knowing it possibly, without claiming it, she stands up for all women." – Maya Angelou

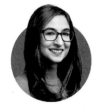

Kanwal L. Haq, M.S. - she/her
Kanwal is a medical anthropologist passionate about creating more connected, more informed, and more equitable systems of care. She specializes in community-based participatory research and builds accessible tools, resources, and programs for women around the globe. Kanwal currently leads the NYC women's health programs at the Arnhold Institute for Global Health at Mount Sinai's Icahn School of Medicine.

72
Mindfulness

Dorothy A. Martin-Neville, Ph.D.

WHAT IS MINDFULNESS?

For millennia, meditation, reflection and prayer have been considered powerful practices that bring us to a place of inner peace and spiritual awareness. In the '80s and '90s, bath and beauty products maker Calgon aired a commercial for their bath soap in which a woman is standing, listening to a crying baby, a barking dog, traffic and a noisy house, when she simply says, "Calgon, take me away." Voila, she is suddenly seen soaking in a gorgeous bubble bath with a nearby glass of champagne. Her focus shifts from the outside world toward herself, an act of mindfulness. However, mindfulness isn't about "getting away" from the potential chaos of your day-to-day life. Rather it involves sitting with an awareness of what is happening within you.

Mindfulness is a way of paying attention to ourselves. Mindfulness offers a process for becoming fully aware of where you are and what you are doing. It does not require you to "stop thinking" or "empty your mind" but rather calmly observe your current state — your thoughts, feelings and sensations as they arise — and then letting those observations "flow" away without judgment.

Developing the practice of mindfulness supports you in becoming connected with yourself. There are different ways of achieving mindfulness, but a key characteristic they have in common is starting with an intention to cultivate awareness. We cultivate this awareness by placing our attention on something tangible (usually our body and breath) so that we can be present in the moment. As we do this, thoughts, feelings and sensations will arise and sometimes we will allow them to pull us away into an experience beyond the present moment. However, we will eventually come back or "wake up" from that experience and realize we got lost from our intention. When this happens, it is our attitude that matters. We can strive to accept what happened with patience, understanding and kindness and then start again with intention, and without judgment. This is the process of mindfulness.

THE IMPACT OF MINDFULNESS ON HEALTH

The field of epigenetics (the study of how our habits and environments affect the way our genes function) has taught us much about how our thoughts and behaviors

Physical benefits

Leads to better sleep

Enhances heart function

Reduces chronic pain

Alleviates digestive problems

Increases energy levels

Mental benefits

Boosts mood

Enhances self-esteem

Reduces stress

Increases concentration

Lowers anxiety

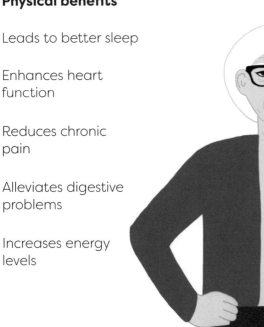

impact our bodies. It has helped us develop an understanding that the stories we tell ourselves, our belief systems and the way we hold stress have immense impact on our health. Rarely do we make up stories about our greatness. Most of the stories we create in our minds reflect a belief in our lack of lovability, our limitedness, our inabilities and our "mistakes."

Take a moment to think about how that feels in your body. It probably causes you to feel tight, defeated or pressured, thus creating vast amounts of stress.

Now imagine feeling the solidness of not only confidence but certainty: Certainty that

you are the best version of yourself that you can be at any given moment; certainty that life happens for you — not to you; and certainty that everything always works out. Imagine how that feels in your body: Calming, powerful and free of stress.

Currently the hectic and unrealistic expectations of modern living have entrenched us so deeply that we are often living in "fight or flight" mode. When high-stress situations become our way of life, mechanisms in our body that should be reserved only for crisis or very rare extreme-stress situations are disrupted. This disruption weakens the immune system and can lead to health conditions based on your body's predispositions (such as heart disease, high blood pressure or anxiety) — predispositions that, with a healthy lifestyle, might not develop into health problems.

Since stress is the major element in disease, minimizing or eliminating it is a key factor in taking care of our health. Mindfulness helps us temporarily separate our internal selves from all the external factors that cause us stress, allowing us to build a more certain sense of well-being. Furthermore, scientists have verified that mindfulness techniques help improve physical health in a number of ways, including:
- Helping relieve stress
- Treating heart disease
- Lowering blood pressure
- Reducing chronic pain
- Improving sleep
- Alleviating gastrointestinal difficulties

Those who practice mindfulness also build other healthy behaviors, such as:
- Eating a healthier diet
- Getting better quality sleep
- Developing an ability to deal with stress before it reaches a panic stage and causes harmful behaviors

WHY IS MINDFULNESS IMPORTANT FOR WOMEN?

As a generalization, women tend to be the ones who others call on most. Women tend to take on far too much, frequently with the belief that if they don't, no one will. This contributes to the fact that women worry more than men, which puts their minds and bodies in "crisis" mode.

However, crisis is a mindset. Notice who stands out in a true crisis. It is the person who detaches from the rush, the panic. This detachment does not mean that the person is ignoring the crisis; she simply is not caught up in the energetic chaos that is immobilizing others. She resonates strength, balance and a clear perspective on how to handle the situation. She doesn't react — she responds. She quickly assesses what resources are available and what needs to get done, and decides the most efficient and effective way to handle the situation. She goes within to respond rather than reacting to what is going on outside.

By momentarily stepping away from seemingly high-stress situations that may surround us, we can see what part we may be playing in the "crisis." We can recognize that we have big problems and little problems but that all problems can be solved. By stepping back, away from the crisis, we can gain a new perspective, another option. We can even immediately stop the crisis, by deciding not to participate in it.

By practicing mindfulness, you begin to see that crisis does not need to be your constant way of living. With mindfulness you learn that you are separate from the life you have created. Mindfulness provides you with agency over your mind and, as a result, agency over your life.

GIVE THIS MINDFULNESS EXERCISE A QUICK TRY

Visualize yourself sitting in a chair. On the far side of the room, far away from you, are all your family members, your children, all your past relationships, past and current friends, the schools you have attended, all the jobs you have held. All of these are simply a part of the life you have created — they are not you.

Do you see the difference?

When you recognize that you are a distinct entity, separate from everything and everyone in your life, you can begin to cultivate the ability to be mindful. Too frequently we get so busy "getting things done" that we have little to no idea exactly what we think or feel about anything. Being so focused on what's happening outside of ourselves, we become lost in the midst of so much activity, so many demands, and disappear into the life we have created.

When you stop running and take the time to sit in your own presence, you become aware of your own experience, of what you feel, what you think, what you want, what you need and what you are willing to do with all this inner knowledge. You discover strengths, fears, needs and wants you hadn't noticed. Slowly, you discover yourself, your values, your core, your essence. You can remember the you that once existed and now recognize the woman she has become.

PEARLS OF WISDOM

Epigenetics confirms that the practice of mindfulness — and the inner peace and contentment it provides — can support our ability to change our perspectives, providing us an opportunity to heal. Our bodies are designed to self-heal, but only when we create the right environment for them. We have the power to do that, but it requires a conscious awareness of what stress feels like when it occurs.

Mindfulness offers us the opportunity to understand what stress looks and feels like in our bodies, how to step away from our stress and see new perspectives, and how to engage in this practice every day to improve our emotional, mental and physical health.

"Inner peace and self-awareness are the best prescriptions for health care."

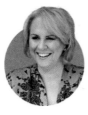

Dorothy A. Martin-Neville, Ph.D. - she/her Dr. Martin-Neville is currently a Business/Life coach working with women to support business success and health, emotionally, spiritually and physically. She specializes in teaching how stress, beliefs and behaviors impact health.

73
Acupuncture

Christina Y. Chen, M.D.

WHAT IS ACUPUNCTURE?

Acupuncture is a component of traditional Chinese medicine (TCM) that originated more than 2,500 years ago. It involves inserting hair-thin, sterile needles into specific points in the body, called acupoints. These points are located along the body's energy meridians, pathways through which your life energy is believed to flow. The philosophy behind TCM focuses on maneuvers to balance this energy, or qi (pronounced "chee"), which is considered vital to general health and function. Qi is often described as blocked, depleted or in excess when disease-specific conditions and symptoms surface.

The goal of acupuncture is to promote and restore the balance of energy and improve overall health and well-being. Thus, acupuncture has been offered as an attractive treatment option for many health conditions because it does not involve the use of drugs to heal but rather focuses on restoring balance and aiding your own healing ability. The practice of acupuncture varies, depending on whether the stimulation of the needles is electrical, if ear acupuncture is also used, how long the needles are retained in the body and how frequently the treatments occur.

HOW DOES ACUPUNCTURE WORK?

How acupuncture works in the body isn't fully understood. For pain control, the procedure likely stimulates pain fibers that close the "pain gates" in the central nervous system, weakening the pain signal transmitted to the brain. Evidence shows that acupuncture also increases the release of endorphins (your body's natural painkillers), such as serotonin, dopamine, neurotrophins and nitric oxide. People experiencing chronic pain due to migraines, back problems, fibromyalgia and other conditions may benefit from acupuncture.

In addition to pain management, acupuncture is used to help treat other symptoms caused by a wide variety of conditions, including:
- Mental health disorders (anxiety, depression)
- Sleep disorders
- Neurological conditions (Parkinson's disease, stroke)
- Digestive issues (nausea, vomiting, constipation, irritable bowel syndrome)
- Chronic inflammatory or degenerative disease (such as rheumatoid arthritis)
- Low white blood cell counts due to chemotherapy

HOW CAN ACUPUNCTURE IMPACT WOMEN?

Acupuncture has been used to treat many health conditions that are specific to or common in women, including those related to fertility, menstrual health, menopause and urinary incontinence.

Fertility

Acupuncture has been offered in the treatment of infertility. For example, studies show that women who undergo in vitro fertilization (IVF) and receive acupuncture around the time of embryo transfer have a higher pregnancy rate and birth rate. However, it's important to note that some of the acupuncture methods used in these studies were not routine and may differ from methods used by other practitioners of acupuncture.

Beyond IVF, acupuncture may promote your natural fertility and reproductive health. Research suggests that acupuncture may affect the secretion of gonadotropin-releasing hormones, which influence the balance of your menstrual cycle and fertility. Acupuncture may stimulate blood flow to the uterus. It may also promote production of endogenous opioids (natural painkillers), which in turn may counter stress hormones known to negatively affect fertility.

Menstrual health

From the perspective of traditional Chinese medicine, a woman's overall health and fertility is intimately related to her menstrual health and the flow of blood. Acupuncture may improve women's health by helping improve menstrual regulation. Research suggests that acupuncture may reduce the symptoms of dysmenorrhea (painful menstruation), although its effectiveness in treating premenstrual syndrome (PMS) is not yet known. Acupuncture may also help treat problems with menstrual regulation caused by an underlying condition, such as polycystic ovary syndrome (PCOS), thyroid dysfunction, ovarian failure or an eating disorder. For example, studies have demonstrated that acupuncture may be helpful in regulating ovulation for women with PCOS and may also improve the function of their endocrine system. Acupuncture may also have a role in reducing pelvic pain caused by endometriosis.

Menopause

Some studies suggest that acupuncture may help relieve hot flashes in perimenopausal and postmenopausal women, but more research is needed. Acupuncture has also been shown to treat hot flashes in women who have undergone treatment for breast cancer. If you're interested in exploring acupuncture treatments for hot flashes or other menopausal symptoms, discuss the option with your primary care clinician or a certified acupuncturist.

Urinary incontinence

Urinary incontinence can cause involuntary leakage in women of all ages, but is most common in middle-aged and older adult women. One type of incontinence is stress incontinence — leakage that occurs when there is a sudden stress on the bladder, such as from a strong sneeze, cough, running or jumping. The overall evidence shows that acupuncture reduces urinary leakage in middle-aged and older adult women who experience stress incontinence. Your clinician may recommend acupuncture as one component of your larger treatment plan.

COMMONLY ASKED QUESTIONS ABOUT ACUPUNCTURE

Are there risks involved?

Overall, the risks of acupuncture are very low if you are treated by a certified acupuncture practitioner. The needles are sterile and disposable to reduce infection risks. Possible side effects include minor issues, such as temporary bruising at the needle sites. Although extremely rare, injury may occur if the needles are pushed in too deeply (particularly around the chest area). However, this only occurs with the use of longer needles. The majority of treatments involve shallow needle insertion. Please let your practitioner know if you are pregnant, have a pacemaker or suffer from any bleeding disorders so your treatments may be designed to your specific needs.

Does acupuncture hurt?

Acupuncture treatments should not be a painful experience. You may initially feel a small prick upon needle insertion. After that, you may feel a sensation of pressure, deep ache or warmth with the needle stimulation. This means that the needle has made contact with the energy, or qi. Typical treatments last from 20 to 30 minutes after all the needles are placed.

What should I expect afterward?

People often report a general sensation of relaxation and rejuvenation after an acupuncture treatment. How frequent the treatment is and how long it lasts typically depends on your condition and the treatment plan agreed upon by you and your practitioner. Typically, chronic conditions may require more frequent treatments, longer courses of treatment or both.

PEARLS OF WISDOM

As with any health decision, consider the risks and benefits of acupuncture to decide if it's an appropriate option for you. Acupuncture is a practice that has been a part of many people's healing journey, guided by trusted clinicians and growing evidence. The purpose of the treatment is to restore your health in a comprehensive fashion and stimulate the body's own abilities to restore balance and harmony. Whether acupuncture is used on its own or along with conventional medicine, the ultimate goal is to promote and maintain your best self — physically, emotionally and mentally — throughout your health journey.

"Women should feel empowered to optimize their well-being through all health care practices, both conventional and integrative."

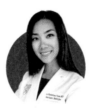

Christina Y. Chen, M.D. - she/her
Dr. Chen is a Geriatrician and acupuncturist at Mayo Clinic in Rochester, Minnesota. Her area of interest is in the role of integrative medicine in the care of older adults and innovative strategies toward promoting healthy aging and cognitive health.

74

Vaccines

Jennifer R. Maynard, M.D., C.A.Q.S.M., and Adrianna D. M. Clapp, M.D.

WHAT ARE VACCINES?

Over 300 years have passed since the development of the smallpox vaccine in 1798. After that first vaccine, science has advanced to create many effective vaccines against bacteria and viruses that could otherwise cause serious illness or death. Ongoing research in vaccinations has allowed for the rapid development and emergency-use approval of multiple vaccines against SARS-CoV-2, the virus that caused the global COVID-19 pandemic.

The human immune system

To gain a complete picture of how vaccines work to fight off disease, it is important to understand the basics of the human immune system. Once germs such as viruses or bacteria enter the human body, their main goal is to replicate, which can cause widespread infection in the body with unpleasant symptoms. For example, bacteria may replicate in the lungs causing pneumonia with cough and fever.

The human immune system is equipped with white blood cells that recognize the whole germ — or a small part of the germ known as an antigen — as a foreign invader. Once they've identified these foreign invaders, white blood cells work hard to prevent replication and infection. During an immune response, some white blood cells (B-cells) produce antibodies that recognize and attack foreign antigens while some (T-cells) attack germ-infected cells. When a germ is first encountered, the immune system may require several days to respond. But a subsequent infection from the same germ will be quickly recognized by the memory cells of the immune system, resulting in faster production of antibodies to fight off the infection.

Natural immunity may be acquired from having had the disease itself, but this is not without risk of serious illness or death. Vaccines imitate an infection, using different techniques to expose the body to certain viruses or bacteria and prepare the immune system's response, but with minimal side effects or risk.

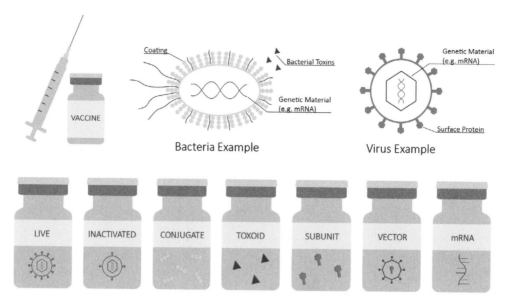

Figure 1: Different vaccine types

TYPES OF VACCINES

There are various types of vaccines designed to fight different types of germs.

Live vaccines
Live, attenuated vaccines — such as the measles, mumps and rubella (MMR) and varicella (chicken pox) vaccines — contain a small amount of the weakened live virus or bacteria. Since these vaccines are the closest to an actual infection, they may have mild side effects that mimic the actual infection. As such, they are not recommended for pregnant women and people with weakened immune systems. Their advantage, however, is that they tend to mount a long-lasting strong immune response.

Inactivated vaccines
Inactivated vaccines, such as the polio or hepatitis A vaccines, introduce a killed version of the germ that is unable to replicate in the body. This way the body learns to recognize the virus or bacteria without getting sick.

Conjugate vaccines
Conjugate vaccines involve antigens such as pieces of the sugar-coating shell that some bacteria use to try to avoid detection by white blood cells. This type of vaccine prevents the bacteria from hiding from the immune system. Examples include Haemophilus influenza (Hib), pneumococcal and meningococcal vaccines.

Toxoid vaccines
Toxoid vaccines work against bacteria that produce toxins and cause infections such as diphtheria and tetanus. The weakened toxin, called a toxoid, is a component of the vaccine and cannot cause actual illness.

Subunit vaccines
Subunit vaccines are similar to conjugate vaccines in that they use an important component of a bacteria or virus that the

immune system recognizes as an antigen — usually a protein, such as a viral surface protein. The pertussis, hepatitis B, shingles and certain influenza vaccines are examples of subunit vaccines.

Vector vaccines

Vector vaccines use a nonreplicating version of a different virus (vector), such as a common cold virus (like adenovirus), to deliver a portion of the target germ's genetic material into the body and stimulate an immune response. A person cannot get sick from the vector virus, nor does this genetic material change a person's own DNA. Historically, these types of vaccines have been developed to fight dangerous diseases, such as Ebola. In addition to other vaccine platforms, adenovirus vector vaccines have been developed to protect against COVID-19 illness.

mRNA vaccines

Although these vaccines have been in scientific development for the past 10 to 15 years, mRNA vaccines are the latest to be deployed for use. They directly introduce strands of genetic material (mRNA) from the germ into the body. These strands act as instructions for the body to build specific antigens that lead to a robust immune response.

It is important to note that mRNA vaccines do not actually change a person's genetic code. The technology that created mRNA vaccines received a great deal of attention in the media when it was used to develop some of the initial vaccines against COVID-19. These mRNA COVID-19 vaccines continue to be incredibly effective for preventing severe disease, hospitalization and death from COVID-19.

WHICH VACCINES ARE NEEDED AND WHEN?

The main purpose of a vaccine is to teach the body to recognize a dangerous virus or bacteria if such a germ is ever encountered. Just as a race car driver revs up the engine before a race, the vaccine's job is to rev up the immune system, so it is ready to go! The following section outlines when to receive various vaccines.

Childhood

Each year, the Advisory Committee of Immunization Practices (ACIP) of the Centers for Disease Control & Prevention (CDC) update their guidance on childhood vaccinations. Vaccines begin at birth to give infants and young children protection before they are exposed to certain life-threatening diseases. Vaccines are responsible for virtually eliminating deadly diseases such as polio and measles in most of the world. Outbreaks of measles in the United States in the past 5 to 10 years are mainly due to pockets of unvaccinated individuals.

Childhood vaccines are typically given in the pediatrician's or family doctor's office during a well-child visit. Recommended vaccines of young childhood include:
- Hepatitis B (Hep B)
- Hepatitis A (Hep A)
- Haemophilus influenza (Hib)
- Diphtheria, tetanus and pertussis (DTaP)
- Rotavirus (Rota)
- Pneumonia (PCV13)
- Measles, mumps and rubella (MMR)
- Polio (IPV)
- Chicken pox (Varicella)

- Influenza (flu)
  › Advised for everyone older than 6 months annually, due to the changing types of virus each year.
- COVID-19 vaccines
  › At the time this book was printed, the CDC recommended that all children age 5 and older get vaccinated against COVID-19 with a 2-dose series of an mRNA vaccine (Pfizer-BioNTech) followed by a booster dose at least 5 months later. The dose given to children between the ages of 5 and 11 is less than that given to older children and adults. However, children have very strong immune systems and will mount a strong immune response to the vaccine. Please check the CDC's website for the latest guidelines on COVID-19 vaccines.

Adolescence

Additional vaccines are recommended for adolescents to protect against bacteria that can cause meningitis and against the human papilloma virus (HPV), a virus that's commonly transmitted through sexual activity and that can cause cervical cancer and genital warts. Booster vaccines for tetanus, diphtheria and pertussis (Tdap vaccine) are also recommended for this age group. Booster vaccines remind the immune system of the characteristics of a particular antigen.

Adulthood

In adults, some of the recommended vaccines are boosters while others are given to prevent illnesses that occur primarily later in life, such as shingles and pneumonia. Some work, school or volunteer programs may require immunity titers — a blood test that measures the amount of antibodies to

certain bacteria or viruses in the blood. Booster shots are given if antibodies are no longer present at adequate levels. Here's a closer look at a few of the vaccines of adulthood and why some are particularly beneficial for women.

Tetanus, diphtheria and pertussis vaccination
Tdap becomes a booster vaccination every 10 years starting after the adolescent dose. For pregnant women, experts now recommend one dose of Tdap during each pregnancy, regardless of the timing of the prior Tdap dose. A mother's antibodies can be transferred to the baby during pregnancy and breastfeeding, but the level of antibodies may wane over time before the next pregnancy. Research has found that giving the Tdap vaccine between 27 and 36 weeks of gestation decreases the risk of whooping cough in babies by 78%.

Human papilloma virus (HPV) vaccine This is a vaccine against cervical cancer. Gardasil-9 protects against the nine most common high-risk types of HPV, which can cause cervical cancer, genital warts and other infections. The vaccine is available starting at age 9 up to age 45 for both women and men. Studies show that this vaccine is safe and highly effective at decreasing cervical cancer rates in women, by nearly 90%.

Herpes Zoster vaccine Because older adults have a higher risk of developing shingles, which is a painful rash, vaccination is recommended for all adults 50 years and older. The original shingles vaccine, Zostavax, was a single-dose live-attenuated vaccine, but it showed decreasing effectiveness with age, down to 38% for those over age 70. Zostavax is no longer available in the U.S. The current shingles vaccine (Shingrix) is a subunit vaccine given in a two-dose series that provides over 90% efficacy in all adults over 50. For the best protection, it is recommended that you consider the Shingrix vaccine even if you have already received Zostavax. Studies have shown that shingles occurs more frequently in women in nearly all age groups, which makes prevention particularly important for women.

Pneumonia vaccine There are two types of pneumonia vaccines that are commonly used: polysaccharide (Pneumovax, PPSV23) and conjugate vaccines (Prevnar13, Vaxneuvance, Prevnar20). In childhood, four doses of PCV13 (Prevnar) are recommended. For those 65 and older whose vaccination history is unknown or who have not previously had a pneumococcal conjugate vaccine, there are several options. Vaxneuvance (PCV15) can be given followed by a PPSV23 vaccine one year later; or a single dose of PCV20 (Prevnar 20) vaccine may be given. For people of all ages with certain medical conditions including chronic heart disease, chronic lung disease, chronic liver disease, diabetes mellitus, spinal fluid leak, cochlear implants, certain blood disorders, kidney disease or immunodeficiency, they should discuss with their clinician whether any additional pneumonia vaccines are needed. Check the CDC vaccines web page for updated guidance on the timing and frequency of pneumococcal vaccination.

COVID-19 vaccines We could write an entire book on the scientific miracle that was the development of safe and effective vaccines for SARS-CoV-2. It is quite remarkable that these vaccines were created in such a rapid,

safe and efficient manner, complete with robust clinical trials! The CDC strongly recommends COVID-19 vaccines for all people ages 5 and up. Several types of vaccines, as discussed earlier in this chapter, are now widely available. These vaccines have various levels of effectiveness overall, but all approved vaccines are very effective for preventing severe disease, hospitalization and death. Due to emerging data on safety and effectiveness, the CDC has stated that the mRNA vaccines are preferred over the adenovirus vector vaccines in the U.S.

It is widely understood that pregnant women may have more severe disease or complications if they catch COVID-19, including harm to the unborn baby. Importantly, all available vaccines are considered safe in women trying to conceive, and women who are pregnant or breastfeeding.

Due to waning immunity over time, initial booster doses for most of the COVID-19 vaccines are recommended 5 months after the initial series is complete. As of spring 2022, a second booster dose of mRNA vaccine is recommended 4 months after the initial booster dose for those individuals over 50 years of age, immunocompromised, or if the initial booster was a vector vaccine. Be sure to monitor CDC recommendations for booster recommendations for specific vaccines as data emerges.

Pregnancy
Ideally, women who are planning to become pregnant will update their vaccinations before pregnancy. During early pregnancy, clinicians typically check the status of women's immunity to certain diseases such

Recommended adult vaccine chart (does not include all childhood vaccines)

Vaccine name/type	Prevention of disease	Ages	
Flu (influenza) Subunit	Flu (influenza)	Everyone 6 mos and up	
DTaP or Tdap Subunit (pertussis) and toxoid (tetanus, diphtheria)	Lockjaw (tetanus); diphtheria; whooping cough (pertussis)	DTaP starting at 2 mos, then Tdap after age 7	
HPV (Gardasil-9) Subunit	Cervical cancer, genital warts due to high-risk human papilloma virus (HPV)	9 to 45 yrs (ideally prior to first sexual encounter)	
MCV4 or MenACWY (Menactra, Menveo or MenQuadfi) Conjugate	Meningitis (meningococcal groups A, C, W, Y)	Starting at 12 yrs*	
MenB (Bexero or Trumenba) Conjugate	Meningitis (meningococcal group B)	16-23 yrs (preferred age 16-18)*	
RZV (Shingrix) Subunit	Shingles (Herpes Zoster)	50 yrs and up	
PPSV23 (Pneumovax) Polysaccharide	Pneumonia caused by Streptococcus pneumonia	At-risk children 2 to 18 yrs**; adults 65 yrs and over or at-risk adults** who've never had PCV vaccine	
PCV13 (Prevnar-13) , PCV 15 (Vaxneuvance), PCV20 (Prevnar20) Conjugate	Pneumonia caused by Streptococcus pneumonia	All infants starting at 2 mos; at-risk children 2 to 18 yrs**; adults 65 yrs and over or at-risk adults**	
Hep A (Havrix, Vaqta, or combined HepA-HepB vaccine called Twinrix) Inactivated vaccine	Liver disease caused by Hepatitis A virus	All infants starting at 12 mos; at-risk adults***	
Hep B (Monovalent vaccines: Engerix-B, Recombivax HB, Heplisav-B; there are also other combination vaccine options) Subunit	Liver disease caused by Hepatitis B virus	All infants; unvaccinated children and adults to 59 yrs; at-risk adults 60 yrs and older****	
COVID-19 mRNA (Pfizer-BioNTech or Moderna) or vector (Johnson & Johnson)	COVID-19 disease caused by SARS-CoV-2 (coronavirus)	See clinician or CDC for latest guidelines	

*, **, ***, ****: See page 436.

Frequency/intervals	Side effects
Single dose annually	Injection site soreness, headache, fever, muscle aches
Childhood series of 5 doses of DTaP; single dose Tdap every 10 yrs and in 3rd trimester of each pregnancy	Injection site soreness, redness, swelling; mild fever; headache; fatigue; nausea, vomiting, stomach pain
2 doses if series starts before age 15 at 0 and 6-12 months; 3 doses if it starts after age 15 or if immunocompromised at 0, 1-2, 6 months	Injection site soreness, redness, or swelling; dizziness; headache; nausea; muscle or joint pain
2 doses; 1st dose age 11-12, 2nd dose age 16	Injection site arm soreness, fatigue, headache
Bexero: 2 doses at least 1 month apart; Trumenba: 3 doses at 0, 1-2, 6 months	Injection site soreness, fatigue, headache
2 doses; 2nd dose 2-6 months after the 1st	Injection site soreness, redness, or swelling; fatigue; muscle pain; headache; fever; stomach pain
See clinician or CDC for recommendations	Injection site soreness or redness; fever; muscle ache
Childhood series of four Prevnar doses starting at 2 mos; see clinician or CDC for at-risk and older adult recommendations	Injection site soreness, redness or swelling; fever; loss of appetite; fatigue; headache
Havrix: 0 and 6-12 mos apart; Vaqta: 0 and 6-18 mos apart; Twinrix (≥18 yrs): 0, 1, 6 mos apart or 0, 7, 21-30 days with booster 12 mos after dose 1	Injection site arm soreness, redness, swelling or hard lump; low fever; nausea; headache; loss of appetite
Engerix-B or Recombivax HB: 3 doses at 0, 2 and 6 mos; Heplisav-B (18 yrs and older): 2 doses at 0 and 1 mo; booster series as adult if low titers	Injection site arm soreness, redness, swelling; headache; fever
See clinician or CDC for latest guidelines	Injection site arm soreness, redness, swelling; fever; fatigue; headache; nausea; muscle pain

Vaccine schedule changes may occur for:

- Certain medical conditions (anatomic or functional asplenia including sickle cell disease, HIV infection, certain immune deficiencies)
- People who may be taking certain medications such as eculizumab or ravulizumab
- People who missed the initial dose at age 11-12 and need a catch-up
- Travelers to areas with hyperendemic or epidemic meningococcal disease
- Microbiologists who routinely work with meningitis isolates
- First-year college students in residential housing
- Military recruits

**A booster or early dose of certain vaccines may be recommended for people with:*

- Chronic heart disease
- Chronic lung disease
- Chronic kidney disease
- Chronic liver disease
- Diabetes mellitus
- Alcohol use disorder
- Current cigarette smoking
- Cerebrospinal fluid leaks
- Cochlear implant(s)
- Solid organ transplants and stem cell transplants

- Sickle cell disease or other hemoglobinopathies
- Certain cancers and immune deficiencies
- HIV infection
- Congenital or acquired asplenia

***At-risk adults may include those with:*

- Chronic liver disease
- Injection drug use
- HIV infection
- Homelessness
- Work in research laboratory with Hepatitis A
- Travel to countries endemic to Hepatitis A
- High risk scenarios (certain workplace environments, pregnancies at risk for infection, men who have sex with men, close contact with international adoptee)

****At-risk adults may include those with:*

- Chronic liver disease
- Injection drug use
- HIV infection
- Sexual exposure risk
- Incarcerated persons
- Risk for exposure to blood
- Travel to countries endemic to Hepatitis B

as Hepatitis B, MMR and varicella. If acceptable immunity to MMR or varicella is not found, it is best to wait until after delivery to be vaccinated against these diseases, since the vaccines contain live viruses. On the other hand, Tdap and influenza vaccines have been found to be safe for mother and baby and are highly recommended during every pregnancy (see more details later in this chapter). It is important that family members and caregivers close to mother and baby are up to date on all vaccines as well.

Travel

If you are planning a trip, talk to your clinician about any necessary vaccinations. It is important to have an informed discussion about where you are traveling, how long you will be there and your planned activities. Different regions of the world may recommend or even require certain vaccines to prevent serious illnesses, such as Yellow Fever in specific parts of South America or Africa. At the time this book is being written, vaccination against COVID-19 before travel is highly recommended or required by many countries to prevent further spread of the virus. Check the CDC's Travel webpage for destination-specific details.

VACCINE SIDE EFFECTS

It is common for mild symptoms to occur after a vaccination. Side effects may include low-grade fever, soreness or redness at injection site, fatigue, and mild body aches. These effects are typically short-lived, lasting less than two or three days. They indicate an appropriate response of the immune system to the vaccine and can be treated with a nonprescription pain reliever such as acetaminophen or ibuprofen. Be sure to check the label and follow dosing instructions carefully in children. Ibuprofen should not be given prior to 6 months of age.

Serious allergic reactions (anaphylaxis) are quite rare and usually occur within 15 to 20 minutes of receiving a vaccine. People who have had a prior allergic reaction to a vaccine should be monitored for at least 30 minutes following injection and have trained staff on hand to administer treatment if needed.

VACCINATION RECORDS

In the United States, there is no central database that contains everyone's updated vaccination records on file. The CDC does, however, provide blank record templates that you can print out and complete with your clinician. Many individual states have central registries for immunizations, but this information may not follow you if you

move to a different state. Be sure to keep a copy of all immunizations that you or your children receive! Or take a picture of your vaccine record and store it in a safe, secure file so that you will not need to worry about lost paper documents.

The CDC has a list of ways you may be able to collect your or your child's vaccine information:
1. Check with your primary care clinician or the clinics where you or your child received vaccines
2. Check baby books or childhood documents
3. Check with high school, college, or past employer health services that may have collected your or your child's immunization records
4. Check your state's health department, as many states maintain vaccine registries where clinicians can enter vaccine administration dates

If you cannot find certain vaccine records, your primary care clinician may order blood tests (titers) to prove immunity, or may re-order missing vaccines, which are safe to get even if you've had them before.

WHY VACCINES MATTER TO WOMEN

The scientific evolution of vaccines has been revolutionary in preventing and nearly eliminating many life-threatening diseases. Childhood vaccinations are imperative to keep children safe and often require boosters in adulthood. Vaccines during pregnancy, including influenza, Tdap, and now COVID-19 vaccine, help protect mother and child.

The development and deployment of safe and effective vaccines against harmful germs, such as SARS-CoV-2, is the cornerstone of ending global pandemics. Women should lead by example and get vaccinated! By getting vaccinated, women can be instrumental in advancing medical and scientific recommendations and promoting healthy choices for generations to come.

PEARLS OF WISDOM

Remember, vaccines have been around for over 300 years and have been proven to be an extremely effective and safe way to prevent and, in some cases, completely eliminate severe or deadly diseases! The CDC and FDA have rigorous protocols in place for monitoring side effects and continue to be transparent in educating the public on potential risks, which are generally greatly outweighed by the benefits of vaccination.

Feel empowered to have an open discussion with your clinician regarding any questions or concerns you may have about vaccines. The transformative science of the most recent vaccines is extraordinary and revolutionary. Women have the unique chance to lead the way in stopping the spread of newer diseases such as COVID-19 by trusting the vaccination recommendations of their clinicians and immunization experts.

ACKNOWLEDGMENT
The authors would like to thank Alyssa Clapp, who designed the graphics for Figure 1.

"Women should feel empowered to ask challenging questions in order to be their own health care advocate."

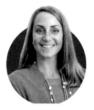

Jennifer R. Maynard, M.D., C.A.Q.S.M. - she/her
Dr. Maynard is the program director of the Primary Care Sports Medicine Fellowship at Mayo Clinic in Jacksonville, Florida. She is an Assistant Professor and dual appointed in the Department of Family Medicine and Orthopedics. As Medical Advisor for the Women's Tennis Association (WTA), her passion lies in the comprehensive care of the female athlete.

"A means to empower women is to support them in their physical and mental health, starting with preventive medicine."

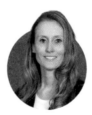

Adrianna D. M. Clapp, M.D. - she/her
Dr. Clapp is a Chief Resident completing her final year in the Family Medicine program at Mayo Clinic in Jacksonville, Florida. She was one of the recipients of the 2021 American Academy of Family Physicians (AAFP) Award for Excellence in Graduate Medical Education in recognition of her leadership, civic involvement, and exemplary patient care. She has an interest in women's preventive health and global health initiatives.

75
Medical research

Carolyn M. Mazure, Ph.D.

WHAT SHOULD I KNOW ABOUT HOW RESEARCH WORKS?

Understanding the basics of medical research is important because biomedical and behavioral research provide the foundation for the treatments that you may eventually receive to prevent or treat medical disorders.

Two major types of medical research are laboratory studies and clinical studies.

Laboratory studies
Laboratory investigations focus mainly on the biology of various conditions, whether at the level of cells, in tissues or within organ systems. Information uncovered in the lab sets the stage for further research that is designed to create treatments, such as new drugs and therapeutic devices, for specific disorders.

Clinical studies
Establishing the safety and effectiveness (efficacy) of newly devised treatments requires testing in human subjects. This is accomplished in scientific studies known as clinical trials. Clinical trials study the safety and efficacy of different therapies in groups of people using protocols that are tightly controlled. Companies use the data from these trials, as well as from the lab, to seek approval from the U.S. Food and Drug Administration (FDA) for the therapy they are seeking to bring to the public. The FDA is the regulatory agency that oversees drugs and medical devices available on the U.S. market.

Importantly, a vast array of other forms of clinical research, which includes investigations of biology, behavior and the intersection of those two areas, is also conducted to uncover the nature of disorders as well as approaches to treatment and prevention.

Data from both laboratory and clinical studies provide critically important information on aspects of health and disease, such as:
- Risk factors that increase the possibility of developing a given disorder
- How a disorder first appears and how it looks over time
- How to reduce risk of a disorder
- How to enhance health outcomes through various treatments and prevention strategies

WHAT IS THE ROLE OF RESEARCH IN RELATION TO WOMEN'S HEALTH?

You may be saying, "OK, I understand a bit more about how research generates the findings that affect my clinical care, but what has this got to do with the health of women?" The answer is, "Quite a bit."

It was not until the mid-1990s that the National Institutes of Health (NIH), the largest single funder of health research in the country and an influential leader in the direction of research, initiated a requirement that women be included as participants in clinical research. Before that time women generally were not studied — with some notable exceptions, such as in female reproductive health. When women were included in clinical trials, it was usually because the research was focused on a disorder that happened to be common in women, such as depression. However, even then, subject data were generally "pooled," or grouped together, meaning that possible differences by sex or gender were not investigated.

Furthermore, it wasn't until 2016 that the NIH began requiring the inclusion of female animals in laboratory studies. This means that the biological underpinnings of health and disease had thus far been based on male physiology and might not apply to females.

Now, however, the NIH requires that the research it funds include the influence of biological sex on study results, with the goal of ensuring a better understanding of how sex affects health processes and outcomes.

The general exclusion of females in identifying and testing new treatments and prevention strategies has left a large knowledge gap concerning the health of women and sex- and gender-specific health differences. Today we are working to fill this gap and ensure that rigorously examined data on the health of both women and men are increasingly available to guide clinical care.

WHAT IS THE DIFFERENCE BETWEEN SEX AND GENDER?

The terms sex and gender have an interesting history. A more detailed understanding of the terms began with a committee convened by the Institute of Medicine — an independent, nonprofit organization focused on advising the nation about health. The committee was charged with evaluating whether laboratory studies needed to consider biological differences between males and females. It responded with a resounding yes in their 2001 report, *Exploring the Biological Contributions to Human Health: Does Sex Matter?*

In conducting their evaluation, the committee wanted to acknowledge both biological and social-behavioral contributions to health. Consequently, they used the term sex to signify the biological classification linked to reproductive organs and the type of chromosomes that a person has at birth, generally male or female. They used the term gender to indicate a person's self-representation, as influenced by social, cultural and personal experience.

Importantly, these were meant to be working definitions that would likely change over time. Today we understand that sex is not always binary and that gender exists on a spectrum — like so much of human behavior.

WHY WEREN'T WOMEN STUDIED?

Two major reasons excluded women from being study participants. The first was based on the commitment to protect women, especially during their childbearing years, from experimental risk. These concerns are legitimate and must be taken seriously, of course, as should protection of all study participants. However, efforts to reduce this risk were very broadly applied, resulting in the exclusion of women generally, even from research on disorders that were leading causes of death in women.

The first trial of estrogen as a preventive therapy for recurrence of heart attack offers a classic example of the overreach of protection commitment. The choice of estrogen as a treatment for preventing another heart attack was well-considered, as it was known that estrogen lowers blood fats associated with heart disease, such as cholesterol and triglycerides. It was also understood that as estrogen declines around menopause, women are more likely to have heart attacks. Yet in this first trial of estrogen for heart attack prevention, over 8,000 men were enrolled — and no women.

The second major reason that women were not included in research was based on the notion that the variability of female hormones would confound or confuse study findings. In fact, this reasoning presents a paradox. If women are not included because they are biologically different from men, then how will the findings drawn from male subjects apply to females? Moreover, this reasoning prompts us to ask a further question: Doesn't this variation actually require the study of both women and men?

I am often asked, "How could this happen in science — that women would be left out?" My answer is that science is embedded within our culture and deeply influenced by societal views. As determined by another committee of the Institute of Medicine, policies designed to protect women do not account for all of the lack of focus on studying women's health. It also may come from biases that exist within society.

HOW HAS RESEARCH CHANGED? ARE WOMEN STUDIED NOW?

Time for some good news. Yes, the historical exclusion of women from medical research has changed. Here are just two examples.

Heart disease
One field in which there have been dramatic changes is in cardiology, the study of diseases of the heart and blood vessels. Increased awareness that cardiovascular disease is the greatest killer of women, as well as men, has spurred investigations resulting in new data to inform approaches to diagnosis and treatment. For example, it is now clear that heart attacks — caused by reduced blood flow to the heart — can produce different symptoms in women and men. And, just as important, these different symptoms signal different causes, such as small vessel constriction in women

compared with artery blockage more commonly seen in men.

Additional research, with more underway, focuses on ensuring that women who may be having a heart attack receive evaluation beyond the routine procedures that look for blockage in the arteries. This approach, coupled with evolving diagnostics, provides an opportunity to ensure that everyone seeking care receives the most appropriate treatment.

Cancer

Another area of research that is changing is cancer studies. Cancers are the second-greatest cause of mortality in women and men, and we now better understand that specific cancers occur at different rates in women than in men and may have different outcomes.

For example, colon cancer is more common in men, yet right-sided colon cancer is more common in women and has a worse outcome. Recent data show that colon cancer cells fuel tumor growth differently in women than in men. This difference is associated with a more aggressive form of tumor growth that occurs more frequently in women. New scientific technologies are being used to investigate how the body converts food and liquids into energy to gain insight into how diseases, including right-sided colon cancer, begin and develop.

Many other examples exist in this book to demonstrate the progress that has been made in including women as participants in clinical research.

WHAT HAVE WE LEARNED? IS MORE RESEARCH NEEDED?

There's a growing recognition that although reproductive health is an essential part of women's health, the scope of what needs to be included in studying the health of women is so much broader. We also now recognize that male and female differences extend beyond reproductive and hormonal issues.

Reflecting on how recently women began to be studied, we can appreciate that we are in the infancy of learning about the health of women and have only touched the surface of learning about differences among women. New research aims to inform improved health and health care strategies for all women, including but not limited to women of color, women across the age span and women with varied psychosocial experiences and histories.

In learning more about the health status of women, we also have developed a good idea of specific conditions and disorders that research can target to advance the health of women. For example, research needs to address why women are more likely to:
- Suffer chronic diseases and disability
- Have acute and chronic pain
- Die following a heart attack
- Have autoimmune disease
- Experience depression and anxiety
- Develop Alzheimer's disease independent of lifespan
- Be prescribed opioids, including for conditions that lack data on opioid efficacy and despite rising rates of opioid overdoses

HOW CAN I STAY INFORMED ABOUT ONGOING RESEARCH?

To stay informed, it is key to develop working relationships with all of your clinicians so that you can ask any questions you may have and receive guidance on additional resources. Establishing a relationship with a clinician may take some initial effort to accomplish but will pay dividends in understanding your care.

Next, remember that understanding study results and health information can be complicated, but this doesn't mean that you can't understand what it means for you and how you can effectively use the information.

An important aspect of staying well informed is to use only legitimate and trusted sources when seeking health information online. Examples of reputable sources include websites of academic health centers and each of the institutes within the NIH. These sites provide up-to-date information on various conditions and ongoing research, including research on the health of women.

Well-known and established nonprofit organizations, such as the American Heart Association and the American Cancer Society, also provide useful information, as do nonprofit foundations focusing on health and health policies, such as the Kaiser Family Foundation.

PEARLS OF WISDOM

- Research is constantly producing new findings that are key to improving health. Stay informed and support efforts to advance health research on women.
- If a health recommendation changes, it does not automatically mean prior information was wrong. New data are signs that research is ongoing and that science is at work.
- Develop relationships with your clinicians so that you can ask them about health information and treatment approaches that are different for women compared to those for men.

"Science is changing to ensure that the health of women is advanced."

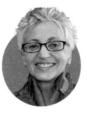

Carolyn M. Mazure, Ph.D. - she/her
Dr. Mazure is the Spungen Bildner Professor in Women's Health Research, Professor of Psychiatry and Psychology at Yale University, and the Director of Women's Health Research at Yale – nationally recognized for launching interdisciplinary research on women and sex and gender differences. She specializes in research on the interplay of stress, resilience, and depression.

76
Personalized medicine

Hetal Desai Marble, Ph.D., and Lauren L. Ritterhouse, M.D., Ph.D.

WHAT IS PERSONALIZED MEDICINE?

The current method in which we practice medicine is primarily based on a one-size-fits-all approach. Personalized medicine — also called precision medicine, individualized medicine, or genomic medicine — is a new approach to change this model, a way to tailor medical treatment specifically to you.

The goal of personalized medicine is to improve health outcomes for each and every person, and to do this by improving personal response to treatments and minimizing side effects. Every person has a genetic makeup that is slightly different from the next person's, which is what makes us unique. This genetic makeup can be the reason why different people with the same disease may respond differently to the same treatment.

The same treatment does not work for everyone. Personalized medicine can help tailor treatment to person-specific factors to figure out which treatment works, who it works for, and when it works.

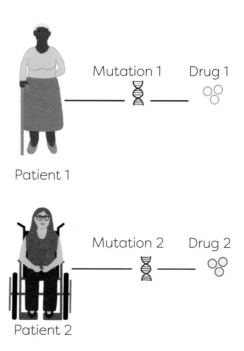

Patient 1 — Mutation 1 — Drug 1

Patient 2 — Mutation 2 — Drug 2

HOW DOES PERSONALIZED MEDICINE WORK?

Personalized medicine tries to take into account the many factors that make a person unique. Genetics is a big factor, but other factors are also important, such as environmental considerations, pre-existing conditions, therapies being taken at the same time (concurrently), and broader considerations such as age, height, weight, race and sex at birth.

Genetics in personalized medicine involves not just the DNA you inherited from your parents but also changes that happen to your DNA. Many of the advances in personalized medicine involve the diagnosis and treatment of cancer, for example. Cancer, at its core, is a genetically driven disease — the uncontrolled growth of cells that is a hallmark of cancer happens because of changes, or mutations, in a cell's genetic code.

The body often produces indicators (biomarkers) that signal genetic and biologic changes within the body. Many biomarkers now exist to diagnose disease earlier, evaluate the risk of death or recurrence, and even predict response to treatment, especially in the setting of cancer.

What is a biomarker?

A biomarker is a measurement of your body or one of its products, such as blood, urine or tissues, that could indicate a deviation from your body's "normal" state. Scientists commonly refer to biomarkers of disease, which you have likely encountered in the form of diagnostic or laboratory tests. For example, a persistently higher-than-normal blood sugar level is a biomarker that indicates the presence of diabetes. Aside from diagnosing conditions, however, biomarkers can also be prognostic or predictive. These categories of biomarkers are especially relevant for personalized medicine and cancer.

What is a prognostic biomarker?

A prognostic biomarker is a measurement that informs clinicians about the course of a disease, the potential for recurrence and the overall outlook for the patient. Prognostic biomarkers can therefore be thought of as indicators of risk. Prognostic biomarkers are critical in cancer treatment since they can tell people what to expect from their diagnosis. Using prognostic biomarkers helps doctors understand what to expect regarding disease course, how aggressive treatment should be, whether there is an increased risk of disease relapse or other complications, and, in some cases, whether the diagnosis is terminal.

There is some discussion as to whether a prognostic biomarker applies only to prognosis — the potential clinical outcome after diagnosis — or whether it can indicate future risk in otherwise healthy people. Personalized genomic medicine enables the evaluation of prognostic biomarkers both before and after diagnosis. Most genomic prognostic biomarkers are used to evaluate gene-related risks in healthy people. Examples of prognostic biomarkers include:

- Changes in BRCA 1 or 2 genes that detail your risk of developing breast or ovarian cancer in the future.
- Blood cholesterol levels in the context of your family history and race to evaluate your risk of heart attack or stroke.

What is a predictive biomarker?

A predictive biomarker is a proxy for your response to specific or targeted therapy. It gives your clinician valuable information about ways to treat your condition. Predictive biomarkers are typically identified in a clinical trial comparing outcomes in biomarker-positive participants who have been given targeted therapy versus standard treatment; if the targeted treatment results in better outcomes for the participants, the predictive biomarker is valid. For solely predictive biomarkers, the biomarker evaluation comes after the disease's initial diagnosis. For biomarkers that are both prognostic and predictive, the biomarker evaluation could come well before the disease's diagnosis.

The primary use of predictive biomarkers lies in tailoring specific treatment regimens to a person's disease characteristics. This is how most people imagine personalized medicine. This goes hand in hand with the recent trend in drug development, especially for cancer, in which drug companies develop therapies targeting vulnerabilities that are only present in the diseased cells. For example, the drug trastuzumab was developed specifically to target HER2, a protein contained in HER2-positive breast cancer cells. Knowing that a woman's breast cancer is HER2- positive allows her health-care team to tailor her treatment to that specific type of breast cancer.

What is a companion diagnostic?

To decide if a targeted therapy, such as trastuzumab, is appropriate for someone, the clinician needs to know if the person will respond to the treatment. The clinician can find out if the treatment is appropriate by checking for the presence of the biomarker tied to the treatment — in the case of trastuzumab, checking for HER2 in breast cancer cells. Drug companies often build the assessment of the predictive biomarker into their FDA approvals in the form of a companion diagnostic, which specifies a device or test that clinicians can use to evaluate the biomarker in their patients. This standardizes the detection of the predictive biomarker and ensures safe and effective administration of the therapy to people who will benefit. Companion diagnostics are a part of the FDA approval of the drug and thereby undergo the same stringent review as the drug.

How are biomarkers assessed?

Diagnostic assessment depends on which biomarker is being tested. For most personalized medicine uses, the focus is typically on genomic biomarkers, which are primarily tested in either tissue samples collected during surgery or in blood or bone marrow samples. Genomic biomarkers are commonly detected via sequencing, which is the systematic assessment of specific stretches of DNA. Sequencing identifies the base sequence of the specified part of your DNA and compares it with the human genome (the complete set of genetic information) to determine if a mutation (an incorrect base or bases) is present. Sequencing can be done using many methods, but all of them evaluate specific regions of your genome to identify patterns of diagnostic, prognostic, or predictive value.

HOW IS PERSONALIZED MEDICINE BEING USED IN CANCER?

Personalized medicine has advanced the most in the diagnosis and treatment of cancer. There is good reason for this. Cancer is primarily a genetic disease, characterized by uncontrolled growth of a tumor due to a genetic (genomic) mutation. Because cancer is driven by mutations, it makes sense to target those same mutations to treat the cancer. In fact, targeting genomic mutations provides superior response rates in several types of cancer and minimizes systemic side effects, such as vomiting, hair loss and fatigue. What's more, certain biomarkers have been identified that apply broadly to all cancer types. Here are some specific examples:

Lung cancer

Lung cancer is the leading cause of cancer-related deaths, making up about 25% of all cancer deaths for both sexes. At the same time, lung cancer, specifically the more commonly occurring non-small cell lung cancer (NSCLC), has seen many advances in diagnosis and treatment. Predictive biomarkers are abundant for NSCLC, including alterations in several genes and gene families such as EGFR, MET, ALK, ROS1, BRAF, RET, and NTRK. NSCLC tumors driven by these gene alterations can be treated with targeted therapies. If you are diagnosed with lung cancer, especially stage III or IV lung cancer, ask your doctor about testing (genotyping) your tumor tissue to identify any targetable alterations. Given the number of genetic vulnerabilities in lung cancer, most lung cancer specimens are genotyped via large sequencing panels to ensure that all potential genetic alterations are assessed.

Breast cancer

Breast cancer is a very common cancer diagnosis. Public awareness campaigns have led to increased screening for breast cancer, which has contributed to early detection of the disease and thereby better outcomes for people with the disease. Breast cancer has numerous prognostic and predictive biomarkers. The most well known are mutations in the genes BRCA1 and BRCA2. These mutations are examples of prognostic genomic biomarkers — they are genetic alterations that serve as a proxy for risk of developing breast cancer.

Other biomarkers in breast cancer are primarily proteins, including estrogen receptor (ER), progesterone receptor (PR), and human epidermal growth factor receptor (HER2). These biomarkers can be both prognostic and predictive. For example, the presence of HER2 in a tumor is a marker of poor prognosis in breast cancer but it also makes HER2 a target for customized treatment. Both ER and HER2 are targets for treatment with specialized drugs, such as the drug tamoxifen, which targets estrogen receptors. You also may have heard of a breast cancer being triple negative, which means the tumor does not make ER, PR or HER2 proteins. In this case, treatments directed at these proteins will not help. Other predictive biomarkers in breast cancer include the mutational status of the estrogen receptor, which can predict resistance to certain anti-estrogen treatment types.

Gynecologic cancers

Gynecologic cancers are a common cause of cancer-related death, especially after menopause. Gynecologic cancers include cancers of the ovary, uterus and cervix. Successful treatment of these cancers requires early diagnosis in combination with targeted treatment. As such, screening measures are used together with laboratory tests to understand risk and to develop treatment regimens after diagnosis.

For example, women are screened for cervical cancer using a Pap smear, which identifies changes in the cells of the cervix that are indicative of cancer. In addition, the cells collected during a Pap smear are genotyped for the presence of high-risk variants of human papilloma virus (HPV). This combination of screening and laboratory testing results in either early diagnosis of cervical cancer, or a more complete understanding of your risk of developing cervical cancer in your lifetime.

Ovarian cancer also uses laboratory testing to understand risk and prognosis. Beyond their usefulness in the diagnosis and treatment of breast cancer, BRCA1 and BRCA2 gene mutations are prognostic indicators of lifetime risk of ovarian cancer and can even predict response to certain chemotherapeutic treatments for ovarian cancer. In addition, ultrasound-based imaging of the ovaries is often combined with the measurement of the CA-125 protein in blood samples to diagnose ovarian cancer. Imaging studies combined with lab tests for specific biomarkers is a powerful method to diagnose and treat most gynecologic cancers.

Pan-cancer biomarkers

Some biomarkers are not restricted to a single cancer type — indeed, they can predict response to therapeutic agents regardless of where the cancer originated. These are called pan-cancer biomarkers. Prior to these biomarkers, the only broad treatments available for cancer relied on cytotoxic chemotherapy, which poisons rapidly growing cancer cells but also kills healthy cells in the body. With the arrival of pan-cancer biomarkers, we are now able to target cancer regardless of its origin in the body if the biomarker indicating vulnerability to specific therapy is present.

The first pan-cancer biomarker to be recognized by the United States Food and Drug Administration is microsatellite instability (MSI). Human genomes have regions of repetitiveness called microsatellites. The rate at which these microsatellites accumulate mutations is a measure of the effectiveness of the genome's proofreading capabilities. In certain instances, due to hereditary or acquired mutations, the ability of the cells to proofread and correct these mutations is poor, leading to an accumulation of mutations that lead to cancer. This means the microsatellite region of the genome is unstable or that MSI is high. Studies show that people whose tumors are unstable or MSI-High respond better to certain therapies that drive the immune system to attack the cancer cells, including therapies such as pembrolizumab (Keytruda). In fact, these therapies are effective in people whose tumors harbor a high number of mutations in general — a measurement called tumor mutational burden (TMB). People who have tumors that are TMB-High are also eligible for these therapies, regardless of their cancer type.

HOW CAN I BE A PART OF PERSONALIZED MEDICINE?

New biomarkers for personalized medicine emerge frequently. Clinical trials are key research tools to evaluate which biomarkers are relevant for human health.

Consider participating in a clinical trial. Participation is entirely voluntary and may be of great benefit to you. Clinical trials are carefully controlled by the doctors who lead them. Before you enroll in a trial, your doctor will go over all of the risks and benefits that apply to you and address your questions. Once you are enrolled, your doctor will monitor you very closely. If at any time you or your doctor no longer feel comfortable with your participation in the trial, you can withdraw and discontinue trial treatment. Trials can offer you specialized treatment early and potentially improve your outcomes, especially if a good treatment doesn't exist for your condition. No one can pressure you to enter a trial, and as a patient you have the right to enroll, or not enroll, in any trial for which you are eligible.

Biomarker clinical trials are especially relevant for cancer, since many new cancer drugs target unique features of cancer, such as mutations. Biomarker-driven trials are becoming more common; even your local hospital may have trials available or may be linked to larger hospitals offering trials. In a biomarker-driven trial, you will be tested for the biomarker in question, usually a genetic mutation. If you have the mutation and you meet all the other eligibility criteria of the trial, you may be asked to participate. As always, this is voluntary, and you will be informed of the risks and benefits before you are asked to consent.

WHY DOES PRECISION MEDICINE MATTER TO WOMEN (AND EVERYONE)?

Throughout history, the practice of medicine has largely been reactive. Even today, we usually wait until a disease develops before trying to treat or cure it. Since the genetic and environmental factors that cause major diseases such as Alzheimer's disease, cancer and diabetes, among many others, aren't fully understood, efforts to treat these diseases are often imprecise, unpredictable and ineffective.

The drugs and treatments currently devised are tested on broad populations and prescribed using statistical averages. Consequently, they work for some people but not for many others, due to genetic differences among the population. On average, any given prescription drug now on the market only works for half of those who take it.

However, a continually growing understanding of genetics and genomics — and how they drive health, disease and drug responses in each person — is helping to provide better disease prevention, more accurate diagnoses, safer drug prescriptions and more effective treatments for the many diseases and conditions that diminish human health. Because personalized medicine is based on each person's unique genetic makeup, it is beginning to overcome the limitations of traditional medicine. Increasingly, it is allowing clinicians to:

- Shift the emphasis in medicine from reaction to prevention
- Predict susceptibility to disease
- Improve disease detection
- Preempt disease progression
- Customize disease-prevention strategies
- Prescribe more effective drugs
- Avoid prescribing drugs with predictable side effects
- Reduce the time, cost and failure rate of pharmaceutical clinical trials
- Eliminate trial-and-error inefficiencies that inflate health care costs and undermine patient care

PEARLS OF WISDOM: THE FUTURE OF PERSONALIZED MEDICINE

As genetic sequencing becomes less expensive and more widely available, genome-linked personalized medicine grows closer to becoming a reality. The field of pharmacogenomics, which predicts your response to drug therapies or the side effects that you may experience based on your genetic code, is a growing area of medical practice that many hope will be the new frontier of medicine.

Soon, your specific genes may dictate treatment of even the most basic condition and may even predict your risk of developing certain conditions. A genetic screen may even become part of your annual physical! In the case of cancer treatment, the future has already arrived, with many treatments targeting and leveraging specific genomic biomarkers for treatment. As research and medicine advance, this targeting of disease traits and prediction of optimal treatment based on your biomarker profile will only become more common and useful.

"Educating ourselves and being our own advocates for our health results in better outcomes for us all."

Hetal Desai Marble, Ph.D. - she/her
Dr. Marble is currently Senior Director, Diagnostic Products at Quanterix Corporation, and was formerly Director of the Translational Research Laboratory at the Center for Integrated Diagnostics/Massachusetts General Hospital. She specializes in the development and clinical implementation of molecular diagnostics and the design of biomarker-driven clinical trials.

"Precision medicine is a key component to improving outcomes in women's health care."

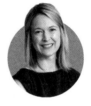

Lauren L. Ritterhouse, M.D., Ph.D. - she/her
Dr. Ritterhouse is the Associate Director of the Center for Integrated Diagnostics at Massachusetts General Hospital in Boston, Massachusetts, and Assistant Professor of Pathology at Harvard Medical School. She is an expert in the translation of emerging biomarkers into clinical practice for the realization of precision medicine.

77

Our connectedness

Mary I. O'Connor, M.D.

"All things are connected like the blood that unites us. We do not weave the web of life; we are merely a strand in it. Whatever we do to the web, we do to ourselves." — Chief Seattle

One critical lesson that we all should have learned from the coronavirus pandemic is how interconnected we are. No one can completely isolate themselves or their families. Everyone is at risk of illness, albeit some more than others. The sicker your community, the greater your risk. The sicker a neighboring community, the greater the risk to yours.

We know that some individuals and communities are at greater risk of illness during a pandemic. The reasons for this are very complex. However, there is a framework, using the example of muscle and joint health, that can help us understand how different factors create these disparities. This framework, called the *Vicious Cycle* (see illustration on page 452), was developed by Movement is Life, a nonprofit multidisciplinary coalition seeking to eliminate racial, ethnic and gender disparities in muscle and joint health by promoting physical mobility to improve quality of life. I have been honored to chair Movement is Life since its inception in 2010.

At the very center of the *Vicious Cycle* is a circle that represents our physical health. Here we see how essential movement is to life!

Women of all ages are more sedentary than men. Joint pain also impacts adult women more than men. Women who do not move — whether because of joint pain, lack of time for physical activity, depression or other factors — tend to gain weight. This often starts the vicious cycle of weight gain leading to increased pressure on joints and creating or increasing joint pain. Joint pain leads to limited mobility, more physical inactivity, greater weight gain and obesity. With obesity and limited physical activity come the development of other conditions such as heart disease, diabetes and depression.

Note that anyone can get trapped in this medical vicious cycle — including affluent white males. However, women — particularly those of lower socioeconomic means— are much more likely to be caught in the loop.

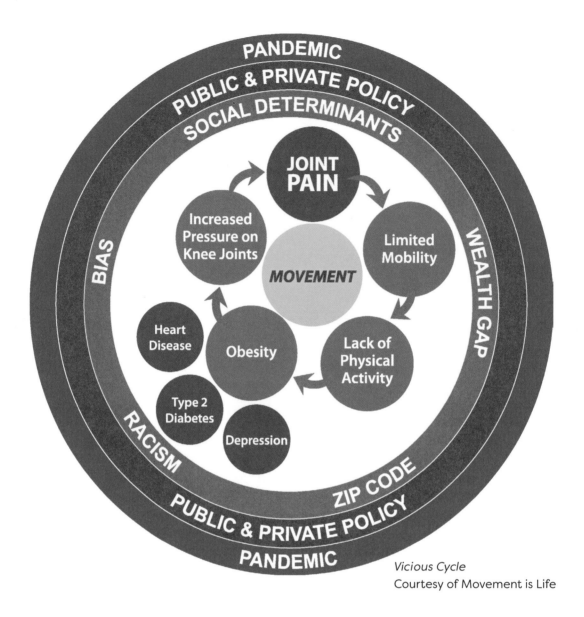

Vicious Cycle
Courtesy of Movement is Life

Why is this? It is because of the influence of the green ring of social determinants of health. We know that women are more likely to earn less money, have greater stress and experience more bias (especially women of color). These social determinants are influenced by the next ring, the blue ring, of public and private policy — think access to health care, the presence of food deserts, safe walking spaces and the quality of education for children in underserved neighborhoods. Policy influences everything! It is important to remember that both public and private policies influence health inequities — and there is much that can be done by nongovernmental groups to address harmful social determinants of health.

In 2019, the world changed with the coronavirus pandemic. We saw the impact of the *Vicious Cycle* in the higher death rates from COVID-19 that struck communities of color and those with underlying medical conditions (obesity, high blood pressure, heart disease, diabetes, lung disease). We saw the cycle's impact on death rates for people whose access to health care was limited to lower-resource hospitals, exemplified in headlines such as, "Low-income COVID-19 patients die needlessly because they are stuck in the wrong hospitals — while the right hospitals too often shut them out." At the same time, we must recognize — as the *Vicious Cycle* illustrates — that there were factors far outside the scope of a hospital or our health care system that influenced the risk of death for many people.

We must all work to break this Vicious Cycle. We must work individually and collectively to address social determinants of health and create positive public and private policies to promote health equity. Remember, we are all connected. The health of each of us influences those around us, and the health of those around us influences our own. By strengthening health in ourselves and our communities we will make our lives and those of our loved ones better — and we will be better positioned to withstand potential future pandemics.

"We are all humans together on one planet. We are all born and we will all die. Let us realize how connected we should be to each other."

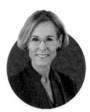 **Mary I. O'Connor, M.D. - she/her**
Dr. O'Connor is co-founder and Chief Medical Officer at Vori Health, an innovative health care enterprise with a mission to empower all people to lead their healthiest lives. She serves as Chair of Movement is Life, a national nonprofit coalition committed to health equity. Dr. O'Connor is a past chair of the Department of Orthopedic Surgery at Mayo Clinic in Jacksonville, Florida, and Professor Emerita of Orthopedics at Mayo Clinic. She specialized in bone and soft tissue tumor surgery and hip and knee replacement surgery.

78

You are a health promoter!

Mary I. O'Connor, M.D., and Kanwal L. Haq, M.S.

Throughout this book we have shared many aspects of health for women — from specific disease conditions to bias against women to specific factors that contribute to women's health. Our purpose in writing this book is to empower women to be better advocates for their own health. Taking care of ourselves is imperative, but we are also a powerful influence on the health of others, those who are in our families and in our communities. We close our book with a call to action — that each of us be health promoters to those around us.

What do we mean by "health promoter?" We mean that, through your actions and your attitudes, you impact those around you to improve their health as well as yours. We say this because we recognize that changing behavior on your own is hard — usually it's really hard! So, what helps a person make healthy behavior change? Emotional support. Health promoters can provide that emotional support.

Mary has seen the power of health promoters through her work as chair of Movement is Life, a multistakeholder coalition committed to health equity. Movement is Life sponsored an 18-week community-based program called Operation Change for underserved women with knee pain and other health issues. Programs were held in various locations across the country, some with groups of African American women, some with Hispanic women and some with rural white women. Each week approximately 40 women would gather for three hours: one hour to learn about a specific health topic (such as arthritis or depression), one hour for movement (such as yoga or line dancing), and one hour for motivational interviewing to try to identify personal barriers to change. The results of the program were impressive: an 18% improvement in walking speed and a nearly 70% improvement in their sense of hopelessness. Yes, hopelessness. We heard women say, "This program saved my life."

When the women of Operation Change were asked what they liked best about the program they did not mention education. After all, they could get the same information from their own clinicians or the internet. They appreciated the hour of movement, as it showed them that they could do such physical activity. They felt that the motivational interviewing was helpful to them as individuals. But what they liked

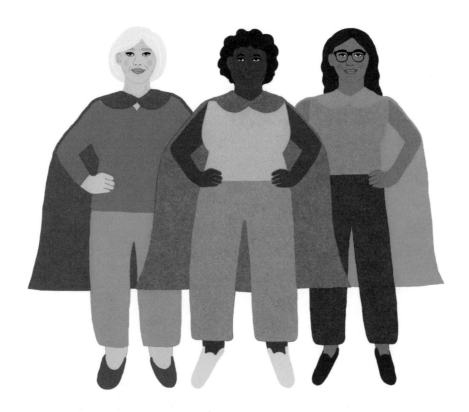

best about the program were the emotional connections they formed with each other. These women had become health promoters for each other! (Learn more via Mary's TEDx talk, "Promoting health — Your secret superpower," on YouTube.)

Women are so powerful. They are natural health promoters for their children, for their families and for each other! A woman who participated in Operation Change shared how she started to cook a healthy dish for herself as part of the family meal. Her husband was not encouraging, but she persisted. Soon the children also started eating the healthy option. Eventually her husband did as well. One woman improved not only her own eating pattern, but that of her entire family. She was a health promoter for her husband and children — like a pebble in a pond, sending ripples out to the shore.

This ripple effect impacts entire communities. In fact, women make 80% of all health care decisions in the United States, making them the most effective agents of health promotion around. Kanwal has witnessed the power of women to promote health again and again through her work as a medical anthropologist and community organizer. One of the initiatives she worked on taught women how to create healthy meals. The participating women appreciated learning how to source and make better meals, but like those who took part in Operation Change, what they valued most on their journey toward health for themselves and their families was having the support of one another — they were a community working toward the same changes.

Similarly, there are endless ways that you can be a health promoter for your community. Here are just a few examples:
- Ask your co-workers to join you for a short walk at lunch or break time
- Suggest a rotation schedule at work for bringing in healthy snacks to share
- Become an accountability buddy to help a loved one get quality sleep, exercise more or eat better
- Set a recurring time with your friends to practice mindfulness to reduce stress
- Add more fruit or vegetables to your family's main meal of the day
- Get your family out for a walk after dinner
- Plant a vegetable garden with your friends

Our hope is that each of you reading this book will make positive health changes in your own lives and support such changes in those around you. We can all be health promoters in our own ways, for our family, friends and colleagues. Together we can promote better health for ourselves and those around us and in so doing, strengthen our communities and our nation. Remember, *illness* can be transformed to *wellness* when we move from *I* to *we*.

"Each of us can give the gift of health promotion to others. We can change our communities and our nation to embrace health."

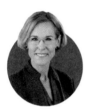

Mary I. O'Connor, M.D. - she/her
Dr. O'Connor is co-founder and Chief Medical Officer at Vori Health, an innovative health care enterprise with a mission to empower all people to lead their healthiest lives. She serves as Chair of Movement is Life, a national nonprofit coalition committed to health equity. Dr. O'Connor is a past chair of the Department of Orthopedic Surgery at Mayo Clinic in Jacksonville, Florida, and Professor Emerita of Orthopedics at Mayo Clinic. She specialized in bone and soft tissue tumor surgery and hip and knee replacement surgery.

"It's time for us to transform ourselves and our communities from ailing patients to thriving agents of health. Women can turn the key, leading the change from reactively treating disease to actively promoting better health!"

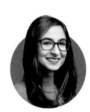

Kanwal L. Haq, M.S. - she/her
Kanwal is a medical anthropologist passionate about creating more connected, more informed, and more equitable systems of care. She specializes in community-based participatory research and builds accessible tools, resources, and programs for women around the globe. Kanwal currently leads the NYC women's health programs at the Arnhold Institute for Global Health at Mount Sinai's Icahn School of Medicine.

Select sources

PART 1 Women and the current health landscape

Chapter 1: The role of social determinants in women's health

Constitution of the World Health Organization. World Health Organization. Accessed June 22, 2021. https://www.who.int/about/governance/constitution

Ducharme J, et al. Your ZIP Code Might Determine How Long You Live — and the Difference Could Be Decades. *Time*. Published online June 17, 2019. Accessed June 22, 2021. https://time.com/5608268/zip-code-health/

Lakhani CM, et al. Repurposing large health insurance claims data to estimate genetic and environmental contributions in 560 phenotypes. *Nature Genetics*. 2019; doi.org/10.1038/s41588-018-0313-7

Hughes LS. Social determinants of health and primary care: Intentionality is key to the data we collect and the interventions we pursue. *Journal of the American Board of Family Medicine*. 2016; doi:10.3122/jabfm.2016.03.160120

America's women and the wage gap. National Partnership for Women & Families. Accessed June 22, 2021. https://www.nationalpartnership.org/our-work/resources/economic-justice/fair-pay/americas-women-and-the-wage-gap.pdf

Risk and protective factors of intimate partner violence. Centers for Disease Control and Prevention. Accessed June 22, 2021. https://www.cdc.gov/violenceprevention/intimatepartnerviolence/riskprotectivefactors.html

Bugiardini R, et al. Delayed care and mortality among women and men with myocardial infarction. *Journal of the American Heart Association*. 2017; doi:10.1161/JAHA.117.005968

Skelding KA, et al. Frequency of coronary angiography and revascularization among men and women with myocardial infarction and their relationship to mortality at one year: an analysis of the Geisinger myocardial infarction cohort. *Journal of Interventional Cardiology*. 2013; doi:10.1111/joic.12009

Infographic: Racial/ethnic disparities in pregnancy-related deaths — United States, 2007-2016. Centers for Disease Control and Prevention. Accessed June 22, 2021. https://www.cdc.gov/reproductivehealth/maternal-mortality/disparities-pregnancy-related-deaths/infographic.html

Fraze TK, et al. Prevalence of Screening for Food Insecurity, Housing Instability, Utility Needs, Transportation Needs, and Interpersonal Violence by US Physician Practices and Hospitals. *JAMA Network Open*. 2019; doi:10.1001/jamanetworkopen.2019.11514

Medicaid Non-Emergency Medical Transportation: Overview and Key Issues in Medicaid Expansion Waivers. Kaiser Family Foundation. Accessed June 22, 2021. https://www.kff.org/medicaid/issue-brief/medicaid-non-emergency-medical-transportation-overview-and-key-issues-in-medicaid-expansion-waivers/

Non-Emergency Medical Transportation. Center for Medicare and Medicaid Services. Published 2020. Accessed June 22, 2021. https://www.cms.gov/Medicare-Medicaid-Coordination/Fraud-Prevention/Medicaid-Integrity-Program/Education/Non-Emergency-Medical-Transport

About Chronic Diseases. Centers for Disease Control and Prevention. Accessed June 22, 2021. https://www.cdc.gov/chronicdisease/about/index.htm

Gundersen C, et al. Food insecurity and health outcomes. *Health Affairs*. 2015; doi:10.1377/hlthaff.2015.0645

Berkowitz SA, et al. Food insecurity, healthcare utilization, and high cost: A longitudinal cohort study. *American Journal of Managed Care*. 2018;24:399-404.

Food Insecurity. *Public Health Reports*. 2016; doi:10.1177/0033354916664154

Downer S, et al. Food is medicine: Actions to integrate food and nutrition into healthcare. *BMJ*. 2020; doi:10.1136/bmj.m2482

Taylor L. Housing and Health: An overview of the literature. *Health Affairs*. doi: 10.1377/hpb20180313.396577

Katch H. Medicaid Can Partner with Housing Providers and Others to Address Enrollees' Social Needs. Center on Budget and Policy Priorities. Accessed June 22, 2021. https://www.cbpp.org/research/health/medicaid-can-partner-with-housing-providers-and-others-to-address-enrollees-social

Tong ST, et al. Clinician experiences with screening for social needs in primary care. *Journal of the American Board of Family Medicine*. 2018; doi:10.3122/jabfm.2018.03.170419

Chapter 2: Challenges faced by women of color

Penner, LA, et al. Reducing racial health care disparities: A social psychological analysis. *Policy insights from the behavioral and brain sciences*. 2014;1:204-212.

Virani SS, et al. Heart disease and stroke statistics—2021 update: a report from the American Heart Association. *Circulation*. 2021; doi:10.1161/CIR.0000000000000950

Melkonian SC, et al. Disparities in cancer incidence and trends among American Indians and Alaska Natives in the United States, 2010-2015. *Cancer Epidemiology and Prevention Biomarkers*. 2019;28:1604-1611.

Notice of Retraction and Replacement: "Health Care Disparity and State-Specific Pregnancy-Related Mortality in the United States, 2005-2014." (Moaddab A, et al.) *Obstetrics & Gynecology*. 2018; doi:10.1097/AOG.0000000000002523

Pregnancy mortality surveillance system. Centers for Disease Control and Prevention. Accessed June 24, 2021. https://www.cdc.gov/reproductivehealth/maternal-mortality/pregnancy-mortality-surveillance-system.htm

National Diabetes Statistics Report, 2020. Centers for Disease Control and Prevention. https://www.cdc.gov/diabetes/pdfs/data/statistics/national-diabetes-statistics-report.pdf

Heart MY, et al. Historical trauma among Indigenous Peoples of the Americas: concepts, research, and clinical considerations. *Journal of Psychoactive Drugs*. 2011; doi:10.1080/02791072.2011.628913

Current Population Survey, 2020: Annual Social and Economic Supplement. U.S. Census Bureau. Accessed July 01, 2021. https://www.census.gov/data/tables/time-series/demo/income-poverty/cps-hi/hi.html

Chapter 3: Special considerations: Sexual and gender minority women

Burkhalter JE, et al. The National LGBT Cancer Action Plan: A White Paper of the 2014 National Summit on Cancer in the LGBT Communities. *LGBT Health*. 2016; doi:10.1089/lgbt.2015.0118

Bruessow D, et al. The Welcoming Environment. In: The GLMA Handbook on LGBT Health, Volume 2, 211-222. Praeger; 2019.

Bruessow DM. Keeping up with LGBT health: Why it matters to your patients. *Journal of the American Academy of Physician Assistants*. 2011;24:14.

Healthy People 2010 Companion Document for Lesbian, Gay, Bisexual and Transgender (LGBT) Health. Gay and Lesbian Medical Association; 2001.

Solarz Al. Lesbian Health: Current assessment and directions for the future. The National Academies Press; 1999. doi:10.17226/6109

Collecting Sexual Orientation and Gender Identity Data in Electronic Health Records: Workshop Summary. The National Academies Press; 2013. doi:10.17226/18260

The Health of Lesbian, Gay, Bisexual and Transgender (LGBT) People: Building a Foundation for Better Understanding. The National Academies Press; 2011. doi:10.17226/13128

James SE, et al. The Report of the 2015 U.S. Transgender Survey. National Center for Transgender Equality; 2016. https://transequality.org/sites/default/files/docs/usts/USTS-Full-Report-Dec17.pdf

Olson KR, et al. Mental health of transgender children who are supported in their identities. *Pediatrics*. 2016; doi:137(3):e20153223

Ryan C, et al. Family acceptance in adolescence and the health of LGBT young adults. *Journal of Child and Adolescent Psychiatric Nursing*. 2010;23:205-213.

Chapter 4: Is Google your first responder?

Hallyburton A, et al. Gender and online health information seeking: A five survey meta-analysis. *Journal of Consumer Health on the Internet*. 2014; doi.org/10.1080/15398285.2014.902268

Online Health Information: Is It Reliable? National Institute on Aging. Accessed Feb. 10, 2022. https://www.nia.nih.gov/health/

online-health-information-it-reliable#where.

Bidmon S, et al. Gender differences in searching for health information on the internet and the virtual patient-physician relationship in Germany: Exploratory results on how men and women differ and why. *Journal of Medical Internet Research*. 2015; doi:10.2196/jmir.4127

Maslen S, et al. "You can explore it more online": a qualitative study on Australian women's use of online health and medical information. *BMC Health Services Research*. 2018; doi.org/10.1186/s12913-018-3749-7

Domain requirements: .gov. Accessed Feb. 10, 2022. https://home.dotgov.gov/registration/requirements/#:~:text=Only%20U.S.%2D-based%20government%20and,government%20or%20a%20state%20government

Fox S, et al. Information Triage. Pew Research Center. Accessed Feb. 10, 2022. https://www.pewresearch.org/internet/2013/01/15/information-triage/

Canelario DM, et al. Completeness, accuracy, and readability of Wikipedia as a reference for patient medication information. *Journal of the American Pharmacists Association*. 2017; doi.org/10.1016/j.japh.2016.12.063

Hints 2017: Women and Health Information Seeking. National Partnership for Women & Families. Accessed Feb. 10, 2022. https://www.nationalpartnership.org/our-work/resources/health-care/hints-2017-women-and-health-info-seeking.pdf

Chapter 5: Who are clinicians? They're not just physicians

Definition of health care provider. Cornell Law School. Accessed Sep. 8, 2021. https://www.law.cornell.edu/cfr/text/29/825.125

Sex, Race and Ethnic Diversity of U.S., Health Occupations (2011-2015). U.S. Department of Health and Human Services. Accessed Sep. 8, 2021. https://bhw.hrsa.gov/sites/default/files/bureau-health-workforce/data-research/diversity-us-health-occupations.pdf

State Practice Environment. American Association of Nurse Practitioners. Accessed Sep. 8, 2021. https://www.aanp.org/advocacy/state/state-practice-environment

DNP Fact Sheet. American Association of Colleges of Nursing. Accessed Sep. 8, 2021. https://www.aacnnursing.org/News-Information/Fact-Sheets/DNP-Fact-Sheet

NONPF DNP Statement May 2018. National Organization of Nurse Practitioner Faculties (NONPF). Accessed Sep. 8, 2021. https://www.nonpf.org/news/400012/NONPF-DNP-Statement-May-2018.htm

Bowie BH, et al. The DNP degree: Are we producing the graduates we intended? *Journal of Nursing Administration*. 2019; doi:10.1097/NNA.0000000000000751

Edwards NE, et al. The impact of the role of doctor of nursing practice nurses on healthcare and leadership. *Medical Research Archives*. 2018; doi:10.18103/mra.v6i4.1734

DNP Education. American Association of Colleges of Nursing. Accessed Sep. 8, 2021. https://www.aacnnursing.org/Nursing-Education-Programs/DNP-Education

Nurse Practitioner Role Grows to More Than 270,000. American Association of Nurse Practitioners. Accessed Sep. 8, 2021. https://www.aanp.org/news-feed/nurse-practitioner-role-continues-to-grow-to-meet-primary-care-provider-shortages-and-patient-demands

Can I See a Nurse Practitioner Instead of a Doctor? Cedars-Sinai. Accessed Sep. 8, 2021. https://www.cedars-sinai.org/blog/difference-nurse-practitioner-vs-doctor.html

Chapter 6: Finding the right clinician

Ammenwerth E, et al. Adult patient access to electronic health records. Cochrane Database of Systematic Reviews. https://www.cochranelibrary.com. 2021. doi: 10.1002/14651858.CD012707.pub2

Alsan M, et al. Does Diversity Matter for Health? Experimental Evidence from Oakland. National Bureau of Economic Research. 2018. https://www.nber.org/system/files/working_papers/w24787/w24787.pdf

Prasad T, et al. Is patient-physician gender concordance related to the quality of patient care experiences? *Journal of General Internal Medicine*. 2021; doi: 10.1007/s11606-020-06411-y

Chapter 7: Shared decision making and you

Epstein NE, et al. 'Unnecessary' spinal surgery: A prospective 1-year study of one surgeon's experience. *Surgical Neurology International*. 2011;2:83.

Centers of Excellence: Walmart, Inc. Catalyst for Payment Reform. https://www.catalyze.org/product/centers-of-excellence-walmart-employer/

Riddle DL, et al. Use of a validated algorithm

to judge the appropriateness of total knee arthroplasty in the United States: A multicenter longitudinal cohort study. 2014. *Arthritis & Rheumatology.* 2014; doi:10.1002/art.38685

Shared Decision Making. National Cancer Institute. https://www.cancer.gov/publications/dictionaries/cancer-terms/def/shared-decision-making

Hargraves I, et al. Shared decision making: The need for patient-clinician conversation, not just information. *Health Affairs.* 2016; doi:10.1377/hlthaff.2015.1354

Cameron KA, et al. Gender disparities in health and healthcare use among older adults. *Journal of Women's Health (Larchmt).* 2010; doi:10.1089/jwh.2009.1701

Borkhoff CM, et al. Influence of patients' gender on informed decision making regarding total knee arthroplasty. *Arthritis Care & Research.* 2013; doi:10.1002/acr.21970

Frosch DL, et al. Authoritarian physicians and patients' fear of being labeled 'difficult' among key obstacles to shared decision making. *Health Affairs.* 2012; doi:10.1377/hlthaff.2011.0576

Patient decision aids. The Ottawa Hospital Research Institute. https://decisionaid.ohri.ca

Gaskin DJ, et al. Potential role of cost and quality of life in treatment decisions for arthritis-related knee pain in African American and Latina women. *Arthritis Care & Research.* 2020; doi:10.1002/acr.23903

Shared Decision Making Tool. Movement is Life. https://www.movementislifecaucus.com/shared-decision-tool/

Chapter 8: Telemedicine: Getting the most out of your care

Telehealth: Defining 21st Century Care. American Telemedicine Association. Accessed May 30, 2021. https://www.americantelemed.org/resource/why-telemedicine/

Bhaskar S, et al. Telemedicine across the globe-position paper from the COVID-19 pandemic health system resilience program (reprogram) international consortium (part 1). Front Public Health. 2020; doi:10.3389/fpubh.2020.556720

Bokol, AJ. Exploring the adoption of telemedicine and virtual software for care of outpatients during and after COVID-19 pandemic. Irish Journal of Medical Science. 2021; doi:10.1007/s11845-020-02299-z

Breen GM, et al. An evolutionary examination of telemedicine: a health and computer-mediated communication perspec-

tive. Social work in public health. 2010; doi:10.1080/19371910902911206

About Telehealth. Center for Connected Health Policy. Accessed June 1, 2021. https://www.cchpca.org

Marin, A. Telemedicine takes center stage in the era of COVID-19. *Science.* 2020; doi:10.1126/science.370.6517.731

Patel, M, et al. Trends in outpatient care delivery and telemedicine during the COVID-19 pandemic in the U.S. *JAMA Internal Medicine.* 2020; doi:10.1001/jamainternmed.2020.5928

Tuckson, RV, et al. Telehealth. *New England Journal of Medicine.* 2017; doi: 10.1056/nejmsr1503323

Chapter 9: Urgent care versus the emergency department

Allen L, et al. (2021). The impact of urgent care centers on nonemergent emergency department visits. *Health Services Research,* 2021; doi:10.1111/1475-6773.13631

Agarwal AK, et al. Online ratings of the patient experience: Emergency departments versus urgent care centers. *Annals of Emergency Medicine,* 2019; doi:10.1016/j.annemergmed.2018.09.029

Buttorff C, et al. Comparison of definitions for identifying urgent care centers in health insurance claims. *Health Services and Outcomes Research Methodology.* 2021; doi:10.1007/s10742-020-00224-6

Carroll G, et al. Examination of EMS decision making in determining suitability of patient diversion to urgent care centers. *Healthcare.* 2019; doi:10.3390/healthcare7010024

Chou SC, et al. Insurance status and access to urgent primary care follow-up after an emergency department visit in 2016. *Annals of Emergency Medicine,* 2018; doi:10.1016/j.annemergmed.2017.08.045

Coster JE, et al. Why do people choose emergency and urgent care services? A rapid review utilizing a systematic literature search and narrative synthesis. *Academic Emergency Medicine.* 2017; doi:10.1111/acem.13220

Ho V, et al. Comparing utilization and costs of care in freestanding emergency departments, hospital emergency departments, and urgent care centers. *Annals of Emergency Medicine.* 2017; doi:10.1016/j.annemergmed.2016.12.006

Lowthian JA, et al. Why older patients of lower clinical urgency choose to attend the emergency department. *Internal Medicine Journal.*

2013; doi:10.1111/j.1445-5994.2012.02842.x

Mnatzaganian G, et al. Sex disparities in the assessment and outcomes of chest pain presentations in emergency departments. *Heart*. 2020; doi:10.1136/heartjnl-2019-315667

Rhodes KV, et al. "Patients who can't get an appointment go to the ER": Access to specialty care for publicly insured children. *Annals of Emergency Medicine*. 2013; doi:10.1016/j.annemergmed.2012.10.030

Siegfried I, et al. Adult emergency department referrals from urgent care centers. *American Journal of Emergency Medicine*. 2019; doi:10.1016/j.ajem.2019.01.029

Timmins L, et al. Pathways to reduced emergency department and urgent care center use: Lessons from the comprehensive primary care initiative. *Health Services Research*. 2020; doi:10.1111/1475-6773.13579

Ward C, et al. Urgent care as intermediary care: How inbound and outbound transport can enhance care of community-based pediatric emergencies. *Clinical Pediatric Emergency Medicine*. 2017; doi:10.1016/j.cpem.2017.02.002

Weinick R, et al. Urgent care centers in the US: Findings from a national survey. *BMC Health Services Research*. 2009; doi:10.1186/1472-6963-9-79

PART 2 Common conditions impacting women

Chapter 10: ACL tears

Musahl V, et al. Anterior cruciate ligament tear. *New England Journal of Medicine*. 2019; doi:10.1056/NEJMcp1805931

Spindler KP, et al. Clinical practice. Anterior cruciate ligament tear. *New England Journal of Medicine*. 2008; doi:10.1056/NEJMco0804745

Taylor JB, et al. Evaluation of the effectiveness of anterior cruciate ligament injury prevention programme training components: A systematic review and meta-analysis. *British Journal of Sports Medicine*. 2015; doi:10.1136/bjsports-2013-092358

Dos'Santos T, et al. The effect of training interventions on change of direction biomechanics associated with increased anterior cruciate ligament loading: A scoping review. *Sports Medicine*. 2019; doi:10/1007/s40279-019-01171-0

Mahapatra P, et al. Anterior cruciate ligament repair: Past, present and future. *Journal of*

Experimental Orthopaedics. 2018; doi:10.1186/s40634-018-0136-6

Cimino F, et al. Anterior cruciate ligament injury: Diagnosis, management, and prevention. *American Family Physician*. 2010;82:917. https://pubmed.ncbi.nlm.nih.gov/20949884/. Accessed January 14, 2021.

Truong LK, et al. Psychological, social and contextual factors across recovery stages following a sport-related knee injury: A scoping review. *British Journal of Sports Medicine*. 2020; doi:10.1136/bjsports-2019-101206

Chapter 11: Anemia

De Benoist B, et al. Worldwide Prevalence of Anaemia 1993-2005. WHO Global Database on Anaemia Geneva, World Health Organization, 2008. Accessed Jan. 3, 2021. https://apps.who.int/iris/bitstream/handle/10665/43894/9789241596657_eng.pdf?ua=1

Iron Fact Sheet for Consumers. National Institutes of Health Office of Dietary Supplements. 2019. Accessed Jan. 3, 2021. https://ods.od.nih.gov/factsheets/Iron-Consumer/

Okam MM, et al. Iron supplementation, response in iron-deficiency anemia: Analysis of five trials. *American Journal of Medicine*. 2017; doi:10.1016/j.amjmed.2017.03.045

Achebe MM, et al. How I treat anemia in pregnancy: Iron, cobalamin, and folate. *Blood*. 2017; doi.org/10.1182/blood-2016-08-672246

Auerbach M, et al. A prospective, multi-center, randomized comparison of iron isomaltoside 1000 versus iron sucrose in patients with iron deficiency anemia; the FERWON-IDA trial. *American Journal of Hematology*. 2019; doi:10.1002/ajh.2556

Crider KS, et al. Folic acid food fortification — its history, effect, concerns, and future directions. *Nutrients*. 2011; doi: 10.3390/nu3030370

Chapter 12: Anxiety

American Psychological Association. What's the Difference between Stress and Anxiety? 2020. https://www.apa.org/topics/stress/anxiety-difference.

American Psychiatric Association. *Diagnostic and Statistical Manual of Mental Disorders*. 5th ed. American Psychiatric Association; 2013.

Hofmann SG, et al. Cross-cultural aspects of anxiety disorders. *Current Psychiatry Reports*. 2014; doi:10.1007/s11920-014-0450-3

Kessler RC, et al. Twelve-month and lifetime

prevalence and lifetime morbid risk of anxiety and mood disorders in the United States. *International Journal of Methods in Psychiatric Research.* 2012; doi:10.1002/mpr.1359

Lewis-Fernandez R, et al. *Depression & Anxiety.* 2010; doi:10.1176/foc.9.3.foc351

Li SH, et al. Why are women so vulnerable to anxiety, trauma-related and stress-related disorders? The potential role of sex hormones. *Lancet Psychiatry.* 2017; doi:10.1016/S2215-0366(16)30358-3

McLean CP, et al. Brave men and timid women? A review of the gender differences in fear and anxiety. *Clinical Psychology Review.* 2009; doi:10.1016/j.cpr.2009.05.003

McLean CP, et al. Gender differences in anxiety disorders: Prevalence, course of illness, comorbidity and burden of illness. *Journal of Psychiatric Research.* 2011; doi:10.1016/j.jpsychires.2011.03.006

Nillni YI, et al. The impact of the menstrual cycle and underlying hormones in anxiety and PTSD: What do we know and where do we go from here? *Current Psychiatry Reports.* 2021; doi:10.1007/s11920-020-01221-9

Schuch, FB, et al. Physical activity protects from incident anxiety: A meta-analysis of prospective cohort studies. *Depression & Anxiety.* 2019; doi:10.1002/da.22915

Chapter 13: Asthma

Aaron SD, et al. Reevaluation of diagnosis in adults with physician-diagnosed asthma. *Journal of the American Medical Association.* 2017; doi:10.1001/jama.2016.19627

Beasley R, et al. Risk factors for asthma: Is prevention possible? *Lancet.* 2015; doi: 10.1016/S0140-6736(15)00156-7

Cloutier MM, et al. Managing asthma in adolescents and adults: 2020 asthma guideline update from the National Asthma Education and Prevention Program. *Journal of the American Medical Association.* 2020; doi:10.1001/jama.2020.21974

Global Initiative for Asthma (GINA). Global Strategy for Asthma Management and Prevention: 2021 GINA Report. Accessed May 2021. ginasthma.org/reports

Triebner K, et al. Menopause as a predictor of new-onset asthma: A longitudinal Northern European population study. *Journal of Allergy and Clinical Immunology.* 2016; doi: 10.1016/j.jaci.2015.08.019

Middleton PG, et al. ERS/TSANZ Task Force Statement on the management of reproduction and pregnancy in women with airways diseases. *European Respiratory Journal.* 2020; doi: 10.1183/13993003.01208-2019

Kogevinas M, et al. Exposure to substances in the workplace and new-onset asthma: an international prospective population-based study (ECRHS-II). *Lancet.* 2007; doi:10.1016/S0140-6736(07)61164-7

Chapter 14: Blood Clots

Greenall, R. Prevention, diagnosis and treatment of venous thromboembolism. *Nursing Older People.* 2017; doi:10.7748/nop.2017.e872

Heit JA, et al. The epidemiology of venous thromboembolism. *Journal of Thrombosis and Thrombolysis.* 2016; doi:10.1007/s11239-015-1311-6

Phang M, et al. Diet and thrombosis risk: Nutrients for prevention of thrombotic disease. *Seminars in Thrombosis and Hemostasis.* 2011; doi:10.1055/s-0031-1273084

Wells PS, et al. Treatment of venous thromboembolism. *Journal of the American Medical Association.* 2014. doi:10.1001/jama.2014.65

Gialeraki A, et al. (2018). Oral contraceptives and HRT risk of thrombosis. *Clinical and Applied Thrombosis/Hemostasis.* 2018. doi:10.1177/1076029616683802

McLean K, et al. Venous thromboembolism and stroke in pregnancy. *Hematology American Society of Hematology Education Program.* 2016. doi:10.1182/asheducation-2016.1.243

Thacker HL. Hormone therapy and the risk of venous thromboembolism. In: *The Cleveland Clinic: Current Clinical Medicine.* 2nd ed. Saunders Elsevier; 2009, 1233 ff.

Canonico M, et al. Obesity and risk of venous thromboembolism among postmenopausal women: Differential impact of hormone therapy by route of estrogen administration. The ESTHER Study. *Journal of Thrombosis and Haemostasis: JTH.* 2006; doi:10.1111/j.1538-7836.2006.01933.x

Vinogradova Y, et al. (2019). Use of hormone replacement therapy and risk of venous thromboembolism: nested case-control studies using the QResearch and CPRD databases. *BMJ (Clinical Research Ed.).* 2019; doi.org/10.1136/bmj.k4810

Speaking of Women's Health. Accessed December 27, 2020. http://www.speakingofwomenshealth.com

Chapter 15: Breast lump

Bleicher, RJ. Management of the palpable breast mass. In: *Diseases of the Breast*, 4th ed. Wolters Kluwer/Lippincott Williams & Wilkins; 2010, Ch. 4.

Morrow M, et al. The evaluation of breast masses in women younger than forty years of age. *Surgery*. 1998;124:634.

Roth MY, et al. Self-detection remains a key method of breast cancer detection for U.S. Women. *Journal of Women's Health*. 2011;20:1135.

Van Dam PA, et al. Palpable solid breast masses: retrospective single- and multimodality evaluation of 201 lesions. *Radiology*. 1988;166:435.

Chapter 16: Breast cancer

Breast Cancer Treatment Information. Moffitt Cancer Center. https://moffitt.org/cancers/breast-cancer/ Accessed Jan 1, 2021.

Breast cancer: Introduction. Cancer.Net Doctor-Approved Patient Information from ASCO. Accessed Jan. 1, 2021. https://www.cancer.net/cancer-types/breast-cancer/introduction

Breast cancer: Types of Treatment. Cancer.Net Doctor-Approved Patient Information from ASCO. Accessed Jan. 1, 2021. https://www.cancer.net/cancer-types/breast-cancer/types-treatment

Can I Lower My Risk of Breast Cancer? American Cancer Society. Accessed Jan. 15, 2021. https://www.cancer.org/cancer/breast-cancer/risk-and-prevention/can-i-lower-my-risk.html

Breast Cancer Risk and Prevention. American Cancer Society. Accessed Jan. 15, 2021. https://www.cancer.org/cancer/breast-cancer/risk-and-prevention.html

Monticciolo DL, et al. Breast cancer screening in women at higher-than-average risk: Recommendations from the ACR. *Journal of the American College of Radiology*. 2018; doi:10.1016/j.jacr.2017.11.034

Chapter 17: Carpal tunnel syndrome

Cranford CS, et al. Carpal tunnel syndrome. *Journal of the American Academy of Orthopaedic Surgeons*. 2007; doi:10.5435/00124635-200709000-00004

Wipperman J, et al. Carpal tunnel syndrome: Diagnosis and management. *American Family Physician*. 2016;94(12):993-999.

Dammers JW, et al. Injection with methylprednisolone in patients with the carpal tunnel syndrome: A randomised double blind trial testing three different doses. *Journal of Neurology*. 2006; doi:10.1007/s00415-005-0062-2

Padua L, et al. Systematic review of pregnancy-related carpal tunnel syndrome. *Muscle & Nerve*. 2010; doi:10.1002/mus.21910

Mondelli M, et al. Prospective study of positive factors for improvement of carpal tunnel syndrome in pregnant women. *Muscle & Nerve*. 2007; doi:10.1002/mus.20863

Ekman-Ordeberg G, et al. Carpal tunnel syndrome in pregnancy. A prospective study. *Acta Obstetricia et Gynecologica Scandinavica*. 1987; doi:10.3109/00016348709020753

Thomson JG. Diagnosis and treatment of carpal tunnel syndrome. *The Lancet Neurology*. 2017; doi:10.1016/s1474-4422(17)30059-5

Chapter 18: Cervical cancer

Siegel RL, et al. Cancer statistics, 2021. *CA: A Cancer Journal for Clinicians*. 2021; doi:10.3322/caac.21654

Schiffman M, et al. Human papillomavirus and cervical cancer. *Lancet*. 2007; doi:10.1016/S0140-6736(07)61416-0

Brianti P, et al. Review of HPV-related diseases and cancers. *New Microbiologica*. 2017;40(2):80.

Drolet M, et al. Population-level impact and herd effects following the introduction of human papillomavirus vaccination programmes: Updated systematic review and meta-analysis. *Lancet*. 2019; doi:10.1016/S0140-6736(19)30298-3

Gee J, et al. Quadrivalent HPV vaccine safety review and safety monitoring plans for nine-valent HPV vaccine in the United States. *Human Vaccines & Immunotherapeutics*. 2016; doi:10.1080/21645515.2016.1168952

Ramirez PT, et al. Minimally invasive versus abdominal radical hysterectomy for cervical cancer. *New England Journal of Medicine*. 2018; doi:10.1056/NEJMoa1806395

Singh GK. Rural-urban trends and patterns in cervical cancer mortality, incidence, stage, and survival in the United States, 1950-2008. *Journal of Community Health*. 2012; doi:10.1007/s10900-011-9439-6

Cohen PA, et al. Cervical cancer. *Lancet*. 2019; doi:10.1016/S0140-6736(18)32470-X

Chapter 19: Chronic fatigue syndrome (myalgic encephalomyelitis)

Institute of Medicine. *Beyond Myalgic Encephalomyelitis/Chronic Fatigue Syndrome: Redefining an Illness*. The National Academies

Press; 2015. doi:10.17226/19012

Lim EJ, et al. Systematic review and meta-analysis of the prevalence of chronic fatigue syndrome/myalgic encephalomyelitis (CFS/ME). *Journal of Translational Medicine.* 2020; doi:10.1186/s12967-020-02269-0

Jason LA. How science can stigmatize: The case of chronic fatigue syndrome. *Journal of Chronic Fatigue Syndrome.* 2007; doi:10.3109/10573320802092146

ME/CFS Road to Diagnosis Survey. Chronic Fatigue and Immune Dysfunction Syndrome (CFIDS) Association of America. 2014. https://solvecfs.org/wp-content/uploads/2014/01/IOM_RoadtoDiagnosisSurveyReport.pdf

Maixner W, et al. Overlapping chronic pain conditions: Implications for diagnosis and classification. *Journal of Pain.* 2016; doi: 10.1016/j.jpain.2016.06.002

Cortes Rivera M, et al. Myalgic encephalomyelitis/chronic fatigue syndrome: A comprehensive review. *Diagnostics.* 2019; doi:10.3390/diagnostics9030091

Komaroff AL, et al. Will COVID-19 lead to myalgic encephalomyelitis/chronic fatigue syndrome? *Frontiers in Medicine.* 2021; doi:10.3389/fmed.2020.606824

Twisk FNM, et al. A review on cognitive behavioral therapy (CBT) and graded exercise therapy (GET) in myalgic encephalomyelitis (ME)/chronic fatigue syndrome (CFS): CBT/GET is not only ineffective and not evidence-based, but also potentially harmful for many patients with ME/CFS. *Neuro Endocrinology Letters,* 2009;30(3):284-299.

Oka T, et al. Changes in fatigue, autonomic functions, and blood biomarkers due to sitting isometric yoga in patients with chronic fatigue syndrome. *BioPsychoSocial Medicine.* 2018; doi:10.1186/s13030-018-0123-2

Chapter 20: Chronic obstructive pulmonary disease

Chapman KR, et al. Gender bias in the diagnosis of COPD. *Chest.* 2001; doi:10.1378/chest.119.6.1691

Demeo DL, et al. Women manifest more severe COPD symptoms across the life course. *International Journal of Chronic Obstructive Pulmonary Disease.* 2018; doi:10.2147/COPD.S160270

Jenkins CR, et al. Improving the management of COPD in women. *Chest.* 2017; doi: 10.1016/j.chest.2016.10.031

Silverman EK, et al. Gender-related differences in severe, early-onset chronic obstructive pulmonary disease. *American Journal of Respiratory and Critical Care Medicine.* 2000; doi:10.1164/ajrccm.162.6.2003112

Sorheim IC, et al. Gender differences in COPD: Are women more susceptible to smoking effects than men? *Thorax.* 2010; doi:10.1136/thx.2009.122002

Chapter 21: Colorectal cancer

Wolf AMD, et al. Colorectal cancer screening for average-risk adults: 2018 guideline update from the American Cancer Society. *CA: A Cancer Journal for Clinicians.* 2018; doi:10.3322/caac.21457

US Preventive Services Task Force. Screening for colorectal cancer. US Preventive Services Task Force Recommendation Statement. *Journal of the American Medical Association,* 2021;325(19). doi:10.1001/jama.2021.6238

National Cancer Institute. Physician Data Query (PDQ). Colorectal Cancer Prevention. 2019. Accessed Feb. 06, 2020. https://www.cancer.gov/types/colorectal/patient/colorectal-prevention-pdq

Surveillance, Epidemiology, and End Results (SEER) Program. SEER*Stat Database: Populations - Total U.S. (1969-2018). Linked to County Attributes - Total U.S., 1969-2018 Counties, National Cancer Institute, DCCPS, Surveillance Research Program. December 2019. http://www.seer.cancer.gov

Aykan NF. Red meat and colorectal cancer. *Oncology Reviews.* 2015; doi:10.4081/oncol.2015.288

Klampfer L. Vitamin D and colon cancer. *World Journal of Gastrointestinal Oncology.* 2014. doi:10.4251/wjgo.v6.i11.430

American Cancer Society. Cancer Statistics Center. Accessed January 31, 2021. http://cancerstatisticscenter.cancer.org

Chapter 22: Constipation

Rao SSC, et al. Diagnosis and management of chronic constipation in adults. *Nature Reviews Gastroenterology & Hepatology.* 2016; doi: 10.1038/nrgastro.2016.53

Sharma A, et al. Constipation: Pathophysiology and current therapeutic approaches. *Handbook of Experimental Pharmacology.* 2017; doi:10.1007/164_2016_111

Chey SW, et al. Exploratory comparative effectiveness trial of green kiwifruit, psyllium, or prunes in US patients with chronic constipation. *American Journal of Gastroenterology*. 2021; doi:10.14309/ajg.0000000000001149

Rao SSC, et al. ANMS-ESNM position paper and consensus guidelines on biofeedback therapy for anorectal disorders. *Neurogastroenterology and Motility*. 2015; doi:10.1111/nmo.12520

Deutsch JK, et al. Complementary and alternative medicine for functional gastrointestinal disorders. *American Journal of Gastroenterology*. 2020; doi:10.14309/ajg.0000000000000539

Moosavi S, et al. Irritable bowel syndrome in pregnancy. *American Journal of Gastroenterology*. 2021; doi:10.14309/ajg.0000000000001124

Klein MC, et al. Relationship of episiotomy to perineal trauma and morbidity, sexual dysfunction, and pelvic floor relaxation. *American Journal of Obstetrics and Gynecology*. 1994; doi:10.1016/0002-9378(94)90070-1

Chapter 23: Dementia

Alzheimer's Association. 2021 Alzheimer's Disease Facts and Figures. Accessed March 6, 2021. https://www.alz.org/alzheimers-dementia/facts-figures

National Institute on Aging. What Causes Alzheimer's Disease? Accessed March 5, 2021. https://www.nia.nih.gov/health/what-causes-alzheimers-disease

Livingston G, et al. Dementia prevention, intervention, and care: 2020 report of the Lancet Commission. *Lancet*. 2020; doi:10.1016/S0140-6736(20)30367-6

Ralph SJ, et al. Increased all-cause mortality by antipsychotic drugs: Updated review and meta-analysis in dementia and general mental health care. *Journal of Alzheimer's Disease Reports*. 2018; doi:10.3233/ADR-170042

Mielke MM, et al. Sex and gender in Alzheimer's disease — Does it matter? *Alzheimer's & Dementia*. 2018; doi:10.1016/j.jalz.2018.08.003

Xiong C, et al. Sex and gender differences in caregiving burden experienced by family caregivers of persons with dementia: A systematic review. *PLoS One*. 2020; doi:10.1371/journal.pone.0231848

Chapter 24: Depression

American Psychiatric Association. *Diagnostic and Statistical Manual of Mental Disorders*. 5th ed. American Psychiatric Association; 2013. doi:10.1176/appi.books.9780890425596

Eid RS, et al. Sex differences in depression: Insights from clinical and preclinical studies. *Progress in Neurobiology*. 2019; doi:10.1016/j.pneurobio.2019.01.006

Grigoriadis S, et al. Gender issues in depression. *Annals of Clinical Psychiatry*. 2007; doi:10.1080/10401230701653294

Kandola A, et al. Physical activity and depression: Towards understanding the antidepressant mechanisms of physical activity. *Neuroscience & Biobehavioral Reviews*. 2019; doi:10.1016/j.neubiorev.2019.09.040

Kellner C, et al. Unipolar major depression in adults: Indications for and efficacy of electroconvulsive therapy (ECT). Accessed April 6, 2021. http://www.uptodate.com

Krishnan R. Unipolar depression in adults: epidemiology, pathogenesis, and neurobiology. Accessed April 6, 2021. http://www.uptodate.com

Muñoz RF, et al. Major depression can be prevented. *American Psychologist*. 2012; doi:10.1037/a0027666

Chapter 25: Diabetes

Centers for Disease Control and Prevention. What is diabetes? Accessed Jan. 25, 2021. https://www.cdc.gov/diabetes/basics/diabetes.html

National Institute of Diabetes and Digestive and Kidney Diseases. Risk Factors for Type 2 Diabetes. Accessed Jan. 25, 2021. https://www.niddk.nih.gov/health-information/diabetes/overview/risk-factors-type-2-diabetes

American College of Obstetricians and Gynecologists. Gestational Diabetes. Accessed Jan. 25, 2021. https://www.acog.org/womens-health/faqs/gestational-diabetes

Evert AB, et al. Nutrition therapy for adults with diabetes or prediabetes: A consensus report. *Diabetes Care*. 2019; doi:10.2337/dci19-0014

Knowler WC, et al. Reduction in the incidence of type 2 diabetes with lifestyle intervention or metformin. *New England Journal of Medicine*. 2002; doi:10.1056/NEJMoa012512

Centers for Disease Control and Prevention. Diabetes and Women. Accessed January 25, 2021. https://www.cdc.gov/diabetes/library/features/diabetes-and-women.html

Chapter 26: Diverticulitis

Feuerstein JD, et al. Diverticulosis and diverticulitis. *Mayo Clinic Proceedings*. 2016; doi:10.1016/j.mayocp.2016.03.012

Jacobs DO. Diverticulitis. *New England Journal of Medicine*. 2007; doi:10.1056/nejmcp073228

Cohan JN. Uncomplicated sigmoid

diverticulitis. *Diseases of the Colon & Rectum.* 2018; doi:10.1097/DCR.0000000000001200

Aldoori WH, et al. A prospective study of alcohol, smoking, caffeine, and the risk of symptomatic diverticular disease in men. *Annals of Epidemiology.* 1992; doi:10.1016/1047-2797(94)00109-7

Böhm SK. Risk factors for diverticulosis, diverticulitis, diverticular perforation, and bleeding: A plea for more subtle history taking. *Viszeralmedizin.* 2015; doi:10.1159/000381867

Desai M, et al. Antibiotics versus no antibiotics for acute uncomplicated diverticulitis: A systematic review and meta-analysis. *Diseases of the Colon & Rectum.* 2019; doi:10.1097/DCR.0000000000001324

Van de Wall BJM, et al. Surgery versus conservative management for recurrent and ongoing left-sided diverticulitis (DIRECT trial): an open-label, multicentre, randomised controlled trial. *Lancet Gastroenterology & Hepatology.* 2017; doi:10.1016/S2468-1253(16)30109-1

Santos A, et al. Comparing laparoscopic elective sigmoid resection with conservative treatment in improving quality of life of patients with diverticulitis: The laparoscopic elective sigmoid resection following diverticulitis (LASER) randomized clinical trial. *JAMA Surgery.* 2020; doi:10.1001/jamasurg.2020.5151

Chapter 27: Endometrial cancer

ACOG Practice Bulletin No. 147: Lynch syndrome. *Obstetrics & Gynecology.* 2014; doi:10.1097/01.AOG.0000456325.50739.72

Aubrey C, et al. Endometrial cancer and bariatric surgery: A scoping review. *Surgery for Obesity and Related Diseases.* 2019; doi:10.1016/j.soard.2018.12.003

DeSantis CE, et al. Cancer statistics for African Americans. *CA: A Cancer Journal for Clinicians.* 2019; doi:10.3322/caac.21555

Doll KM, et al. Assessment of prediagnostic experiences of Black women with endometrial cancer in the United States. *JAMA Network Open.* 2020; doi:10.1001/jamanetworkopen.2020.4954

Kim MK, et al. Comparison of dilatation & curettage and endometrial aspiration biopsy accuracy in patients treated with high-dose oral progestin plus levonorgestrel intrauterine system for early-stage endometrial cancer. *Gynecologic Oncology.* 2013; doi:10.1016/j.ygyno.2013.06.035

Lewin SN, et al. Comparative performance of the 2009 International Federation of Gynecology and Obstetrics' staging system for uterine corpus cancer. *Obstetrics & Gynecology.* 2010; doi:10.1097/AOG.0b013e3181f39849

Clarke MA, et al. Hysterectomy-corrected uterine corpus cancer incidence trends and differences in relative survival reveal racial disparities and rising rates of nonendometrioid cancers. *Journal of Clinical Oncology.* 2019; doi:10.1200/JCO.19.00151

Chapter 28: Endometriosis

Taylor HS, et al. Chapter 32: Endometriosis. In: *Speroff's Clinical Gynecologic Endocrinology and Infertility.* 9th ed. Wolters Kluwer; 2020.

Llarena NC, et al. Fertility preservation in women with endometriosis. *Clinical Medicine Insights: Reproductive Health.* 2019; doi:10.1177/1179558119873386

Schwartz K, et al. The role of pharmacotherapy in the treatment of endometriosis across the lifespan. *Expert Opinion on Pharmacotherapy.* 2020; doi:10.1080/14656566.2020.1738386

Hur C, et al. (2021). Robotic treatment of bowel endometriosis. *Best Practice & Research. Clinical Obstetrics & Gynaecology.* 2021; doi:10.1016/j.bpobgyn.2020.05.012

Bulun SE, et al. (2019). Endometriosis. *Endocrine Reviews.* 2019; doi:10.1210/er.2018-00242

Marsh EE, et al. Endometriosis in premenarcheal girls who do not have an associated obstructive anomaly. *Fertility and Sterility.* 2005; doi:10.1016/j.fertnstert.2004.08.025

Hsu AL, et al. (2010). Invasive and noninvasive methods for the diagnosis of endometriosis. *Clinical Obstetrics and Gynecology.* 2010; doi:10.1097/GRF.0b013e3181db7ce8

Chapter 29: Fibromyalgia

Yunus MB. Fibromyalgia and overlapping disorders: The unifying concept of central sensitivity syndromes. *Seminars in Arthritis and Rheumatism.* 2007; doi:10.1016/j.semarthrit.2006.12.009

Martinez-Martinez LA, et al. Sympathetic nervous system dysfunction in fibromyalgia, chronic fatigue syndrome, irritable bowel syndrome, and interstitial cystitis: a review of case-control studies. *Journal of Clinical Rheumatology.* 2014; doi:10.1097/RHU.0000000000000089

Gota CE. What you can do for your fibromyalgia patient. *Cleveland Clinic Journal of Medicine.* 2018; doi:10.3949/ccjm.85gr.18002

Gota CE, et al. The impact of depressive and bipolar

symptoms on socioeconomic status, core symptoms, function and severity of fibromyalgia. *International Journal of Rheumatic Diseases.* 2015; doi:10.1111/1756-185X.12603

Arnold LM, et al. Fibromyalgia and chronic pain syndromes: A white paper detailing current challenges in the field. *Clinical Journal of Pain.* 2016; doi:10.1097/AJP.0000000000000354

Macfarlane GJ, et al. EULAR revised recommendations for the management of fibromyalgia. *Annals of the Rheumatic Diseases.* 2017; doi:10.1136/annrheumdis-2016-209724

Hauser W, et al. Fibromyalgia as a chronic primary pain syndrome: Issues to discuss. *Pain.* 2019; doi:10.1097/j.pain.0000000000001686

Martinez-Lavin M. Fibromyalgia as a sympathetically maintained pain syndrome. *Current Pain and Headaches Report.* 2004; doi:10.1007/s11916-996-0012-4

Arnold LM, et al. Fibromyalgia syndrome: practical strategies for improving diagnosis and patient outcomes. *American Journal of Medicine.* doi:10.1016/j.amjmed.2010.04.001

Wolfe F, et al. The development of fibromyalgia - I: Examination of rates and predictors in patients with rheumatoid arthritis (RA). *Pain.*2011; doi:10.1016/j.pain.2010.09.027

Yunus MB. Gender differences in fibromyalgia and other related syndromes. *Journal of Gender Specific Medicine.* 2002;5(2):42-47.

Chapter 30: Gastroesophageal reflux disease

Clarett D, et al. Gastroesophageal reflux disease (GERD). *Missouri Medicine.* 2018;115(3): 214-8.

Schizas D, et al. LINX reflux management system to bridge the "treatment gap" in gastroesophageal reflux disease: a systematic review of 35 studies. *World Journal of Clinical Cases.* 2020; doi:10.12998/wjcc.v8.i2.294

Ka Seng Thong B, et al. Proton pump inhibitors and fracture risk: A review of current evidence and mechanisms involved. *International Journal of Environmental Research and Public Health.* 2019; doi:10.3390/ijerph16091571

Nochaiwong S, et al. The association between proton pump inhibitor use and risk of adverse kidney outcomes: A systematic review and meta-analysis. *Nephrology, Dialysis, Transplantation.* 2018; doi:10.1093/ndt/gfw470

Su B, et al. Use of impedance planimetry (Endoflip) in Foregut Surgery Practice: Experience of more than 400 cases. *Journal of the American College of Surgeons.* 2020; doi:10.1016/j.jamcollsurg.2020.02.017

Chapter 31: Hand and thumb pain

Giladi AM, et al. Corticosteroid or hyaluronic acid injections to the carpometacarpal joint of the thumb joint are associated with early complications after subsequent surgery. *Journal of Hand Surgery, European Volume.* 2018; doi:10.1177/1753193418805391

Armstrong AL, et al. The prevalence of degenerative arthritis of the base of the thumb in post-menopausal women. *Journal of Hand Surgery.* 1994; doi:10.1016/0266-7681(94)90085-x

Jónsson H, et al. Hypermobility associated with osteoarthritis of the thumb base: a clinical and radiological subset of hand osteoarthritis. *Annals of Rheumatic Diseases.* 1996; doi:10.1136/ard.55.8.540

Wolf JM, et al. Male and female differences in musculoskeletal disease. *Journal of the American Academy of Orthopaedic Surgeons.* 2015; doi:10.5435/JAAOS-D-14-00020

Chapter 32: Heart disease

Facts about women and heart disease. American Heart Association. Accessed Dec. 12, 2021. https://www.goredforwomen.org/en/about-heart-disease-in-women/facts

Mozaffarian D, et al. Heart disease and stroke statistics—2015 update: A report from the American Heart Association. *Circulation.* 2015; doi:10.1161/CIR.0000000000000152

Balfour Jr PC, et al. Cardiovascular disease in Hispanics/Latinos in the United States. *Journal of Latina/o Psychology.* 2016; doi:10.1037/lat0000056

Volgman AS, et al. Atherosclerotic cardiovascular disease in South Asians in the United States: Epidemiology, risk factors, and treatments: A scientific statement from the American Heart Association. *Circulation.* 2018; doi: 10.1161/CIR.0000000000000580

Spatz ES, et al. The variation in recovery: Role of gender on outcomes of young AMI patients (VIRGO) classification system: A taxonomy for young women with acute myocardial infarction. *Circulation.* 2015; doi:10.1161/circulationaha.115.016502

Honigberg MC, et al. Heart failure in women with hypertensive disorders of pregnancy: insights from the cardiovascular disease in Norway project. *Hypertension.* 2020; doi:10.1161/hypertensionaha.120.15654

Gunderson EP, et al. Gestational diabetes history and glucose tolerance after pregnancy associated with coronary artery calcium in women during midlife: the CARDIA study. *Circulation*. 2021; doi: 10.1161/circulationaha.120.047320

Gianturco L, et al. Cardiovascular and autoimmune diseases in females: the role of microvasculature and dysfunctional endothelium. *Atherosclerosis*. 2015; doi:10.1016/j.atherosclerosis.2015.03.044

Garcia M, et al. Cardiovascular disease in women: Clinical perspectives. *Circulation Research*. 2016; doi:10.1161/circresaha.116.307547

Lichtman JH, et al. Sex differences in the presentation and perception of symptoms among young patients with myocardial infarction: Evidence from the VIRGO study (variation in recovery: role of gender on outcomes of young AMI patients). *Circulation*. 2018; doi:10.1161/circulationaha.117.031650

McSweeney JC, et al. Cluster analysis of women's prodromal and acute myocardial infarction symptoms by race and other characteristics. *The Journal of Cardiovascular Nursing*. 2010; doi:10.1097/JCN.0b013e3181cfba15

Chapter 33: Hepatitis C

Bradley H, et al. Hepatitis C Virus prevalence in 50 U.S. states and D.C. by sex, birth cohort, and race: 2013-2016. *Hepatology Communications*. 2020; doi:10.1002/hep4.1457

Kaplan DE. Hepatitis C virus. *Annals of Internal Medicine*. 2020; doi:10.7326/AITC202009010

Terrault NA, et al. Sexual transmission of hepatitis C virus among monogamous heterosexual couples: The HCV partners study. *Hepatology*. 2013; doi:10.1002/hep.26164

Benova L, et al. Vertical transmission of hepatitis C virus: Systematic review and meta-analysis. *Clinical Infectious Diseases*. 2014; doi:10.1093/cid/ciu447

Bravi F, et al. Coffee reduces risk for hepatocellular carcinoma: An updated meta-analysis. *Clinical Gastroenterology & Hepatology*. 2013; doi:10.1016/j.cgh.2013.04.039

Chen CM, et al. Alcohol and hepatitis C mortality among males and females in the United States: A life table analysis. *Alcoholism, Clinical and Experimental Research*. 2007; doi:10.1111/j.1530-0277.2006.00304.x

Chapter 34: High blood pressure

Whelton PK, et al. ACC/AHA/AAPA/ABC/ACPM/AGS/APhA/ASH/ASPC/NMA/APCNA Guideline for the prevention, detection, evaluation, and management of high blood pressure in adults. A Report of the American College of Cardiology/American Heart Association Task Force on Clinical Practice Guidelines. *Hypertension* 2018; doi:10.1161/HYP.0000000000000065

Julius S, et al. Feasibility of treating prehypertension with an angiotensin-receptor blocker. *New England Journal of Medicine*. 2006; doi:10.1056/NEJMoa060838

Brook RD, et al. Beyond medications and diet: Alternative approaches to lowering blood pressure: A scientific statement from the American Heart Association. *Hypertension*. 2013; doi:1161/HYP.)b13e318293645f

Rasmussen CB, et al. Dietary supplements and hypertension: Potential benefits and precautions. Journal of Clinical Hypertension. 2012; doi:10.1111/j.1751-7176.2012.00642.x

Virani SS, et al. Heart Disease and Stroke Statistics 2021 Update. *Circulation*. 2021; doi:10.1161/CIR.0000000000000950

Ji H, et al. Sex differences in blood pressure associations with cardiovascular outcomes. *Circulation*. 2021; doi:10.1161/circulationaha.120.049360.

Cameron N, et al. Pre-pregnancy hypertension among women in rural and urban areas of the United States. *Journal of the American College of Cardiology*. 2020; doi:10.1016/j.jacc2020.09601

Chapter 35: High cholesterol

American Heart Association. What is Cholesterol? Accessed Apr 9, 2021. https://www.heart.org/en/health-topics/cholesterol/about-cholesterol

Grundy SM, et al. 2018 AHA / ACC/ AACVPR/ AAPA/ ABC/ ACPM/ ADA/ AGS/ APhA/ ASPC/NLA/PCNA Guideline on the Management of Blood Cholesterol: A report of the American College of Cardiology/American Heart Association Task Force on Clinical Practice Guidelines. *Circulation*. 2019; doi:10.1161/CIR.0000000000000625

National Center for Complementary and Integrative Health. High Cholesterol and Natural Products: What the Science Says. Accessed Apr 9, 2021. www.nccih.nih.gov/health/providers/digest/high-cholesterol-and-natural-products-science

Palmisano BT, et al. Role of estrogens in the regulation of liver lipid metabolism. *Advances in Experimental Medicine and Biology*. 2017; doi:10.1007/978-3-319-70178-3_12

Peters SAE, et al. Sex differences in the prevalence of, and trends in, cardiovascular risk factors, treatment, and control in the United States, 2001 to 2016. *Circulation.* 2019; doi:10.1161/circulationaha.118.035550

Chapter 36: Hip osteoarthritis
Cowie JG, et al. Return to work and sports after total hip replacement. *Archives of Orthopaedic and Trauma Surgery.* 2013; doi: 10.1007/s00402-013-1700-2

Chapter 37: Hip labral tear
Frank JM, et al. Prevalence of femoroacetabular impingement imaging findings in asymptomatic volunteers: A systematic review. *Arthroscopy.* 2015; doi:10.1016/j.arthro.2014.11.042
Hammoud S, et al. The recognition and evaluation of patterns of compensatory injury in patients with mechanical hip pain. *Sports Health.* 2014; doi:10.1177/1941738114522201
Lynch TS, et al. Outcomes after diagnostic hip injection. *Arthroscopy.* 2016; doi:10.1016/j.arthro.2016.02.027
Nepple JJ, et al. Decision-making in the borderline hip. *Sports Medicine and Arthroscopy Review.* 2021; doi:10.1097/JSA.0000000000000298
Pascual-Garrido C, et al. The pattern of acetabular cartilage wear is hip morphology-dependent and patient demographic-dependent. *Clinical Orthopaedics and Related Research.* 2019; doi:10.1097/CORR.0000000000000649
Saadat AA, et al. Prevalence of generalized ligamentous laxity in patients undergoing hip arthroscopy: A prospective study of patients' clinical presentation, physical examination, intraoperative findings, and surgical procedures. *American Journal of Sports Medicine.* 2019; doi:10.1177/0363546518825246
Maldonado DR, et al. Achieving successful outcomes of hip arthroscopy in the setting of generalized ligamentous laxity with labral preservation and appropriate capsular management: A propensity matched controlled study. *American Journal of Sports Medicine.* 2020; doi:10.1177/0363546520914604
Zimmerer A, et al. Osteoarthrosis, advanced age and female sex are risk factors for inferior outcomes after hip arthroscopy and labral debridement for FAI Syndrome - Case Series with minimum 10-year follow-up. *Arthroscopy.* 2021; doi:10.1016/j.arthro.2021.01.024
Yacovelli S, et al. High risk of conversion to THA after femoroacetabular osteoplasty for femoroacetabular impingement in patients older than 40 years. *Clinical Orthopaedics and Related Research.* 2020; doi:10.1097/CORR.0000000000001554

Chapter 38: Irritable bowel syndrome
Billings W, et al. Potential benefit with complementary and alternative medicine in irritable bowel syndrome: A systematic review and meta-analysis. *Clinical Gastroenterology and Hepatology.* 2020; doi:10.1016/j.cgh.2020.09.035
Ford AC, et al. Irritable bowel syndrome. *Lancet.* 2020; doi:10.1016/S0140-6736(20)31548-8
Harer KN, et al. Irritable bowel syndrome: Food as a friend or foe? *Gastroenterology Clinics of North America.* 2021; doi:10.1016/j.gtc.2020.10.002
Kim YS, et al. Sex-gender differences in irritable bowel syndrome. *Journal of Neurogastroenterology and Motility.* 2018; doi:10.5056/jnm18082
Irritable Bowel Syndrome. Mayo Clinic. Accessed March 7, 2021. https://www.mayoclinic.org/diseases-conditions/irritable-bowel-syndrome/symptoms-causes/syc-20360016

Chapter 39: Knee osteoarthritis
Marcum ZA, et al. Recognizing the risks of chronic nonsteroidal anti-inflammatory drug use in older adults. *Annals of Long-Term Care.* 2010;18(9):24-27.
Pan Q, et al. Characterization of osteoarthritic human knees indicates potential sex differences. *Biology of Sex Differences.* 2016; doi:10.1186/s13293-016-0080-z
Hanna FS, et al. Women have increased rates of cartilage loss and progression of cartilage defects at the knee than men: A gender study of adults without clinical knee osteoarthritis. *Menopause.* 2009; doi:10.1097/gme.0b013e318198e30e
Packiasabapathy S, et al. Gender, genetics, and analgesia: Understanding the differences in response to pain relief. *Journal of Pain Research.* 2018; doi:10.2147/JPR.S94650
O'Connor MI. Implant survival, knee function, and pain relief after TKA: Are there differences between men and women? *Clinical Orthopaedics and Related Research.* 2011; doi:10.1007/s11999-011-1782-5

Chapter 40: Knee meniscus injury
Abdülkadir Sari, et al. Meniscus tears and review of the literature. In: *Meniscus of the Knee: Function, Pathology and Management.* IntechOpen; 2019,

Ch. 1. doi:10.5772/intechopen.82009

Brindle T, et al. The meniscus: Review of basic principles with application to surgery and rehabilitation. *Journal of Athletic Training.* 2001;36(2):160-169

Raj MA, et al. Knee meniscal tears. In: StatPearls. StatPearls Publishing; 2020. https://www.ncbi.nlm.nih.gov/books/NBK431067/

Chapter 41: Low back pain

Chou R, et al. Diagnosis and treatment of low back pain: a joint clinical practice guideline from the American College of Physicians and the American Pain Society. *Annals of Internal Medicine.* 2007; doi:10.7326/0003-4819-147-7-200710020-00006

Barr KP, et al. Low back pain. In: *Physical Medicine and Rehabilitation.* 4th ed. Elsevier Saunders; 2011, 871-912.

Choi B, et al. Exercises for prevention of recurrences of low-back pain. *Cochrane Database of Systematic Reviews.* 2010; doi:10.1002/14651858

Calcium and vitamin D requirements. *American Bone Health.* https://americanbonehealth.org/nutrition/how-much-calcium-and-vitamin-d-do-you-need/

Qaseem A, et al. Noninvasive treatments for acute, subacute, and chronic low back pain: a clinical practice guideline from the American College of Physicians. *Annals of Internal Medicine.* 2017; doi:10.7326/M16-2367

Tuakli-Wosornu YA, et al. Lumbar intradiscal platelet-rich plasma (PRP) injections: a prospective, double-blind, randomized controlled study. PM&R. 2016; doi:10.1016/j.pmrj.2015.08.010

National Institutes of Health. Low back pain. Accessed Dec. 13, 2020. https://www.ninds.nih.gov/Disorders/All-Disorders/Back-Pain-Information-Page

Wang Yx, et al. Menopause as a potential cause for higher prevalence of low back pain in women than in age-matched men. *Journal of Orthopaedic Translation.* doi:10.1016/j.jot.2016.05.012

Chapter 42: Lung cancer

Dang TP, et al. Cancer of the lung. In: *DeVita, Hellman, and Rosenberg's Cancer: Principles & Practice of Oncology.* 8th ed. Lippincott, Williams & Wilkins; 2008, Ch. 37.

ASCO-SEP Medical Oncology Self-Evaluation Program. 6th ed. ASCO (American Society of Clinical Oncology) University; 2018.

Centers for Disease Control and Prevention. Current cigarette smoking among adults in the United States. Accessed Apr 10, 2021. https://www.cdc.gov/tobacco/data_statistics/fact_sheets/adult_data/cig_smoking/index.htm

Smith K, et al. Household air pollution from solid cookfuels and its effects on health. In: *Injury Prevention and Environmental Health.* 3rd ed. The International Bank for Reconstruction and Development / The World Bank; 2017. doi:10.1596/978-1-4648-0522-6_ch7

World Health Organization. Household air pollution and health. Accessed Mar 31, 2021. https://www.who.int/news-room/fact-sheets/detail/household-air-pollution-and-health

Torres-Duque C, et al. Biomass fuels and respiratory diseases: A review of the evidence. *Proceedings of the American Thoracic Society.* 2008; doi:10.1513/pats.200707-100RP

Connellan SJ. Lung diseases associated with hydrocarbon exposure. *Respiratory Medicine.* 2017; doi:10.1016/j.rmed.2017.03.021

Callaghan RC, et al. Marijuana use and risk of lung cancer: A 40-year cohort study. *Cancer Causes & Control.* 2013; doi:10.1007/s10552-013-0259-0

American Cancer Society. Cancer Prevention and Early Detection Facts and Figures 2021. Accessed Mar. 27, 2021. https://www.cancer.org/research/cancer-facts-statistics/all-cancer-facts-figures/cancer-facts-figures-2021.html

Shankar A, et al. Environmental and occupational determinants of lung cancer. *Translational Lung Cancer Research.* 2019; doi:10.21037/tlcr.2019.03.05

Fehringer G, et al. Alcohol and lung cancer risk among never smokers: A pooled analysis from the international lung cancer consortium and the SYNERGY study. *International Journal of Cancer.* 2017; doi:10.1002/ijc.30618

Chao C, et al. Alcoholic beverage intake and risk of lung cancer: the California Men's Health Study. *Cancer Epidemiology, Biomarkers & Prevention.* 2008; doi:10.1158/1055-9965.EPI-08-0410

Troche J, et al. The association between alcohol consumption and lung carcinoma by histological subtype. *American Journal of Epidemiology.* 2016; doi:10.1093/aje/kwv170

Gallicchio L, et al. Carotenoids and the risk of developing lung cancer: A systematic review. *American Journal of Clinical Nutrition.* 2008; doi:10.1093/ajcn/88.2.372

Karp DD, et al. Randomized, double-blind, placebo-controlled, phase III chemoprevention trial of selenium supplementation in patients with resected stage I non-small-cell lung cancer: ECOG 5597. *Journal of Clinical Oncology*. 2013; doi:10.1200/JCO.2013.49.2173

Andersen AH, et al. Do patients with lung cancer benefit from physical exercise? *Acta Oncologica*. 2011; doi:10.3109/0284186X.2010.529461

Bade BC, et al. Increasing physical activity and exercise in lung cancer: reviewing safety, benefits, and application. *Journal of Thoracic Oncology*. 2015; doi:10.1097/JTO.0000000000000536 Erratum in: *Journal of Thoracic Oncology*. 2015; doi: 10.1097/JTO.0000000000000681

Rutkowska A, et al. Exercise training in patients with non-small cell lung cancer during in-hospital chemotherapy treatment: A randomized controlled trial. *Journal of Cardiopulmonary Rehabilitation and Prevention*. 2019; doi:10.1097/HCR.0000000000000410

John Hopkins Medicine. Lung Cancer Risk Factors. Accessed Apr. 2, 2021. https://www.hopkinsmedicine.org/health/conditions-and-diseases/lung-cancer/lung-cancer-risk-factors

American Cancer Society. Lung cancer. Accessed Apr 2, 2021. https://www.cancer.org/cancer/lung-cancer.html

American Cancer Society. Cancer Facts & Figures for African Americans 2019-2021. Accessed Mar 27, 2021. https://www.cancer.org/content/dam/cancer-org/research/cancer-facts-and-statistics/cancer-facts-and-figures-for-african-americans/cancer-facts-and-figures-for-african-americans-2019-2021.pdf

American Lung Association. Trends in Lung Cancer Morbidity and Mortality. Accessed Apr 10, 2021. https://www.lung.org/getmedia/ee16997d-52d9-4d05-a967-ddf90d209922/lc-trend-report.pdf.pdf

Chapter 43: Lupus

Gronhagen CM, et al. Cutaneous lupus erythematosus and the association with systemic lupus erythematosus: a population-based cohort of 1088 patients in Sweden. *British Journal of Dermatology*. 2011; doi: 10.1111/j.1365-2133.2011.10272

Drenkard, C. and S.S. Lim. Update on lupus epidemiology: advancing health disparities research through the study of minority populations. *Current Opinion in Rheumatology*. 2019; doi:10.1097/BOR.0000000000000646

Alunno A, et al. Diet in rheumatoid arthritis versus systemic lupus erythematosus: Any differences? *Nutrients*. 2021; doi:10.3390/nu13030772

Chowdhary VR. Broad concepts in management of systemic lupus erythematosus. *Mayo Clinic Proceedings*. 2017; doi:10.1016/j.mayocp.2017.02.007

Ruiz-Irastorza G, et al. Update on antimalarials and systemic lupus erythematosus. *Current Opinion in Rheumatology*. 2020; doi:10.1097/BOR.0000000000000743

Navarrete-Navarrete N, et al. Efficacy of cognitive behavioural therapy for the treatment of chronic stress in patients with lupus erythematosus: A randomized controlled trial. *Psychotherapy and Psychosomatics*. 2010; doi:10.1159/000276370

Duffy EM, et al. The clinical effect of dietary supplementation with omega-3 fish oils and/or copper in systemic lupus erythematosus. *Journal of Rheumatology*. 2004;31:1551.

Clowse, M.E., Grotegut C. Racial and ethnic disparities in the pregnancies of women with systemic lupus erythematosus. *Arthritis Care & Research (Hoboken)*. 2016; doi:10.1002/acr.22847

Chapter 44: Migraines

Ashina M. Migraine. *New England Journal of Medicine*. 2020; doi:10.1056/NEJMra1915327

Biller J. *Practical Neurology*. 5th ed. Lippincott Williams & Wilikins; 2017.

Mauskop A. Nonmedication, alternative, and complementary treatments for migraine. *Continuum: Lifelong Learning in Neurology*. 2012; doi:10.1212/01.CON.0000418643.24408.40

Najib U, et al. Neuromodulation therapies for headache. *Practical Neurology*. 2019. Accessed Dec 28, 2020. https://practicalneurology.com/articles/2019-may/neuromodulation-therapies-for-headache/pdf

Schwedt TJ. Preventative therapy of migraine. *Continuum: Lifelong Learning in Neurology*. 2018; doi:10.1212/CON.0000000000000635

Vargas BB. Acute Treatment of Migraine. *Continuum: Lifelong Learning in Neurology*. 2018; doi:10.1212/CON.0000000000000639

Chapter 45: Multiple sclerosis

McGinley MP, et al. Diagnosis and treatment of multiple sclerosis: A review. *Journal of the American Medical Association*. 2021; doi:10.1001/jama.2020.26858

Lublin FD, et al. Defining the clinical course of multiple sclerosis: The 2013 revisions. *Neurology*. 2014; doi:10.1212/WNL.0000000000000560

Brown JWL, et al. Association of initial disease-modifying therapy with later conversion to secondary progressive MS. *Journal of the American Medical Association.* 2019; doi:10.1001/jama.2018.20588

Hauser SL, et al. Treatment of multiple sclerosis: A review. *American Journal of Medicine.* 2020; doi:10.1016/j.amjmed.2020.05.049

Faissner S, et al. Progressive multiple sclerosis: from pathophysiology to therapeutic strategies. *Nature Reviews Drug Discovery.* 2019; doi:10.1038/s41573-019-0035-2

Stankiewicz JM, et al. An argument for broad use of high efficacy treatments in early multiple sclerosis. *Neurology Neuroimmunology & Neuroinflammation.* 2020; doi:10.1212/NXI.0000000000000636

Kalincik T, et al. Sex as a determinant of relapse incidence and progressive course of multiple sclerosis. *Brain.* 2013; doi:10.1093/brain/awt281

Ribbons KA, et al. Male sex is independently associated with faster disability accumulation in relapse-onset MS but not in primary progressive MS. *PLoS One.* 2015; doi:10.1371/journal.pone.0122686

Krysko KM, et al. Association between breastfeeding and postpartum multiple sclerosis relapses: A systematic review and meta-analysis. *JAMA Neurology.* 2020; doi:10.1001/jamaneurol.2019.4173

Chapter 46: Neck pain

Binder AI. Neck pain. *BMJ Clinical Evidence.* 2008;2008:1103. https://www.ncbi.nlm.nih.gov/pmc/articles/PMC2907992/

Chen X, et al. Modifiable individual and work-related factors associated with neck pain in 740 office workers: A cross-sectional study. *Brazilian Journal of Physical Therapy.* 2018; doi:10.1016/j.bjpt.2018.03.003

Chapter 47: Nonalcoholic fatty liver disease

Han MAT, et al. Diversity in NAFLD: A review of manifestation of nonalcoholic fatty liver disease in different ethnicities globally. *Journal of Clinical and Translational Hepatology.* 2021; doi:10.14218/JCTH.2020.00082

Kumar R, et al. Non-alcoholic fatty liver disease: Growing burden, adverse outcomes and associations. *Journal of Clinical and Translational Hepatology.* 2020; doi:10.14218/JCTH.2019.00051

Lonardo A, et al. NAFLD in some common endocrine diseases: Prevalence, pathophysiology, and principles of diagnosis and management.

International Journal of Molecular Science. 2019; doi:10.3390/ijms20112841

Sarkar M, et al. NAFLD cirrhosis is rising among childbearing women and is the most common cause of cirrhosis in pregnancy. *Clinical Gastroenterology and Hepatology.* 2021; doi:10.1016/j.cgh.2021.01.022

Sherif ZA, et al. Global epidemiology of nonalcoholic fatty liver disease and perspectives on US minority populations. *Digestive Diseases and Sciences.* 2016; doi:10.1007/s10620-016-4143-0

Summart U, et al. Gender differences in the prevalence of nonalcoholic fatty liver disease in the Northeast of Thailand: A population-based cross-sectional study. *F1000Research.* 2017; doi:10.12688/f1000research.12417.2

Younossi ZM, et al. From NAFLD to MAFLD: Implications of a premature change in terminology. *Hepatology.* 2020; doi:10.1002/hep.31420

Kwak MS, et al. Nonalcoholic fatty liver disease is associated with breast cancer in nonobese women. *Digestive and Liver Disease.* 2019; doi:10.1016/j.dld.2018.12.024

Allen AM, et al. Women with nonalcoholic fatty liver disease lose protection against cardiovascular disease: A longitudinal cohort study. *American Journal of Gastroenterology.* 2019; doi:10.14309/ajg.0000000000000401

Chapter 48: Obesity and metabolic syndrome

Cheung L, et al. Obesity Prevention Source. Harvard T. H. Chan. Accessed Dec. 16, 2021. www.hsph.harvard.edu/obesity-prevention-source

Centers for Disease Control and Prevention. Defining Adult Overweight and Obesity. 2017; https://www.cdc.gov/obesity/adult/defining.html

Hales C, et al. Prevalence of Obesity Among Adults: United States, 2017-2018. NCHS Data Brief. 2020; https://www.cdc.gov/nchs/data/databriefs/db360-h.pdf

Anekwe CV, et al. Socioeconomics of obesity. *Current Obesity Reports.* 2020; doi:10.1007/s13679-020-00398-7

Ali YS, Kelly C. How to Prevent Obesity. Verywell Health. Accessed Nov. 29, 2021. https://www.verywellhealth.com/obesity-prevention-4014175

Creagan ET. How do I control stress-induced weight gain? Mayo Clinic. Accessed Nov. 29, 2021. https://www.mayoclinic.org/healthy-lifestyle/stress-management/expert-answers/stress/faq-20058497

Tauqeer Z, et al. Obesity in women: Insights for the clinician. *Journal of Women's Health (Larchmt).* 2018; doi:10.1089/jwh.2016.6196

Palmisano GL, et al. Life adverse experiences in relation with obesity and binge eating disorder: A systematic review. *Journal of Behavioral Addictions.* 2016; doi:10.1556/2006.5.2016.018

Kyle T, et al. Prescription Medications & Weight Gain - What You Need to Know. Obesity Action Coalition. 2013; https://www.obesityaction.org/resources/prescription-medications-weight-gain/

King K, et al. Weight Bias: Does it Affect Men and Women Differently? Obesity Action Coalition. 2013; http://www.obesityaction.org/wp-content/uploads/Weight-Bias-in-Men-and-Women.pdf

Hales CM, et al. Prevalence of obesity and severe obesity among adults: United States, 2017–2018. National Center for Health Statistics. 2020. Accessed Dec. 16, 2021. www.cdc.gov/nchs/products/databriefs/db360.htm

Chapter 49: Osteoporosis

NIH Consensus Development Panel on Osteoporosis Prevention, Diagnosis, and Therapy. Osteoporosis prevention, diagnosis, and therapy. *JAMA.* 2001; doi:10.1001/jama.285.6.785

National Osteoporosis Foundation. Accessed May 11, 2021. https://www.nof.org/.

University of Sheffield, United Kingdom. FRAX Fracture Risk Assessment Tool. Accessed May 11, 2021. https://www.sheffield.ac.uk/FRAX/.

Weaver CM, et al. Nutrition and osteoporosis. In: *Primer on the Metabolic Bone Diseases and Disorders of Mineral Metabolism.* 8th ed. American Society for Bone and Mineral Research; 2013. doi:10.1002/9781118453926.ch42

Cosman F, et al. Clinician's guide to prevention and treatment of osteoporosis. *Osteoporosis International.* 2014; doi:10.1007/s00198-014-2794-2

Ross AC, et al. Dietary reference intakes for calcium and vitamin D. The National Academies Press; 2011. doi:10.17226/13050

Curry SJ, et al. Screening for osteoporosis to prevent fractures: US preventive services task force recommendation statement. *Journal of the American Medical Association.* 2018; doi:10.1001/jama.2018.7498

Centers for Disease Control and Prevention. STEADI – Older Adult Fall Prevention. Accessed May 11, 2021. https://www.cdc.gov/steadi/patient.html

2019 American Geriatrics Society Beers Criteria Update Expert Panel. American Geriatrics Society 2019 Updated AGS Beers Criteria for Potentially Inappropriate Medication Use in Older Adults. *Journal of American Geriatric Society.* 2019; doi:10.1111/jgs.15767

Gourlay ML, et al. Bone-density testing interval and transition to osteoporosis in older women. *New England Journal of Medicine.* 2012; doi:10.1056/NEJMoa1107142

Chapter 50: Ovarian cancer

American Cancer Society. Cancer Facts & Figures 2021. https://www.cancer.org/research/cancer-facts-statistics/all-cancer-facts-figures/cancer-facts-figures-2021.html

Howlader N, et al. Lifetime Risk (Percent) of Being Diagnosed with Cancer by Site and Race/Ethnicity; Males, 18 SEER Areas, 2012-2014. SEER Cancer Statistics Review, 1975-2014. April 2017. National Cancer Institute. https://seer.cancer.gov/csr/1975_2014/

Salvador S, et al. The fallopian tube: primary site of most pelvic high-grade serous carcinomas. *International Journal of Gynecological Cancer.* 2009; doi:10.1111/IGC.0b013e318199009c

Fleming GF, et al. Epithelial ovarian cancer. In: *Principles and Practice of Gynecologic Oncology.* 7th ed. Lippincott Williams & Wilkins; 2017.

Chapter 51: Painful sex

Bornstein J, et al. 2015 ISSVD, ISSWSH and IPPS consensus terminology and classification of persistent vulvar pain and vulvodynia. *Obstetrics and Gynecology.* 2016; doi:10.1097/AOG.0000000000001359

Goldstein AT, et al. *Female Sexual Pain Disorders: Evaluation and Management.* John Wiley & Sons Ltd.; 2020. doi:10.1002/9781119482598

Jahshan-Doukhy O, et al. Long-Term Efficacy of Physical Therapy for Localized Provoked Vulvodynia. *International Journal of Women's Health.* 2021; doi:10.2147/IJWH.S297389

Zolnoun D, et al. Patient perceptions of vulvar vibration therapy for refractory vulvar pain. *Sexual and Relationship Therapy.* 2008; doi:10.1080/14681990802411685

Pagano R, et al. Use of amitriptyline cream in the management of entry dyspareunia due to provoked vestibulodynia. *Journal of Lower Genital Tract Disease.* 2012; doi:10.1097/LGT.0b013e3182449bd6

Diomande I, et al. Subcutaneous botulinum toxin type A injections for provoked vestibulodynia:

a randomized placebo-controlled trial and exploratory subanalysis. *Archives of Gynecology and Obstetrics*. 2019; doi:10.1007/s00404-019-05043-w

Reed BD, et al. Treatment of vulvodynia with tricyclic antidepressants: efficacy and associated factors. *Journal of Lower Genital Tract Disease*. 2006; doi:10.1097/01.lgt.0000225899.75207.0a

Chapter 52: Pelvic inflammatory disease

Sufrin, CB et al. Neisseria gonorrhea and Chlamydia trachomatis screening at intrauterine device insertion and pelvic inflammatory disease. *Obstetrics and Gynecology*. 2012; doi:10.1097/aog.0b013e318273364c

Shafer MA, et al. Pelvic inflammatory disease in adolescent females. *Adolescent Medicine*. 1990;1:545.

Tarr ME, et al. Sexually transmitted infections in adolescent women. *Clinical Obstetrics and Gynecology*. 2008;51:306.

Sutton MY, et al. Trends in pelvic inflammatory disease hospital discharges and ambulatory visits, United States, 1985- 2001. *Sexually Transmitted Diseases*. 2005; doi:10.1097/01.olq.0000175375.60973.cb

Chapter 53: Pelvic organ prolapse

Barber MD, et al. Epidemiology and outcome assessment of pelvic organ prolapse. *International Urogynecology Journal*. 2013; doi:10.1007/s00192-013-2169-9

American College of Obstetricians and Gynecologists. Practice Bulletin No. 214: Pelvic Organ Prolapse. *Obstetrics & Gynecology*. 2019; doi:10.1097/AOG.0000000000003519

Haylen BT, et al. An International Urogynecological Association (IUGA)/International Continence Society (ICS) joint report on the terminology for female pelvic organ prolapse (POP). *International Urogynecology Journal*. 2016; doi:10.1007/s00192-015-2932-1

Bump RC, et al. The standardization of terminology of female pelvic organ prolapse and pelvic floor dysfunction. *American Journal of Obstetrics and Gynecology*. 1996; doi:10.1016/s0002-9378(96)70243-0

Walters MD, et al. *Urogynecology and Reconstructive Pelvic Surgery*. 4th ed. Saunders; 2014.

Chapter 54: Peripheral arterial disease

Mascarenhas JV, et al. Peripheral arterial disease. *Endocrinology and Metabolism Clinics of North America*. 2014; doi:10.1016/j.ecl.2013.09.003

Pollak AW. PAD in women: the ischemic continuum. *Current Atherosclerosis Reports*. 2015; doi:10.1007/s11883-015-0513-x

Firth C, et al. Discordant values in lower extremity physiologic studies predict increased cardiovascular risk. *Journal of American Heart Association*. 2020; doi:10.1161/JAHA.119.015398

Conte SM, et al. Peripheral arterial disease. *Heart, Lung and Circulation*. 2018; doi:10.1016/j.hlc.2017.10.014

Firnhaber JM, et al. Lower extremity peripheral artery disease: diagnosis and treatment. *American Family Physician*. 2019;99:362.

Chapter 55: Polycystic ovary syndrome

Raperport C, et al. The source of polycystic ovarian syndrome. *Clinical Medicine Insights: Reproductive Health*. 2019; doi:10.1177/1179558119871467

Osibogun O, et al. Polycystic ovary syndrome and cardiometabolic risk: Opportunities for cardiovascular disease prevention. *Trends in Cardiovascular Medicine*. 2020; doi:10.1016/j.tcm.2019.08.010

Barber TM, et al. Obesity and polycystic ovary syndrome. *Clinical Endocrinology*. 2021; doi:10.1111/cen.14421

Jiskoot G, et al. A three-component behavioural lifestyle program for preconceptional weight-loss in women with polycystic ovary syndrome (PCOS): A protocol for a randomized controlled trial. *Reproductive Health*. 2017; doi:10.1186/s12978-017-0295-4

Shishehgar F, et al. Does a restricted energy low glycemic index diet have a different effect on overweight women with or without polycystic ovary syndrome? *BMC Endocrine Disorders*. 2019; doi:10.1186/s12902-019-0420-1

Mackowiak K, et al. Dietary fiber as an important constituent of the diet. *Advances in Hygiene and Experimental Medicine*. 2016; doi:10.5604/17322693.1195842

Wright H. *The PCOS Diet Plan*. 2nd ed. Ten Speed Press; 2010.

Chaudhari AP, et al. Anxiety, depression, and quality of life in women with polycystic ovarian syndrome. *Indian Journal of Psychological Medicine*. 2018; doi:10.4103/IJPSYM.IJPSYM_561_17

Yildiz BO. Approach to the patient: Contraception in women with polycystic ovary syndrome. *The Journal of Clinical Endocrinology and Metabolism*. 2015; doi:10.1210/jc.2014-3196

Eunice Kennedy Shriver National Institute of Child Health and Human Development. Polycystic Ovary Fibrosis. Accessed Feb 15, 2021. http://

www.nichd.nih.gov/health/topics/factsheets/pcos

Chapter 56: Rheumatoid arthritis

Agca R, et al. EULAR recommendations for cardio-vascular disease risk management in patients with rheumatoid arthritis and other forms of inflammatory joint disorders: 2015/2016 update. *Annals of the Rheumatic Diseases.* 2017; doi:10.1136/annrheumdis-2016-209775

Peterson LS. Mayo Clinic Guide to Arthritis: Managing joint pain for an active life. Mayo Clinic; 2020.

Rheumatoid arthritis. Mayo Clinic. Accessed Apr. 15, 2021. https//www.mayoclinic.org/diseases-conditions/rheumatoid-arthritis/symptoms-causes/syc-20353648

Arthritis Foundation. Rheumatoid arthritis: Causes, symptoms, treatments and more. Accessed Apr. 15, 2021. https//www.arthritis.org/diseases/rheumatoid-arthritis

Singh JA, et al. 2015 American College of Rheumatology Guideline for the treatment of rheumatoid arthritis. *Arthritis Care & Research.* 2015; doi: 10.1002/acr.22783

Vermeer M, et al. Implementation of a treat-to-target strategy in very early rheumatoid arthritis: results of the Dutch Rheumatoid Arthritis Monitoring remission induction cohort study. *Arthritis & Rheumatism.* 2011; doi:10.1002/art.30494

Chapter 57: Shoulder pain

Bonsell S, et al. The relationship of age, gender, and degenerative changes observed on radiographs of the shoulder in asymptomatic individuals. *Journal of Bone and Joint Surgery.* 2000; doi:10.1302/0301-620X.82B8.10631

Friedman RJ, et al. Are age and patient gender associated with different rates and magnitudes of clinical improvement after reverse shoulder arthroplasty? *Clinical Orthopaedics and Related Research.* 2018; doi:10.1007/s11999.0000000000000270

Greenberg DL. Evaluation and treatment of shoulder pain. *Medical Clinics of North America.* 2014; doi:10.1016/j.mcna.2014.01.016

Hanvold TN, et al. Long periods with uninterrupted muscle activity related to neck and shoulder pain. IOS Press; 2012: doi:10.3233/WOR-2012-0494-2535

Kirsch Micheletti J, et al. Association between lifestyle and musculoskeletal pain: Cross-sectional study among 10,000 adults from the general working population. *BMC Musculoskeletal Disorders.* 2019; doi:10.1186/s12891-019-3002-5

Meroni R, et al. Shoulder disorders in female working-age population: A cross sectional study. *BMC Musculoskeletal Disorders.* 2014; doi:10.1186/1471-2474-15-118

Razmjou H, et al. Sex and gender disparity in pathology, disability, referral pattern, and wait time for surgery in workers with shoulder injury. *BMC Musculoskeletal Disorders.* 2016; doi:10.1186/s12891-016-1257-7

Sansone V, et al. Women performing repetitive work: Is there a difference in the prevalence of shoulder pain and pathology in supermarket cashiers compared to the general female population? *International Journal of Occupational Medicine and Environmental Health.* 2014; doi:10.2478/s13382-014-0292-6

Valencia C, et al. Stability of conditioned pain modulation in two musculoskeletal pain models: Investigating the influence of shoulder pain intensity and gender. *BMC Musculoskeletal Disorders.* 2013; doi:10.1186/1471-2474-14-182

Wong SE, et al. The effect of patient gender on outcomes after reverse total shoulder arthroplasty. *Journal of Shoulder and Elbow Surgery.* 2017; doi:10.1016/j.jse.2017.07.013

Chapter 58: Stroke

Saver JL. Time is brain – quantified. *Stroke.* 2005; doi:10.1161/01.STR.0000196957.55928.ab

Kleindorfer DO, et al. 2021 Guideline for the prevention of stroke in patients with stroke and transient ischemic attack: A guideline from the American Heart Association/American Stroke Association. *Stroke.* 2021; doi:10.1161/STR.0000000000000375

Flach C, et al. Risk and secondary prevention of stroke recurrence. *Stroke.* 2020; doi:10.1131/strokeaha.120.028992

Schurks M, et al. Migraine and cardiovascular disease: systematic review and meta-analysis. *British Medical Journal.* 2009; doi:10.1136/bmj.b3914

Demaerschalk BM, et al. Scientific rationale for the inclusion and exclusion criteria for intravenous alteplase in acute ischemic stroke. *Stroke.* 2015; doi:10.1161/STR.0000000000000086

Christensen H, et al. Stroke in women. *Continuum.* 2010; doi:10.1012/CON.0000000000000836

Powers WJ, et al. Stroke 2018 guidelines for the early management of patients with acute ischemic stroke. *Stroke.* 2018; doi: 10.1161/STR.0000000000000158

Carcel C, et al. Sex differences in treatment and outcome after stroke: Pooled analysis including 19,000 participants. *Neurology*. 2019; doi:10.1212/WNL.0000000000008615

Bruce SS, et al. Differences in diagnostic evaluation in women and men after acute ischemia stroke. *Journal of American Heart Association*. 2020; doi:10.1161/JAHA.119.015625

Kenmuir CL, et al. Cerebral venous sinus thrombosis in users of a hormonal vaginal ring. *Obstetrics and Gynecology*. 2015; doi:10.1097/AOG.0000000000000931

Chapter 59: Thyroid disease

Department of Health and Human Services, Office on Women's Health. Fact Sheet, Thyroid Disease. Accessed Mar. 27, 2021. www.womenshealth.gov/a-z-topics/thyroid-disease

The Endocrine Society. Hashimoto Disease. Accessed April 1, 2021. www.hormone.org/diseases-and-conditions/hashimoto-disease

American Thyroid Association. Graves Disease FAQs. Accessed Dec. 17, 2021. www.thyroid.org/graves-disease/

American Thyroid Association. Thyroid Nodule FAQs. Accessed April, 2021. www.thyroid.org/nodules.

Jonklaas J, et al. Guidelines for the treatment of hypothyroidism: Prepared by the American Thyroid Association Task Force on Thyroid Hormone Replacement. *Thyroid*. 2014; doi:10.1089/thy.2014.0028

Santini F, et al. Treatment of hypothyroid patients with L-thyroxine plus triiodothyronine sulfate. A phase II, open-label, single center, parallel groups study on therapeutic efficacy and tolerability. *Frontiers in Endocrinology*. 2019; doi:10.3389/fendo.2019.00826

Douglas RS, et al. Teprotumumab for the treatment of active thyroid eye disease. *New England Journal of Medicine*. 2020; doi:10.1056/NEJMoa1910434

Chapter 60: Urinary incontinence

Coyne KS, et al. National community prevalence of overactive bladder in the United States stratified by sex and age. *Urology*. 2011; doi:10.1016/j.urology.2010.08.039 Accessed 2/28/2021.

Wing RR, et al. Improving urinary incontinence in overweight and obese women through modest weight loss. *Obstetrics and Gynecology*. 2010; doi:10.1097/aog.0b013e3181e8fb60

Woodley SJ, et al. Pelvic floor muscle training for preventing and treating urinary and faecal incontinence in antenatal and postnatal women. *Cochrane Database of Systematic Reviews*. 2020; doi:10.1002/14651858.CD007471.pub4

Mobley D, et al. Smoking: Its Impact on Urologic Health. *Reviews in Urology*. 2015;17:220

Hershorn S, et al. A population-based study of urinary symptoms and incontinence: The Canadian urinary bladder survey. BJU International. 2008; doi:10.1111/j.1464-410X.2007.07198.x

Al-Shaikh G, et al. Pessary use in stress urinary incontinence: A review of advantages, complications, patient satisfaction, and quality of life. *International Journal of Women's Health*. 2018; doi:10.2147/IJWH.S152616

Thom DH, et al. Prevalence of postpartum urinary incontinence: A systematic review. *Acta Obstetricia et Gynecologica Scandinavica*. 2010; doi:10.3109/00016349.2010.526188

Chapter 61: Urinary tract infection

Foxman B. Epidemiology of urinary tract infections: incidence, morbidity, and economic costs. *American Journal of Medicine*. 2002; doi:10.1016/s0002-9343(02)01054-9

Beerepoot M, et al. Non-antibiotic prophylaxis for urinary tract infections. *Pathogens*. 2016; doi:10.3390/pathogens5020036

Lee BS, et al. Methenamine hippurate for preventing urinary tract infections. *Cochrane Database of Systematic Reviews*. 2012; doi:10.1002/14651858.CD003265.pub3

Ahmed H, et al. Long-term antibiotics for prevention of recurrent urinary tract infection in older adults: systematic review and meta-analysis of randomised trials. *BMJ Open*. 2017; doi:10.1136/bmjopen-2016-015233

Aydin A, et al. Recurrent urinary tract infections in women. *International Urogynecology Journal*. 2015; doi:10.1007/s00192-014-2569-5

Gupta K, et al. International clinical practice guidelines for the treatment of acute uncomplicated cystitis and pyelonephritis in women: A 2010 update by the Infectious Diseases Society of America and the European Society for Microbiology and Infectious Diseases. *Clinical Infectious Diseases*. 2011; doi:10.1093/cid/ciq257

Nicolle LE, et al. Clinical practice guideline for the management of asymptomatic bacteriuria: 2019 update by the Infectious Diseases Society of America. *Clinical Infectious Diseases*. 2019; doi:10.1093/cid/ciy1121. PMID: 30895288

Hooton TM, et al. A prospective study of risk factors for symptomatic urinary tract infection in young women. *New England Journal of Medicine.* 1996; doi:10.1056/NEJM199608153350703

Scholes D, et al. Risk factors for recurrent urinary tract infection in young women. *Journal of Infectious Diseases.* 2000; doi:10.1086/315827

Chapter 62: Uterine fibroids

Baird DD, et al. High cumulative incidence of uterine leiomyoma in black and white women: ultrasound evidence. *American Journal of Obstetrics and Gynecology.* 2003; doi:10.1067/mob.2003.99

Ghant MS, et al. An altered perception of normal: Understanding causes for treatment delay in women with symptomatic uterine fibroids. *Journal of Women's Health.* 2016; doi:10.1089/jwh.2015.5531

Hartmann KE, et al. Management of UTERINE FIBROIDS. Comparative Effectiveness Review No. 195. Agency for Healthcare Research and Quality; 2017; doi:10.23970/AHRQEPCCER195

Laughlin-Tommaso SK, et al. Moving toward individualized medicine for uterine leiomyomas. *Obstetrics and Gynecology.* 2018; doi:10.1097/AOG.0000000000002785

Laughlin-Tommaso SK, et al. Cardiovascular and metabolic morbidity after hysterectomy with ovarian conservation: A cohort study. *Menopause.* 2018; doi:10.1097/GME.0000000000001043

Stewart EA. *Uterine Fibroids: The Complete Guide.* Johns Hopkins University Press; 2007.

Stewart EA. Clinical practice. Uterine fibroids. *New England Journal of Medicine.* 2015; doi:10.1056/NEJMcp1411029

Stewart EA, et al. Moving beyond reflexive and prophylactic gynecologic surgery. *Mayo Clinic Proceedings.* 2021; doi:10.1016/j.mayocp.2020.05.012

Wallace K, et al. Comparative effectiveness of hysterectomy versus myomectomy on one-year health-related quality of life in women with uterine fibroids. *Fertility and Sterility.* 2020; doi:10.1016/j.fertnstert.2019.10.028

Wise LA, et al. Epidemiology of uterine fibroids: From menarche to menopause. *Clinical Obstetrics and Gynecology.* 2016; doi:10.1097/GRF.0000000000000164

Chapter 63: Vaginal bleeding (abnormal)

Munro MG, et al. The two FIGO systems for normal and abnormal uterine bleeding symptoms and classification of causes of abnormal uterine bleeding in the reproductive years: 2018 revisions. *International Journal of Gynecology & Obstetrics.* 2018; doi:10.1002/ijgo.12666

National Collaborating Centre for Women's and Children's Health (UK). *Heavy Menstrual Bleeding.* RCOG Press; 2007.

Lieng M, et al. Treatment of endometrial polyps: A systematic review. *Acta Obstetricia Gynecologica Scandinavica.* 2010; doi:10.3109/00016349.2010.493196

Lee SC, et al. The oncogenic potential of endometrial polyps: A systematic review and meta-analysis. *Obstetrics and Gynecology.* 2010; doi:10.1097/AOG.0b013e3181f74864

Kimura T, et al. Abnormal uterine bleeding and prognosis of endometrial cancer. *International Journal of Gynaecology and Obstetrics.* 2004; doi:10.1016/j.ijgo.2003.12.001

Chapter 64: Vaginal infections

Brown H, et al. Improving the diagnosis of vulvovaginitis: Perspectives to align practice, guidelines, and awareness. *Population Health Management.* 2020; doi:10.1089/pop.2020.0265

Paladine HL, et al. Vaginitis: Diagnosis and treatment. *American Family Physician.* 2018;97:321.

Nyirjesy P. Management of persistent vaginitis. *Obstetrics & Gynecology.* 2014; doi:10.1097/AOG.0000000000000551

Anderson MR, et al. Evaluation of vaginal complaints. *Journal of the American Medical Association.* 2004; doi:10.1001/jama.291.11.1368

Workowski KA, et al. Sexually Transmitted Diseases Treatment Guidelines, 2015. Morbidity and Mortality Weekly Report. 2015. Accessed June 18, 2021. https://www.cdc.gov/mmwr/preview/mmwrhtml/rr6403a1.htm

St. Cyr S, et al. Update to CDC's Treatment Guidelines for Gonococcal Infection, 2020. Morbidity and Mortality Weekly Report. 2020; doi:10.15585/mmwr.mm6950a6

Chapter 65: When your illness is a mystery

Spillmann RC, et al. A window into living with an undiagnosed disease: Illness narratives from the Undiagnosed Diseases Network. *Orphanet Journal of Rare Diseases.* 2017; doi:10.1186/s13023-017-0623-3

Lipsitt DR, et al. Medically unexplained symptoms: Barriers to effective treatment when nothing is the matter. *Harvard Review of Psychiatry.* 2015; doi:10.1097/HRP.0000000000000055

Isaac ML, et al. Medically unexplained symptoms. *Medical Clinics of North America.* 2014; doi:10.1016/j.mcna.2014.01.013

Husain M, et al. Medically unexplained symptoms: Assessment and management. *Clinical Medicine.* 2021; doi:10.7861/clinmed.2020-0947

Leaviss J, et al. Behavioural modification interventions for medically unexplained symptoms in primary care: Systematic reviews and economic evaluation. *Health Technology Assessment.* 2020; doi:10.3310/hta24460

PART 3 Taking care of you

Chapter 66: What contributes to your health?

World Health Organization. Constitution of the World Health Organization. *Basic Documents,* 45th ed. Supplement. 2006; https://www.who.int/governance/eb/who_constitution_en.pdf

Beauvais, Joel. (April 26, 2016). "Moving Forward for America's Drinking Water." *EPA Blog.* U.S. Environmental Protection Agency (EPA). Accessed Nov. 22, 2021. https://news-sciences-10.blogspot.com/2016/04/moving-forward-for-americas-drinking.html

Watson K, et al. Clean drinking water a bigger global threat than climate change, EPA's Wheeler says. Mar 20, 2019. CBS News. https://www.cbsnews.com/news/epa-administrator-andrew-wheeler-exclusive-interview

Rao M, et al. Do healthier foods and diet patterns cost more than less healthy options? A systematic review and meta-analysis. *BMJ Open.* 2013; doi:10.1136/bmjopen-2013-004277

Chapter 69: Physical activity

Centers for Disease Control and Prevention. Benefits of physical activity. https://www.cdc.gov/physicalactivity/basics/pa-health/index.htm

Mayo Clinic. Alzheimer's disease: Can exercise prevent memory loss? https://www.mayoclinic.org/diseases-conditions/alzheimers-disease/expert-answers/alzheimers-disease/faq-20057881

Harvard Health Publishing. Exercising to relax. https://www.health.harvard.edu/staying-healthy/exercising-to-relax

Schnell S, et al. The 1-year mortality of patients treated in a hip fracture program for elders. *Geriatric Orthopaedic Surgery & Rehabilitation.* 2010; doi:10.1177/2151458510378105

Tang VL, et al. Rates of recovery to pre-fracture function in older persons with hip fracture: An observational study. *Journal of General Internal Medicine.* 2017; doi:10.1007/s11606-016-3848-2

U.S. Department of Health and Human Services. *Physical Activity Guidelines for Americans,* 2nd ed. 2018. https://health.gov/sites/default/files/2019-09/Physical_Activity_Guidelines_2nd_edition.pdf

Chapter 70: Purposeful activity

Coventry PA, et al. The mental health benefits of purposeful activities in public green spaces in urban and semi-urban neighbourhoods: A mixed-methods pilot and proof of concept study. *International Journal of Environmental Research and Public Health.* 2019; doi:10.3390/ijerph16152712

Takeda F, et al. How possibly do leisure and social activities impact mental health of middle-aged adults in Japan?: An evidence from a national longitudinal survey. *PLoS One.* 2015; doi:10.1371/journal.pone.0139777

Tomioka K, et al. Relationship of having hobbies and a purpose in life with mortality, activities of daily living, and instrumental activities of daily living among community-dwelling elderly adults. *Journal of Epidemiology.* 2016; doi:10.2188/jea.JE20150153

Fancourt D, et al. How leisure activities affect health: A narrative review and multi-level theoretical framework of mechanisms of action. *Lancet Psychiatry.* 2021; doi:10.1016/S2215-0366(20)30384-9

Pressman SD, et al. Association of enjoyable leisure activities with psychological and physical well-being. *Psychosomatic Medicine.* 2009; doi:10.1097/PSY.0b013e3181ad7978

Tominaga K, et al. Family environment, hobbies and habits as psychosocial predictors of survival for surgically treated patients with breast cancer. *Japanese Journal of Clinical Oncology.* 1998; doi:10.1093/jjco/28.1.36

Hughes TF, et al. Engagement in reading and hobbies and risk of incident dementia: The MoVIES Project. *American Journal of Alzheimer's Disease and other Dementias.* 2010; doi:10.1177%2F1533317510368399

Roe B, et al. Coffee, Cake & Culture: Evaluation of an art for health programme for older people in the community. *Dementia.* 2014; doi:10.1177%2F1471301214528927

Mills S, et al. Health and social determinants and

outcomes of home cooking: A systematic review of observational studies. *Appetite.* 2017; doi:10.1016/j.appet.2016.12.022

Corkhill B, et al. Knitting and well-being. *Textile.* 2015; doi:10.2752/175183514x13916051793433

Carlson MC, et al. Evidence for neurocognitive plasticity in at-risk older adults: the Experience Corps program. *Journals of Gerontology.* 2009; doi:10.1093/gerona/glp117

Frith CD. The social brain? *Philosophical Transactions of the Royal Society B.* 2007; doi:10.1098/rstb.2006.2003

Bickart KC, et al. Amygdala volume and social network size in humans. *Nature Neuroscience.* 2011; doi:10.1038/nn.2724

Chapter 71: Social relationships

Social Isolation and Loneliness in Older Adults: Opportunities for the Health Care System. The National Academies Press. 2020; doi. org/10.17226/25663

Carr, D, et al. Advances in families and health research in the 21st century. *Journal of Marriage and Family.* 2010; doi.org/10.1111/j.1741-3737.2010.00728.x

Harvard Health Publishing. The health benefits of strong relationships. https://www.health.harvard.edu/staying-healthy/the-health-benefits-of-strong-relationships

Duncan GJ, et al. Cleaning up their act: The effects of marriage and cohabitation on licit and illicit drug use. *Demography.* 2006; doi:10.1353/dem.2006.0032

Bernstein AB, et al. Marital status is associated with health insurance coverage for working-age women at all income levels, 2007. Centers for Disease Control and Prevention. https://www.cdc.gov/nchs/products/databriefs/db11.htm

Horn EE, et al. Accounting for the physical and mental health benefits of entry into marriage: A genetically informed study of selection and causation. *Journal of Family Psychology.* 2013; doi:10.1037/a0029803

Wong CSK, et al. Marital status and risk of cardiovascular diseases: A systematic review and meta-analysis. *Heart.* 2018; doi:10.1136/heartjnl-2018-313005

Cardoso-Moreno MJ, et al. The influence of perceived family support on post surgery recovery. *Psychology, Health & Medicine.* 2017; doi:10.1080/13548506.2016.1153680

Welch JD, et al. Social support, loneliness, eating, and activity among parent–adolescent dyads. *Journal of Behavioral Medicine.* 2019; doi:10.1007/s10865-019-00041-4

Ryan C, et al. Family acceptance in adolescence and the health of LGBT young adults. *Journal of Child and Adolescent Psychiatric Nursing.* 2010; doi:10.1111/j.1744-6171.2010.00246.x

National Institutes of Health. Do social ties affect our health? Exploring the biology of relationships. https://newsinhealth.nih.gov/2017/02/do-social-ties-affect-our-health

Prang KH, et al. Recovery from musculoskeletal injury: The role of social support following a transport accident. *Health and Quality of Life Outcomes.* 2018; doi:10.1186/s12955-015-0291-8

Shakya HB, et al. Association of Facebook use with compromised well-being: A longitudinal study. *American Journal of Epidemiology.* 2017; doi:10.1093/aje/kww189

Westergren, T, et al. A nested case–control study: Personal, social and environmental correlates of vigorous physical activity in adolescents with asthma. *Journal of Asthma.* 2015; doi:10.3109/02770903.2014.955190

Christakis NA, et al. The collective dynamics of smoking in a large social network. *New England Journal of Medicine.* 2008; doi:10.1056/NEJMsa0706154

Guan S-SA, et al. Parental support buffers the association of depressive symptoms with cortisol and C-reactive protein during adolescence. *Brain, Behavior & Immunity.* 2016; doi:10.1016/j.bbi.2016.03.007

Steeves ETA, et al. Social influences on eating and physical activity behaviours of urban, minority youths. *Public Health Nutrition.* 2016; doi:10.1017/S1368980016001701

Pattussi MP, et al. Workplace social capital, mental health and health behaviors among Brazilian female workers. *Social Psychiatry and Psychiatric Epidemiology.* 2016; doi:10.1007/s00127-016-1232-5

Valente MSS, et al. Depressive symptoms and psychosocial aspects of work in bank employees. *Occupational Medicine.* 2016; doi:10.1093/occmed/kqv124

Suls J. Toxic affect: Are anger, anxiety, and depression independent risk factors for cardiovascular disease? *Emotion Review.* 2018; doi:10.1177/1754073917692863

Uchino BN, et al. Integrative pathways linking close family ties to health: A neurochemical perspective. *American Psychologist.* 2017; doi:10.1037/amp0000049

Leschak CJ, et al. Social connection and immune

processes. *Psychosomatic Medicine.* 2019; doi:10.1097/PSY.0000000000000685

Donoho CJ, et al. Marital quality, gender, and markers of inflammation in the MIDUS cohort. *Journal of Marriage & Family.* 2013; doi:10.1111/j.1741-3737.2012.01023.x

Choi H, et al. Marital quality, socioeconomic status, and physical health. *Journal of Marriage & Family.* 2013; doi:10.1111/jomf.12044

Rodriguez AJ, et al. Wives' and husbands' cortisol reactivity to proximal and distal dimensions of couple conflict. *Family Process.* 2013; doi:10.1111/famp.12037

Smokowski PR, et al. The effects of positive and negative parenting practices on adolescent mental health outcomes in a multicultural sample of rural youth. *Child Psychiatry and Human Development.* 2015; doi:10.1007/s10578-014-0474-2

Forbes MK, et al. Depression, anxiety, and peer victimization: Bidirectional relationships and associated outcomes transitioning from childhood to adolescence. *Journal of Youth and Adolescence.* 2019; doi:10.1007/s10964-018-0922-6

Robles TF, et al. The physiology of marriage: Pathways to health. *Physiology of Behavior.* 2003; doi:10.1016/s0031-9384(03)00160-4

Wang C, et al. Associations of job strain, stressful life events, and social strain with coronary heart disease in Women's Health Initiative Observational Study. *Journal of the American Heart Association.* 2021; doi:10.1161/JAHA.120.017780

Christakis NA, et al. The spread of obesity in a large social network over 32 years. *New England Journal of Medicine.* 2007; doi:10.1056/NEJMsa066082

Ford MT. Perceived unfairness at work, social and personal resources, and resting blood pressure. *Stress & Health.* 2014; doi:10.1002/smi.2491

Ortega A, et al. One-year prospective study on the effect of workplace bullying on long-term sickness absence. *Journal of Nursing Management.* 2011; doi:10.1111/j.1365-2834.2010.01179.x

Lorenz FO, et al. The short-term and decade-long effects of divorce on women's midlife health. *Journal of Health and Social Behavior.* 2006; doi:10.1177/002214650604700202

Dahl SA, et al. His, her, or their divorce? Marital dissolution and sickness absence in Norway. *Journal of Marriage and Family.* 2015; doi:10.1111/jomf.12166

Lee, S, et al. Effects of marital transitions on changes in dietary and other health behaviors in US women. *International Journal of Epidemiology.* 2005; doi:10.1093/ije/dyh258

King M, et al. Death following partner bereavement: A self-controlled case series analysis. *PLoS One.* 2017; doi:10.1371/journal.pone.0173870

Cooney TM, et al. End-of-life care planning: The importance of older adults' marital status and gender. *Journal of Palliative Medicine.* 2019; doi:10.1089/jpm.2018.0451

Holt-Lunstad, J, et al. Social relationships and mortality risk: A meta-analytic review. *PLoS Medicine.* 2010; doi:10.1371/journal.pmed.1000316

DiJulio B, et al. Loneliness and social isolation in the United States, the United Kingdom, and Japan: An international survey. Kaiser Family Foundation. 2018; https://www.kff.org/other/report/loneliness-and-social-isolation-in-the-united-states-the-united-kingdom-and-japan-an-international-survey/

Krampe H, et al. Social relationship factors, preoperative depression, and hospital length of stay in surgical patients. *International Journal of Behavioral Medicine.* 2018; doi:10.1007/s12529-018-9738-8

Relationship Institute. Differences between men and women. Accessed August 25, 2021. https://relationship-institute.com/differences-between-men-and-women

Umberson D, et al. Physical illness in gay, lesbian, and heterosexual marriages: Gendered dyadic experiences. *Journal of Health and Social Behavior.* 2016; doi:10.1177/0022146516671570

American Psychological Association. Gender and stress. Accessed August 25, 2021. https://www.apa.org/news/press/releases/stress/2010/gender-stress#

Kessler RC, et al. Sex differences in vulnerability to undesirable life events. *American Sociological Review.* 1984; doi:10.2307/2095420

Chapter 73: Acupuncture

Zheng CH, et al. Effects of acupuncture on pregnancy rates in women undergoing in vitro fertilization: A systematic review and meta-analysis. *Fertility and Sterility.* 2012; doi: 10.1016/j.fertnstert.2011.12.007

Kang HS, et al. The use of acupuncture for managing gynaecologic conditions: An overview of systematic reviews. *Maturitas.* 2011; doi:10.1016/j.maturitas.2011.02.001

Al-Inany H. Acupuncture for infertility: A recently released evidence. *Middle East Fertility Society Journal.* 2008;13:67.

Ferin M, et al. Endogenous opioid peptides and the control of the menstrual cycle. *European Journal of Obstetrics, Gynecology, and Reproductive Biology*. 1984; doi:10.1016/0028-2243(84)90059-5

Han JS, et al. Effect of low- and high-frequency TENS on Met-enkephalin-Arg-Phe and dynorphin A immunoreactivity in human lumbar CSF. *Pain*. 1991; doi:10.1016/0304-3959(91)90218-M

Smith CA, et al. Acupuncture to treat common reproductive health complaints: An overview of the evidence. *Autonomic Neuroscience*. 2010; doi:10.1016/j.autneu.2010.03.013

Liu ZC, et al. Effect of acupuncture on insulin resistance in non-insulin dependent diabetes mellitus. *Journal of Acupuncture and Tuina Science*. 2004; doi:10.1007/BF02848387

Pastore LM, et al. True and sham acupuncture produced similar frequency of ovulation and improved LH to FSH ratios in women with polycystic ovary syndrome. *Journal of Clinical Endocrinology and Metabolism*. 2011; doi:10.1210/jc.2011-1126

Xu Y, et al. Effects of acupuncture for the treatment of endometriosis-related pain: A systematic review and meta-analysis. *PLoS One*. 2017; doi:10.1371/journal.pone.0186616

Lesi G, et al. Acupuncture as an integrative approach for the treatment of hot flashes in women with breast cancer: A prospective multicenter randomized controlled trial (AcCliMaT). *Journal of Clinical Oncology*. 2016; doi:10.1200/JCO.2015.63.2893

Ee C, et al. Acupuncture for menopausal hot flashes: Clinical evidence update and its relevance to decision making. *Menopause*. 2017; doi:10.1097/GME.0000000000000850

Yang N, et al. Efficacy of acupuncture for urinary incontinence in middle-aged and elderly women: A systematic review and meta-analysis of randomized controlled trials. *European Journal of Obstetrics, Gynecology, and Reproductive Biology*. 2021; doi:10.1016/j.ejogrb.2020.11.001

Chapter 74: Vaccines

Plotkin S. History of vaccination. *Proceedings of the National Academy of Sciences*. 2014; doi:10.1073/pnas.1400472111

Centers for Disease Control and Prevention. Vaccines and Immunizations. Accessed May 15, 2021. https://www.cdc.gov/vaccines/index.html.

Lei J, et al. HPV vaccination and the risk of invasive cervical cancer. *The New England Journal of Medicine*. 2020; doi:10.1056/NEJMoa1917338

Sly JR et al. Recombinant zoster vaccine (Shingrix) to prevent herpes zoster. *Nursing for Women's Health*. 2018; doi:10.1016/j.nwh.2018.07.004

Fleming DM, et al. Gender difference in the incidence of shingles. *Epidemiology and Infection*. 2014; doi:10.1017/s0950268803001523

Centers for Disease Control and Prevention. National Vital Statistics Report - Deaths: Leading Causes for 2017. Accessed May 25, 2021. https://www.cdc.gov/nchs/data/nvsr/nvsr68/nvsr68_06-508.pdf

Polack FP, et al. Safety and efficacy of the BNT162b2 mRNA COVID-19 vaccine. *New England Journal of Medicine*. 2020; doi:10.1056/nejmoa2034577

Baden LR, et al. Efficacy and safety of the mRNA-1273 SARS-CoV-2 vaccine. *New England Journal of Medicine*. 2021; doi:10.1056/nejmoa2035389

Sadoff J, et al. Safety and efficacy of single-dose Ad26.COV2.S vaccine against COVID-19. *New England Journal of Medicine*. 2021; doi:10.1056/nejmoa2101544

Voysey M, et al. Safety and efficacy of the ChAdOx1 nCoV-19 vaccine (AZD1222) against SARS-CoV-2: An interim analysis of four randomised controlled trials in Brazil, South Africa, and the UK. *The Lancet*. 2021; doi:10.1016/s0140-6736(20)32661-1

Chapter 75: Research and women

NIH Office of Research on Women's Health. NIH Policy on Sex as a Biological Variable. Accessed May 21, 2021. https://orwh.od.nih.gov/sex-gender/nih-policy-sex-biological-variable

Institute of Medicine (US) Committee on Understanding the Biology of Sex and Gender Differences. *Exploring the Biological Contributions to Human Health: Does Sex Matter?* National Academies of Science; 2001.

Goetz TG, et al. Women, opioid use and addiction. *The FASEB Journal*. 2021; doi:10.1096/fj.202002125R

The Coronary Drug Project Research Group. The Coronary Drug Project: Design, methods, and baseline results. *Circulation*. 1973; doi:10.1161/01.CIR.47.3S1.I-1

Mastroianni AC, et al. *Women and Health Research: Ethical and Legal Issues of Including Women in Clinical Studies*. Volume 1. National Academies Press; 1994. doi:10.17226/2304

Bairey Merz CN, et al. Ischemia and no obstructive coronary artery disease (INOCA): Developing evidence-based therapies and research agenda for the next decade. *Circulation*. 2017; doi:10.1161/circulationaha.116.024534

Cai Y, et al. Sex differences in colon cancer metabolism reveal a novel subphenotype. *Scientific Reports*. 2020; doi:10.1038/s41598-020-61851-0

Clayton JA. Applying the new SABV (sex as a biological variable) policy to research and clinical care. *Physiology & Behavior*. 2018; doi:10.1016/j.physbeh.2017.08.012

Mazure CM, et al. Sex differences in Alzheimer's disease and other dementias. *The Lancet Neurology*. 2016; doi:10.1016/S1474-4422(16)00067-3

Women's Health Research at Yale. Accessed May 21, 2021. https::// medicine.yale.edu/whr

Chapter 77: Our connectedness

Movement is Life Caucus. https://www.movementislifecaucus.com

University of Exeter. Lifelong Gender Difference in Physical Activity Revealed. *ScienceDaily*, 8 January 2009. www.sciencedaily.com/releases/2009/01/090105190740.htm

Sanyaolu A, et al. Comorbidity and its impact on patients with COVID-19. *SN Comprehensive Clinical Medicine*. 2020; doi:10.1007/s42399-020-00363-4

Low-income COVID-19 patients die needlessly because they are stuck in the wrong hospitals—while the right hospitals too often shut them out. *Health Affairs Blog*. Posted April 2, 2021. doi:10.1377/hblog20210401.95800

Chapter 78: You are a health promoter!

Movement is Life Caucus. https://www.movementislifecaucus.com

Matoff-Stepp S, et al. Women as health care decision-makers: Implications for health care coverage in the United States. *Journal of Health Care for the Poor and Underserved*. 2014; doi:10.1353/hpu.2014.0154

If you take the 'I' out of illness, and add 'We,' you end up with wellness. https://quoteinvestigator.com/2020/05/03/wellness

About the authors

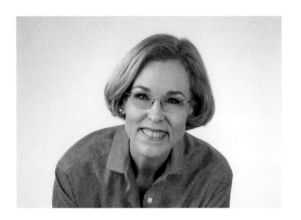

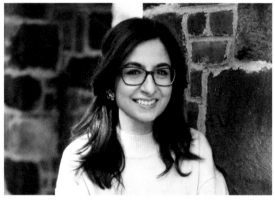

Mary I. O'Connor, M.D., is an internationally recognized orthopedic surgeon and health equity leader. She is co-founder and Chief Medical Officer of Vori Health, a virtual musculoskeletal medical practice delivering an innovative model of patient care to empower humanity to better health.

In a profession dominated by white males, Dr. O'Connor broke numerous glass ceilings. Her distinguished academic career includes more than 200 peer-reviewed publications and 350+ academic presentations. Dr. O'Connor is Professor Emerita at Mayo Clinic, where she served as the Chair of the Orthopedic Department at Mayo Clinic in Florida and was awarded the Distinguished Clinician Award. She is past Professor of Orthopaedics and Rehabilitation at Yale School of Medicine and directed Yale's Center for Musculoskeletal Care.

Dr. O'Connor's championing of women began as an undergraduate at Yale. In 1976, she and her rowing teammates protested the lack of women's facilities at the boathouse in what has been heralded as the first Title IX stand for gender equality in college athletics. In 1979, Dr. O'Connor went on to stroke the Yale Women's Varsity Eight to a national championship and the U.S. National Team Women's Eight to a bronze medal at the World Rowing Championships. She was a member of the 1980 U.S. Olympic Team (Women's Rowing).

Having seen the bias that women, people of color, and other marginalized groups experience in healthcare, Dr. O'Connor has fought tirelessly to advocate for quality care for all. She has led Movement is Life, a national non-profit health equity coalition, since its inception in 2010. Next to caring for the patients she has had the privilege to serve, she considers her greatest professional achievements to be advancing health equity and diversity in medicine.

Kanwal L. Haq, M.S., has been a fierce advocate for change long before she knew what such terms meant. In kindergarten, she repeatedly threw away her uncle's hidden cigarettes; when he tried to divert her cause with a visit to SeaWorld, she used the entire trip to protest "Free Willy!" ... and then threw away her uncle's cigarettes.

Since then Kanwal has learned to use more successful approaches to effect change. She completed her B.S. in biological sciences from the University of Missouri, her M.S. in medical anthropology from Boston University School of Medicine, and worked at the Centre Hospitalier Universitaire de Kigali; Americorps; the United Nations; and Yale School of Medicine. Kanwal currently leads the NYC women's health programs at Mount Sinai Icahn School of Medicine's Arnhold Institute for Global Health.

An applied-research scientist dedicated to education and health equity, Kanwal utilizes community-based participatory research and implementation science to build more effective, efficient and equitable systems of care for women across the world. Her desire to build accessible tools that bridge the gap between academic knowledge and community resources, served as the catalyst for *Taking Care of You*.

Acknowledgments

This book is the result of inspiration and support from so many to whom I am deeply grateful. My dedication to patients comes from my mother, who first taught me about disparities when sharing her victories and defeats as a nurse in providing what we now call "patient-centered care." My self-confidence to be a trailblazer came from my father. His unwavering belief in me — that I could do anything I set my mind to — has never left me. My five siblings first taught me the power of community.

I am indebted to my patients, who showed me why this book is needed. Thank you to my mentors, past partners and residency colleagues at Mayo Clinic, who trained and nurtured me as an orthopedic surgeon and medical leader. In particular, Franklin H. Sim, M.D., profoundly supported my early career. My national work in health equity was made possible by two visionaries at ZimmerBiomet, Inc.: David Dvorak (then CEO) and Verona Brewton (Director of Minority Initiatives). My Vori Health family, especially my co-founder and CEO, Ryan Grant, M.D., share my passion for quality care for all. I would also like to acknowledge David Wilk at Booktrix for pitching our idea to Mayo Clinic Press; the entire Mayo Clinic Press team, especially Rachel Haring Bartony for her excellent editing skills; all our amazing contributors; and my incredible co-author, Kanwal Haq, M.S., for her dedication and belief in our book, and her friendship.

Finally, I want to express my gratitude and love for my husband, Thomas McCormick, and our children, Moira Kathleen, Roarke Patrick and Riona Carlin. Throughout my journey, my path has been brighter because of you.

— Mary I. O'Connor

I have been blessed to learn from great institutions, but even greater individuals. I am forever grateful to my grandparents and parents, who uprooted their lives and immigrated to Poplar Bluff, Missouri, in search of a better life for their children. Their sacrifices made it possible for me to become the first university-educated woman in our family.

I am indebted to a number of remarkable individuals. Dr. Teresa Cooney encouraged my desire to learn and introduced me to the field of qualitative research. Dr. Thomas Phillips introduced me to the world of medical anthropology and the words of Paul Farmer: "The idea that some lives matter less is the root of all that is wrong with the world." He taught me to think critically and challenge harsh realities. Dr. Marilyn James-Kracke guided me to keep going when things get tough and to remember "Hope has two beautiful daughters; their names are Anger and Courage. Anger at the way things are, and Courage to see that they do not remain as they are." (Saint Augustine). Representative Jeanne Kirkton and LA Myra Rosskopf Wolfe showed me what a kickass duo looks like and to "Never doubt that a small group of thoughtful, committed citizens can change the world; indeed, it's the only thing that ever has." (Margaret Mead). Dr. Linda Barnes taught me to aim for "progress, not perfection" and to show myself grace along the way.

I am sincerely grateful to everyone who helped bring this project to life including powerhouse David Wilk and the entire Booktrix team, Mayo Clinic Press editor-in-chief Nina Weiner who always made time to answer my numerous questions and provide her sincere guidance, publisher Dan Harke who believed in our vision and got all the wheels turning to make it happen, and especially our editor turned dear friend Rachel Haring Bartony, who supported us in every possible way and made this book a reality, along with the entire Mayo Clinic Press Team.

I want to also acknowledge all of our fantastic contributors; our illustrator, Margot Sarkozy for not only her artistic talents but her friendship and wisdom beyond her years; and especially my co-author and mentor Dr. Mary O'Connor. She is as kind as she is brilliant, and my personal north star for living a life dedicated to uplifting others.

A special thank-you to my family, friends, and especially my husband, Shiraz who supported me every step of the way. This book was truly a labor of love.

— Kanwal L. Haq

Index